Illustrated Manual of Orthognathic Surgery

Peter Kessler • Nicolas Hardt
Kensuke Yamauchi
Editors

Illustrated Manual of Orthognathic Surgery

Osteotomies of the Mandible

SORG

Springer

Editors
Peter Kessler
Department of Cranio-Maxillofacial Surgery
Maastricht University Medical Center
Maastricht, The Netherlands

Nicolas Hardt
Kantonsspital Lucerne
Clinic and Policlinic
of Cranio-Maxillofacial Surgery
Lucerne, Switzerland

Kensuke Yamauchi
Department of Oral & Maxillofacial Surgery
Tohoku University Sendai
Sendai, Miyagi, Japan

ISBN 978-3-031-06977-2 ISBN 978-3-031-06978-9 (eBook)
https://doi.org/10.1007/978-3-031-06978-9

This Springer imprint is published by the registered company Springer Nature Switzerland AG
The registered company address is: Gewerbestrasse 11, 6330 Cham, Switzerland

Preface

The aim of orthognathic surgery is to correct developmental or acquired skeletal deformities of the viscerocranium, the skeleton of the face and jaws.

Over the last decades, significant progress has been made in the surgical technique of the various approaches to correct the jaw position, as well as in the fixation of the osteotomized segments by plate and screw osteosynthesis including instrumentation and intraoperative quality control by various forms of guided surgery.

Although the basic surgical principles have remained more or less unchanged, numerous new computer-based planning techniques have been introduced, as well as new technical procedures, which have refined the surgical methods and significantly improved and facilitated the treatment of complex maxillofacial deformities.

Detailed surgical planning is essential for a successful clinical outcome. Treatment includes a precise treatment plan, the right choice of instruments for a particular surgical procedure, a thorough surgical routine and adherence to the surgical guidelines and detailed surgical steps.

Although similar treatment objectives exist, there are important differences between osteotomy techniques. It is important that the surgeon interested is aware of these differences to ensure an effective and safe surgical routine in the care of patients with facial deformities.

The choice of an optimal osteotomy method depends on many factors, the indication, the therapeutic goal, the medical conditions, the experience of the surgeon, and the extent of the surgical procedure.

The main objective of this manual is to present practical guidelines for the most commonly used surgical osteotomy techniques in the mandible, including a complete and detailed description of the individual surgical steps in these surgical procedures. Techniques such as bilateral sagittal split osteotomy (BSSO), bilateral vertical osteotomies, segmental mandibular osteotomies, and chin osteotomies are discussed in detail.

In addition—depending on the surgical procedure—the variable and various surgical risks are listed and the most frequent surgical complications and their avoidance through careful and precise surgical approaches are presented.

The manual focuses on the anatomical prerequisites that place high demands on the surgeon and lead to the indications for the various osteotomy procedures.

The presented surgical guidelines and advice are based on the current literature as well as on the personal, long-term surgical experience of the authors.

We thank all co-authors for their excellent contributions. We would like to thank the S.O.R.G., which has always benevolently supported the financial framework of this project.

We especially thank Mr. Keisuke Koyama, DDS, who contributed the perfect illustrations. Special thanks to Mrs. Rachael Kessler, who with infinite patience did the layout in English.

Maastricht, The Netherlands — Peter Kessler
Luzern, Switzerland — Nicolas Hardt
Sendai, Japan — Kensuke Yamauchi

Contents

Part I

Introduction to Orthognathic Surgery in the Mandible

Evolution of the Surgical Standard Techniques

1

Peter Kessler and Nicolas Hardt

Contents

Abstract

The correction of mandibular prognathia, first performed by *Vilray Blair* more than 100 years ago in the United States, was the beginning of dysgnathia surgery (Blair, Cosmos 1906;48:817-820; Surg Gynecol Obstet. 1907;4:67-78; Int J Orthodont 1915;1(8)1:395–432). As early as the beginning of the twentieth century, various surgical procedures were developed for the correction of mandibular malocclusions in the horizontal mandibular body and in the ascending ramus. Between 1914 and 1945 there was no significant progress in dysgnathia surgery, until rapid development began in the 1950s. Both in Central Europe and in the United States, new surgical techniques were introduced into dysgnathia surgery of the mandible, but also for the upper jaw and midface.

In *1955*, *H. Obwegeser* initiated a major progress in orthognathic surgery with the bilateral sagittal splitting of the ascending ramus of the lower jaw to treat mandibular prognathism. The surgical method underwent continuous modifications, such as the enlargement of the bone attachment surface and the associated application of the sagittal splitting technique even in cases of mandibular retrognathism. Bone splitting and segment stabilization have also been significantly modified and improved, allowing complete mobilization of the fragments without compromising the supplying soft tissue structures on the one hand and functionally stable osteosynthesis of the segments on the other

P. Kessler (✉)
Department of Cranio-Maxillofacial Surgery, Maastricht University Medical Center, Maastricht, The Netherlands
e-mail: peter.kessler@mumc.nl

N. Hardt (✉)
Kantonsspital Lucerne, Clinic and Policlinic of Cranio-Maxillofacial Surgery, Lucerne, Switzerland

P. Kessler et al. (eds.), *Illustrated Manual of Orthognathic Surgery*,
https://doi.org/10.1007/978-3-031-06978-9_1

(Bell et al., Surgical correction of dentofacial deformities Vol. 1-3. Saunders;1980; Bell, J Oral Maxillofac Surg. 2018;76(12):2466-2481; Kashani and Rasmusson, A Textbook of Advanced Oral and Maxillofacial Surgery–Volume 3. IntechOpen;2016).

Keywords

Evolution of mandibular osteotomy and splitting techniques · Classification of dysgnathias · Development of orthognathic surgery · Basic osteotomy procedures · Classification of surgical corrections · Ramus osteotomies · Sagittal mandibular split · Bilateral sagittal split osteotomy · BSSO · Segment osteotomies · Chin osteotomies · Genioplasty · Complications

The modern surgical development of transoral sagittal splitting of the mandibular ramus for the treatment of mandibular growth disorders (dysgnathia) was preceded in the first half of the twentieth century by various surgical procedures with extraoral and later intraoral accesses [1–4].

Review of Surgical Procedures

- Horizontal Ramus Osteotomy
- Subcondylar Osteotomy
- Oblique Osteotomy
- Vertical Oblique Osteotomy
- Shaped Osteotomy

After first attempts to correct mandibular growth deficiency by step and sliding osteotomies in the body of the mandible (Fig. 1.1) [5, 6], the focus of correction of mandibular growth impair-

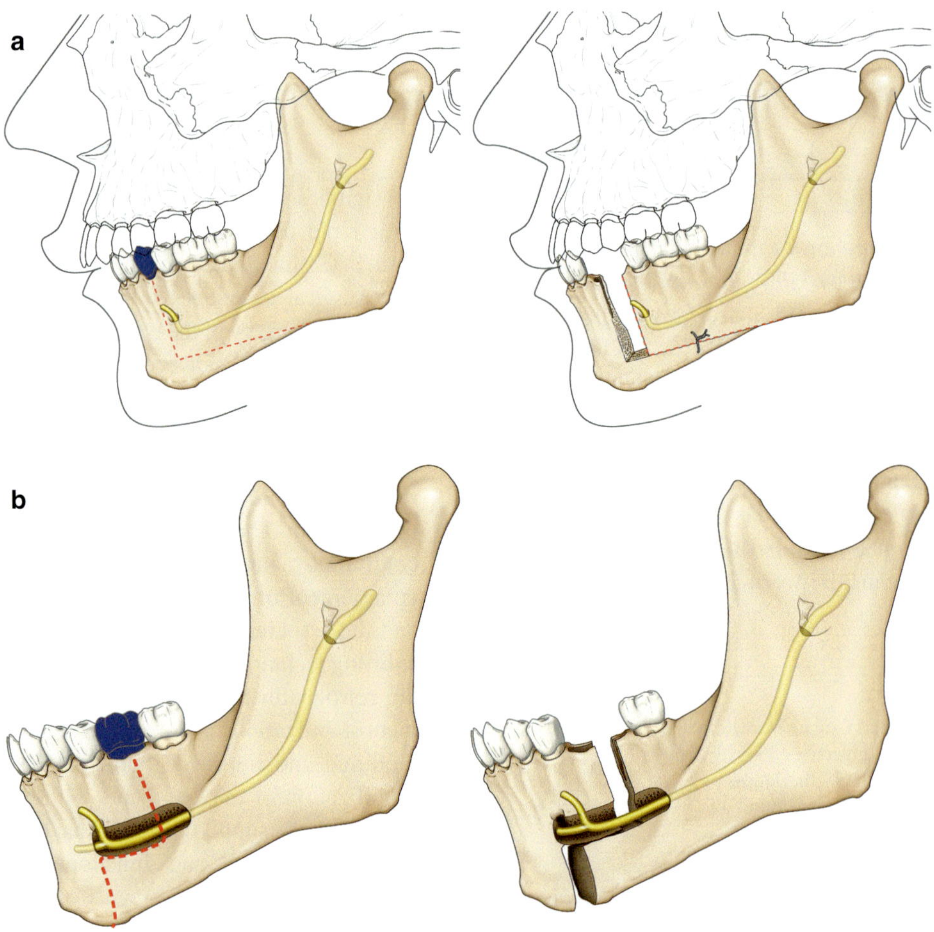

Fig. 1.1 Surgical correction of retrognathia (**a**) Sliding osteotomy of the body of the mandible (Angle) (**b**) Subapical step osteotomy in the mandibular body (v. Eiselsberg) ©Copyright Keisuke Koyama 2020. All rights reserved

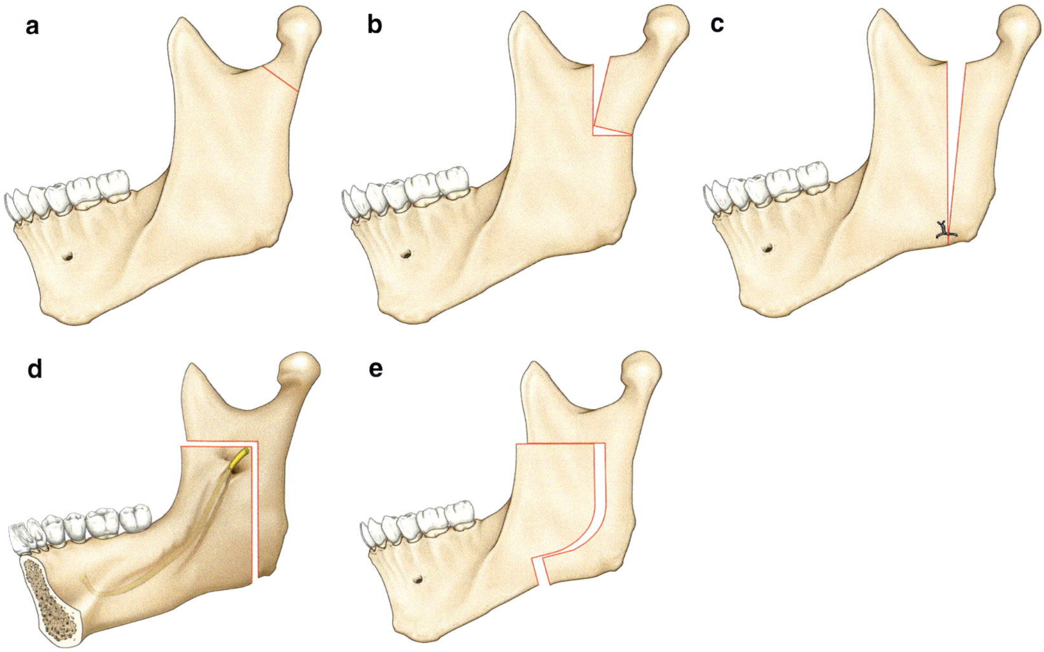

Fig. 1.2 Development of oblique/vertical mandibular osteotomy—according to Bell et al. [1, 51] (**a**) Subcondylar osteotomy by Blair (**b**) Oblique osteotomy by Limberg (**c**) Oblique osteotomy by Robinson et al. (**d**) "Inverted L" osteotomy by Wassmund (**e**) "C" osteotomy by Caldwell et al.

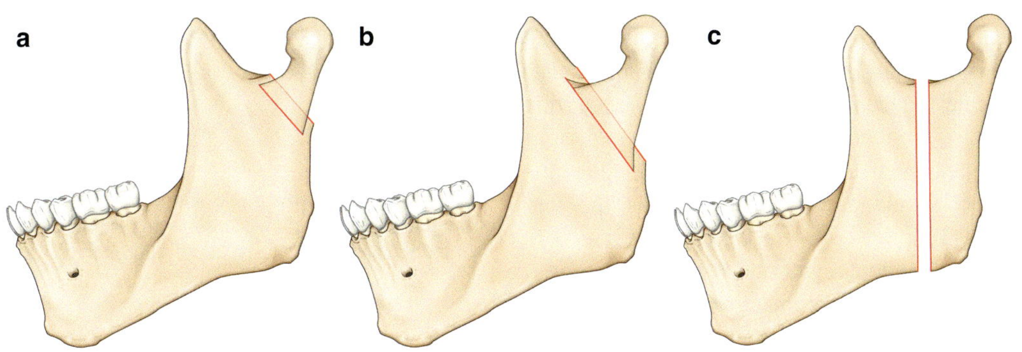

Fig. 1.3 The development from the subcondylar osteotomy to the vertical osteotomy. Different lengths of intraoral vertical ramus osteotomies (IVRO) (**a**) (Blair [29]; Blair [30]) (**b**) Perthes [34] (**c**) Winstanley (1968)

ment soon shifted to the area of the ascending ramus of the mandible. *Blair* in *1906* performed the first osteotomy of the mandibular body for the correction of horizontal mandibular excess and described three distinct problems [7]:

- Cutting of the bone.
- Replacing the segment to a new position.
- Fixation of the segments.

Subsequently, numerous variants of mandibular ramus osteotomies were published, including various modifications of the sliding osteotomies in different planes (Fig. 1.2) [8–11].

In Europe, *Berger* performed the first *horizontal condylectomies* in *1892*. *Dufourmentel et al. 1921/1932* and *Kostecka in 1926/1934* preferred the *subcondylar osteotomies* for the correction of mandibular prognathias. All surgeons chose for a preauricular approach [12–15].

Subsequently subcondylar osteotomies had undergone numerous variations which finally led to the development of the *intraoral vertical ramus osteotomy (IVRO)* (Fig. 1.3).

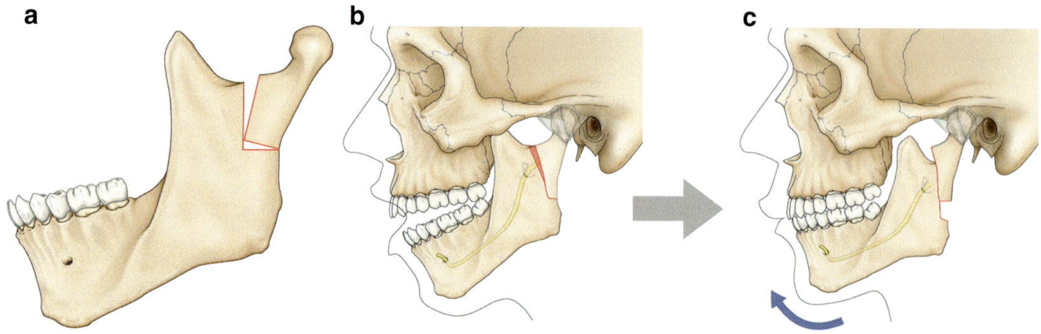

Fig. 1.4 First oblique vertical ramus osteotomy according to Limberg [11]. Extraoral-cervical approach for correction of mandibular retrognathia and open bite (**a**) Osteotomy (**b**) Rotational movement of the mandible (**c**) Situation after correction with anterior open bite

In *1925 Limberg* was the first to develop an *oblique vertical osteotomy* of the mandibular ramus by an extraoral-cervical approach to correct mandibular retrognathia with an open bite (Fig. 1.4) [11].

Due to unpredictable stability of the osteotomized segments, e.g., displacement of the proximal segment through the temporal and medial pterygoid muscles, sagging of the posterior segment due to stripping of the masseter and medial pterygoid muscles, modifications of the IVRO were developed. Longer osteotomy lines starting at the sigmoid notch and ending in the region of the mandibular angle with lesser muscular dissection should prevent dislocation of the segments [16].

Oblique vertical and true vertical ramus osteotomy variants were inaugurated by *Hinds* in *1958*, *Robinson* in *1957/1958*, and *Caldwell and Letterman* in *1954*. All surgeons performed the osteotomy by an extraoral approach. The development led to the first intraoral vertical osteotomy performed by *Hebert et al.* in *1970*.

The development culminated in the first intraoral vertical osteotomy (IVRO) performed in *1968* by *Winstanley* with a dental drill. A significant advance in the IVRO technique was reported by *Herbert et al.* in *1970* with the use of the motorized oscillating saw [17].

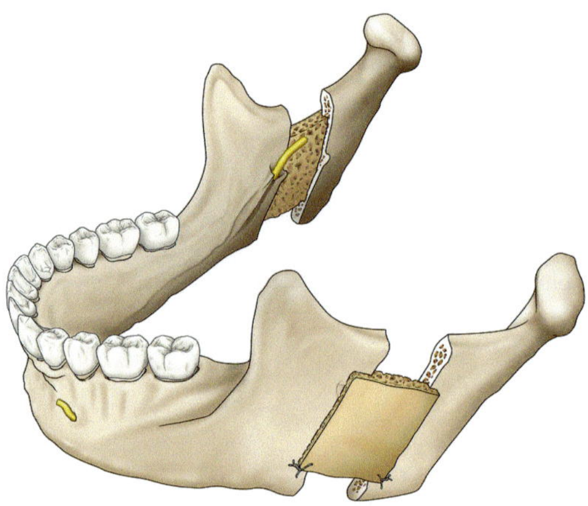

Fig. 1.5 Vertical oblique osteotomy with cortico-cancellous bone graft according to Robinson [19]

The work of *Hall et al.* and *Hall and McKenna* in the 1970s further popularized the procedure, and Hall's work in the 1980s helped quantify clinical outcomes and proposed technique refinements to minimize proximal segment "sag" [1, 18].

For vertical osteotomies, *Robinson* first integrated iliacal cortico-cancellous bone grafts into the osteotomy gap in *1957* (Fig. 1.5). This was especially necessary in cases where mandibular advancement was indicated. The bone transplants

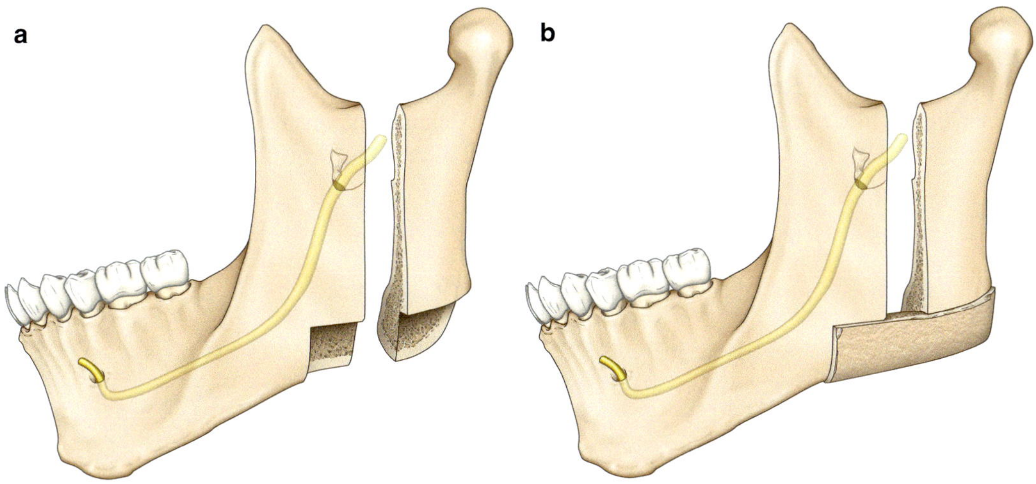

Fig. 1.6 (**a**) Vertical osteotomy with partial decortication (**b**) Integration of cortico-cancellous graft into the osteotomy defect [20]

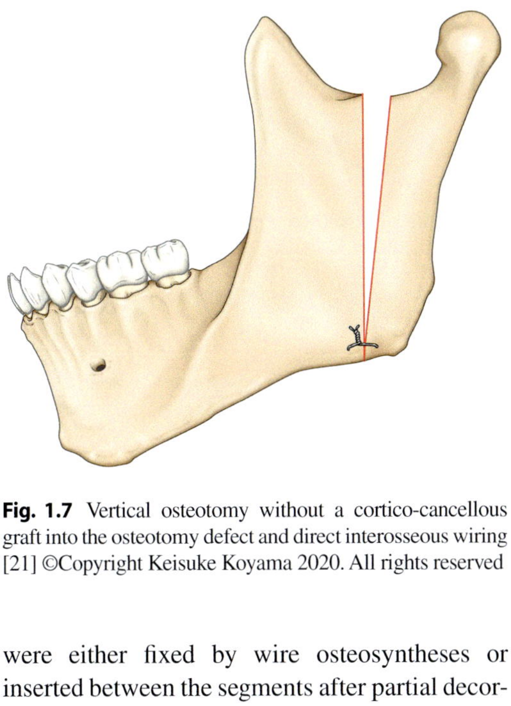

Fig. 1.7 Vertical osteotomy without a cortico-cancellous graft into the osteotomy defect and direct interosseous wiring [21]

were either fixed by wire osteosyntheses or inserted between the segments after partial decortication (Fig. 1.6) [20].

In *1957 Robinson and Lytle* refrained from additional intersegmental bone grafting and performed only direct interosseous osteosynthesis of the proximal fragment (Fig. 1.7).

1 Inverted L Osteotomy and C Osteotomy

Variants of the *oblique vertical osteotomy* were the *modified C-shaped osteotomies.*

These were first described in *1927* by *Wassmund*, who performed an arcuate osteotomy of the ramus in the form of a C-shaped arch with simultaneous mandibular advancement and simultaneous closure of an open bite.

The *C-shaped osteotomy* and the *inverted L osteotomy* were primarily operated via a transfacial approach (Fig. 1.8) [22–28].

Hawkinson published the *arcing osteotomy* in the ascending ramus in *1968*. By doing this he improved the bone-to-bone contact in the osteotomy area. This osteotomy was recommended for dysgnathia where additional mandibular rotations were required in contrast to straight or linear mandibular movements [23].

The vertical component of the *inverted L osteotomy* resembled a *subcondylar ramus osteotomy* with an additional lower oblique and an upper horizontal component to achieve greater apposition of the bone (Fig. 1.9).

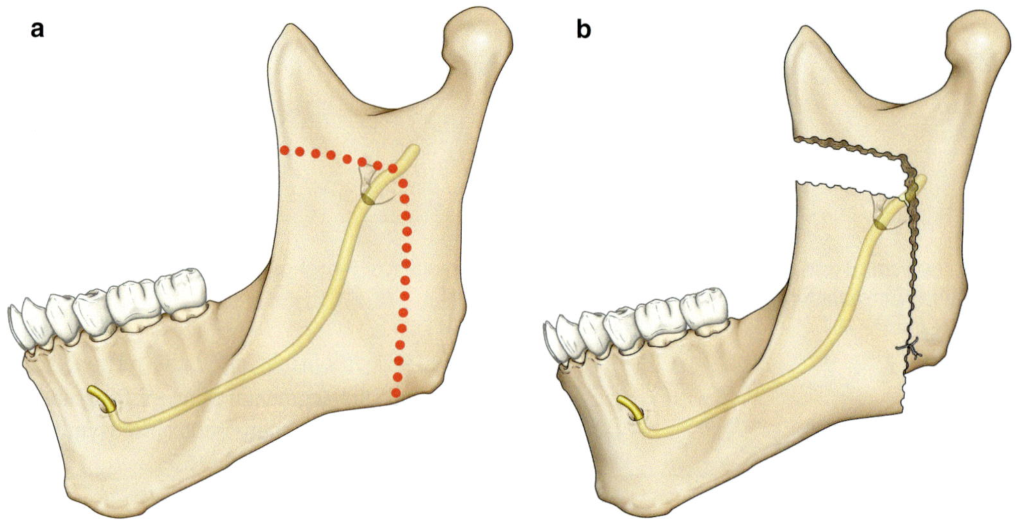

Fig. 1.8 C-shaped osteotomy of the ramus by Wassmund [43] (**a**) Outline of the osteotomy (**b**) Osteotomy and relocation of the distal segment

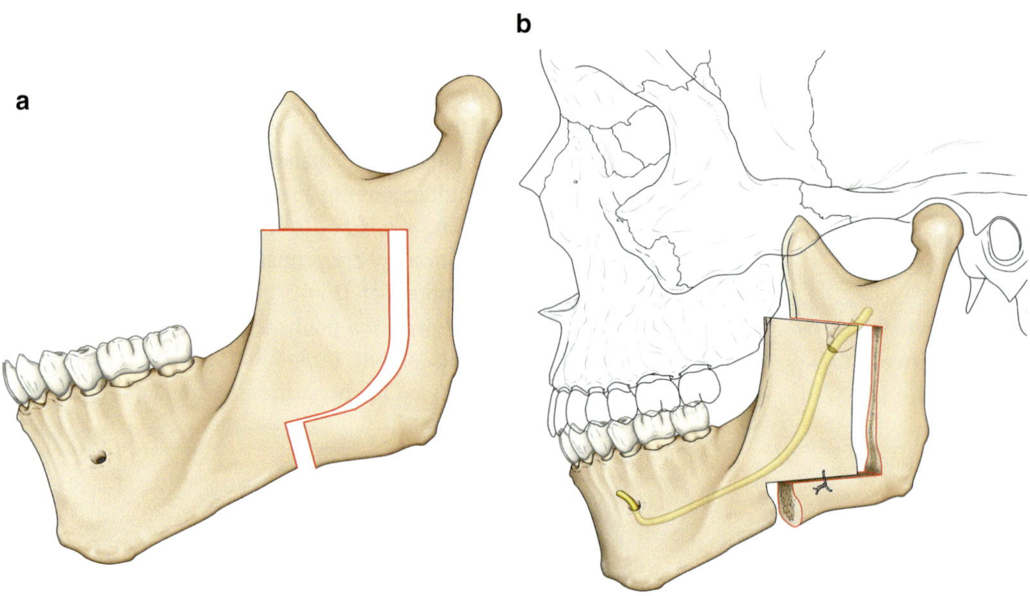

Fig. 1.9 The C osteotomy and the inverted vertical L osteotomy [22] (**a**) Osteotomy design (**b**) Relocation of the distal segment, wire osteosynthesis

2 The Development of Horizontal Ramus Osteotomies to Extended Sagittal Ramus Splitting

The basic development of the sagittal split has led from a purely horizontal osteotomy [29–34] to an oblique sagittal osteotomy [10], through a partially stepped sagittal split osteotomy [25–27], to a complete and longer stepped osteotomy of the ramus [35]. Later extended splitting variants were presented by *Obwegeser*, and finally the long stepped sagittal split was inaugurated by *Dal-Pont* (Fig. 1.10) [1, 4].

As *Bloomquist* stated in *1992*, the sagittal split ramus osteotomy (SSRO) is perhaps the most significant development among the numerous mandibular osteotomies of the vertical ramus [36].

The earliest documented sagittal ramus osteotomy, however, was published by *Perthes* already in *1924* (Fig. 1.11). Then still the transfacial approach was used.

In *1959 Kazanjian and Converse* contributed to the technical development of the mandibular ramus split by performing a sagittal oblique ramus osteotomy from the proximal-medial side to the caudal-lateral aspect to obtain the widest possible bone contact between the segments, but still used an extraoral approach [10].

With regard to the transoral approach *Ernst* was the first to present a set of instruments to that end (special cheek retractors and a long, straight handsaw and a screwed guide channel, *1927*) and cut the ramus horizontally above the foramen as early as in 1934 [31–33]. The transoral approach by *Ernst* was a groundbreaking advance, but it took almost 20 years before the intraoral approach became the surgical standard [37].

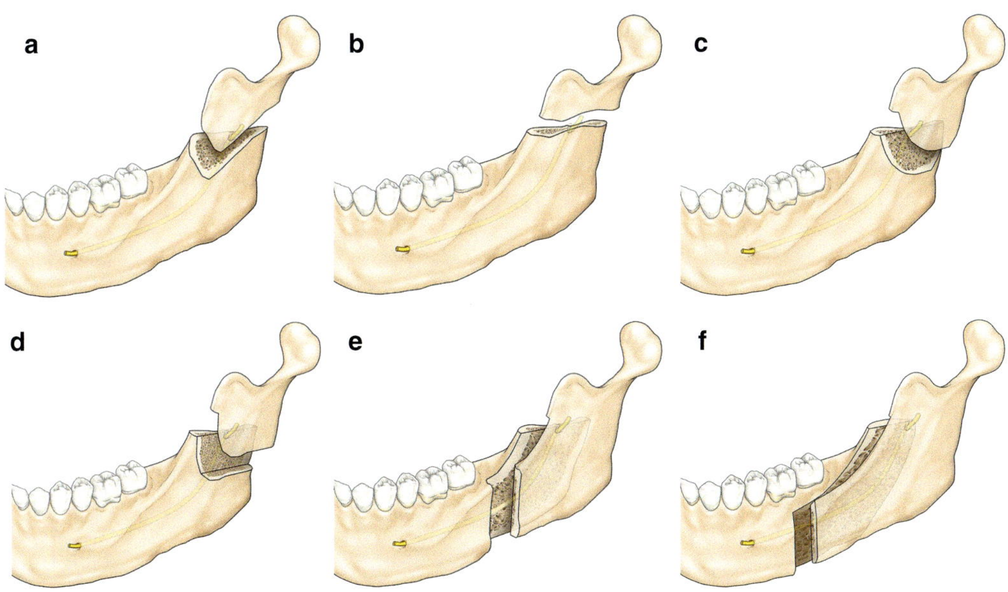

Fig. 1.10 Development of the sagittal split osteotomy (**a**) Perthes osteotomy (1924) (**b**) Kazanjian and Converse (1951) (**c**) Schuchardt [26] (**d**) Trauner & Obwegeser [35] (**e**) Dal Pont [44] (**f**) Hunsuck [45]

According to *Bell, Schuchardt* was the first who created a proximal-medial bone step in the ramus from an intraoral approach in *1955*, from which the oblique sagittal splitting of the ramus took place (Fig. 1.12) [1, 38].

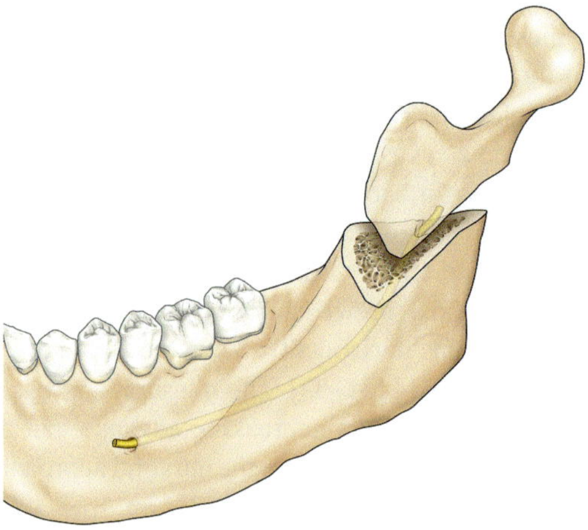

Fig. 1.11 Earliest depiction of the sagittal split osteotomy of the Ramus by Perthes [34] (transfacial approach)

Trauner and Obwegeser performed the two-stage osteotomy in *1955* by relocating the second osteotomy deliberately into the lateral buccal aspect of the mandibular ramus, thereby prolonging the sagittal split and forming a broad bone contact (Fig. 1.13).

Two years later, in *1957*, *Trauner and Obwegeser* located the lateral-horizontal osteotomy line more caudally into the region of the mandibular angle to improve bone-to-bone contact/overlap and enhance the stability of the lateral segment.

In *1959, Obwegeser* adjusted the lateral osteotomy line as a vertical bone cut in the preangular region and suggested the use of this surgical approach for both the prognathic and retrognathic mandible.

In *Obwegeser's* original description of his technic in *1959* the lateral osteotomy is shown distal of the second molar. The lingual osteotomy line lies about 8–10 mm below the sigmoid notch (Fig. 1.14).

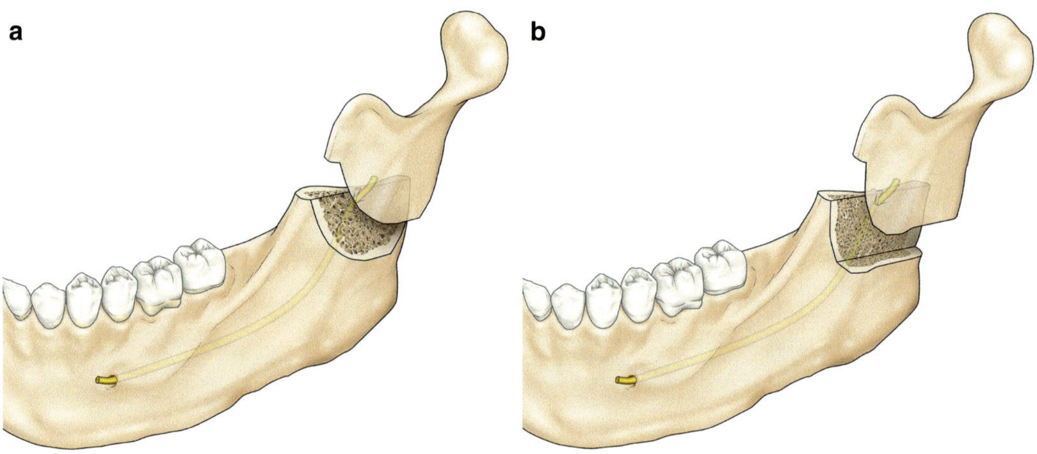

Fig. 1.12 The development of the sagittal split osteotomy from Schuchardt (**a**) to the Trauner/Obwegeser technique (**b**) (intraoral approach)

Dal Pont modified *Obwegeser's* sagittal splitting technique in 1959 by locating the lateral/buccal osteotomy incision forward into the region of the second molar to further increase the bone overlap (Figs. 1.14, 1.15 and 1.16). This technique has been published in English only in 1961. The original publication of 1959 is in Italian language [39–42].

1. The *sagittal retromolar osteotomy*, in which a sufficiently thick cancellous bone layer between the two cortical plates allows a con-

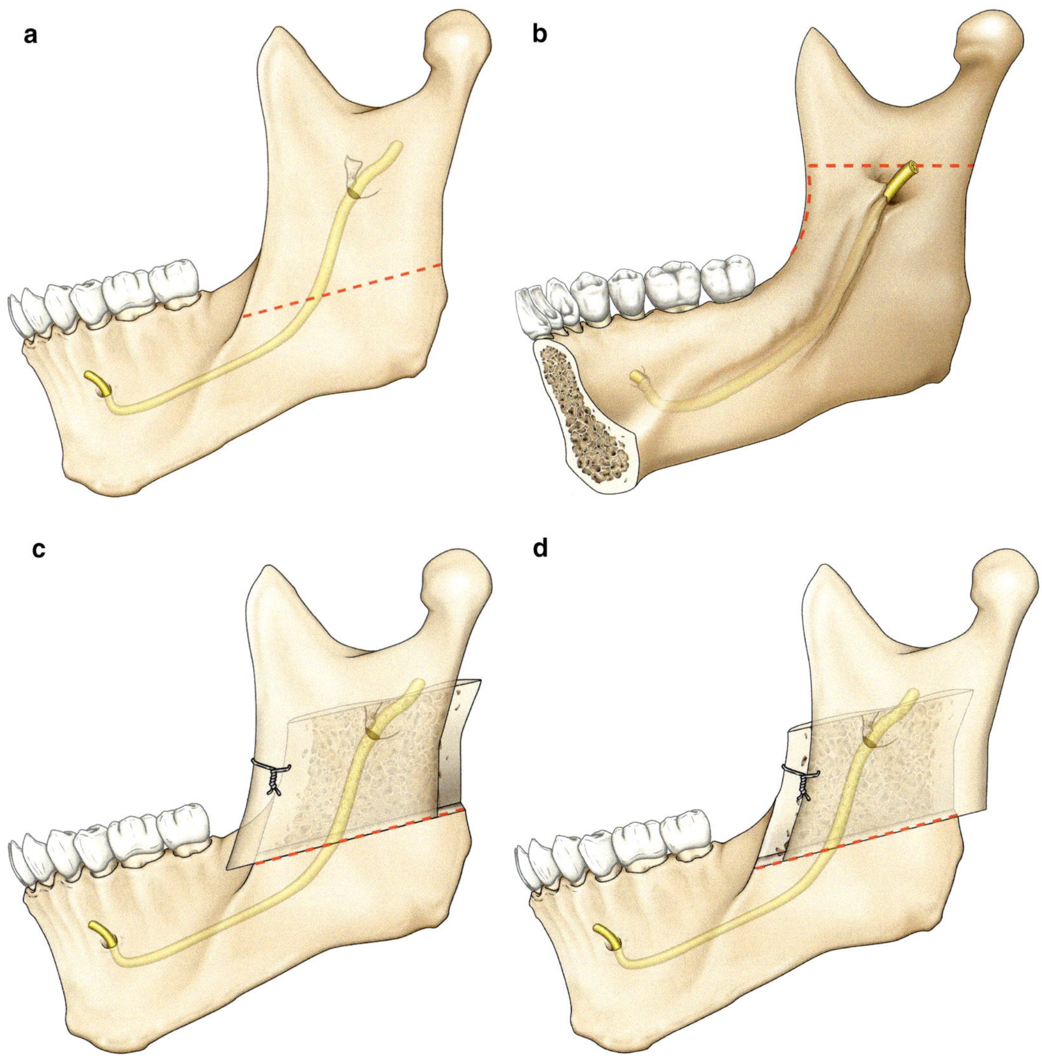

Fig. 1.13 Complete and extended stepped osteotomy of the ramus according to Trauner and Obwegeser (1955) (**a**) buccal osteotomy (**b**) lingual osteotomy (**c**) mandibular setback (**d**) mandibular advancement

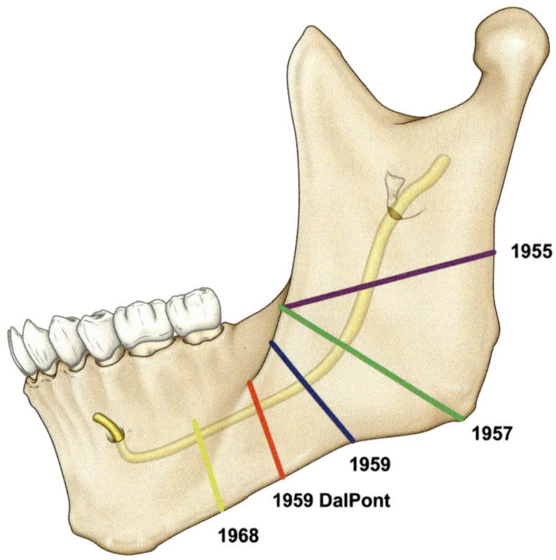

Fig. 1.14 Extended splitting variants on the buccal side by Obwegeser [39, 40] and DalPont [41] ©Copyright Keisuke Koyama 2020. All rights reserved

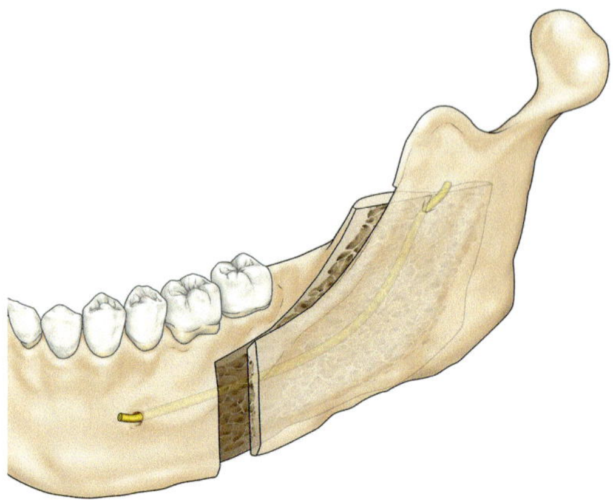

Fig. 1.15 Dal Pont distinguished in 1959 two sagittal osteotomy forms depending on the intercortical cancellous bone mass ©Copyright Keisuke Koyama 2020. All rights reserved

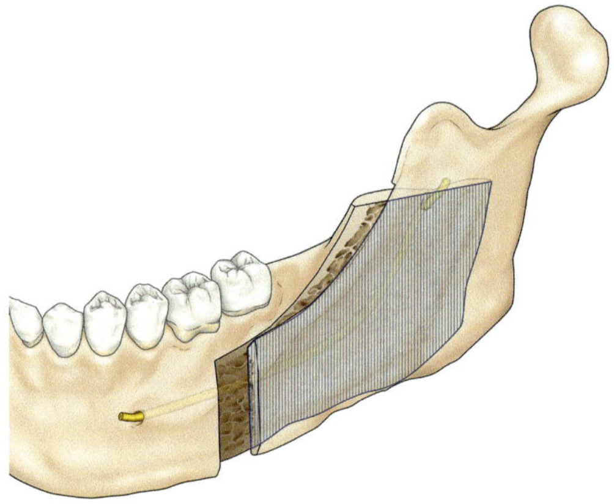

Fig. 1.16 Sagittal retromolar osteotomy The ramus of the mandible is split between the medial and lateral cortical plates. The split extends to the posterior border of the mandible (as indicated by the shaded lines) ©Copyright Keisuke Koyama 2020. All rights reserved

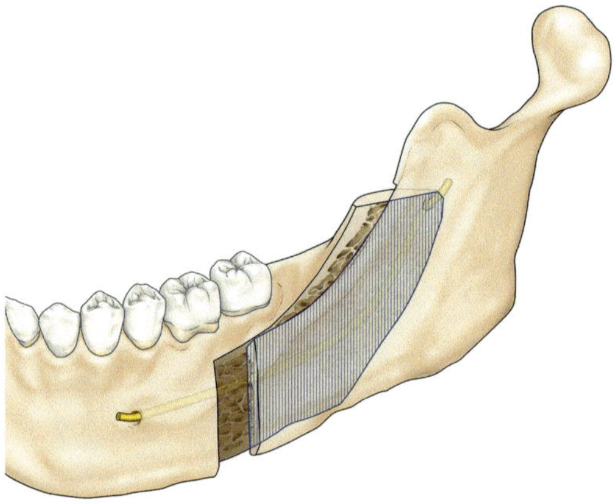

Fig. 1.17 The sagittal split on the lingual side ends in the region of the lingula ©Copyright Keisuke Koyama 2020. All rights reserved

tinuous splitting of the ramus up to the posterior edge of the ascending ramus. Notice the wide overlap of both segments (Fig. 1.16).

2. The *retromolar osteotomy,* in which there is insufficient cancellous bone volume, so that a safe splitting may be limited.

In this situation *Dal Pont* advocated splitting of the medial segment anterior to the posterior margin of the ramus and pleaded for a lingual split just below the mandibular nerve-vessel bundle, an aspect later emphasized by *Hunsuck* in *1968* (Fig. 1.17).

3 Oblique Retromolar Osteotomy

The split in the ramus does not extend to the posterior border, usually because there is little cancellous bone between the two cortical plates.

In order to reduce the unpredictable and uncontrollable course of the sagittal split in the lower-inferior cleavage region (so-called *Hunsuck* effect), *Hunsuck* proposed in *1968* to fundamentally limit the extent of the lingual osteotomy posterior to the mandibular foramen so that the split will be just below the mandibular foramen in order to reduce subperiosteal exposure of the ramus and surgical trauma to the neurovascular vessel bundle on the one hand, and to limit undesirable splitting complications on the other (Fig. 1.18).

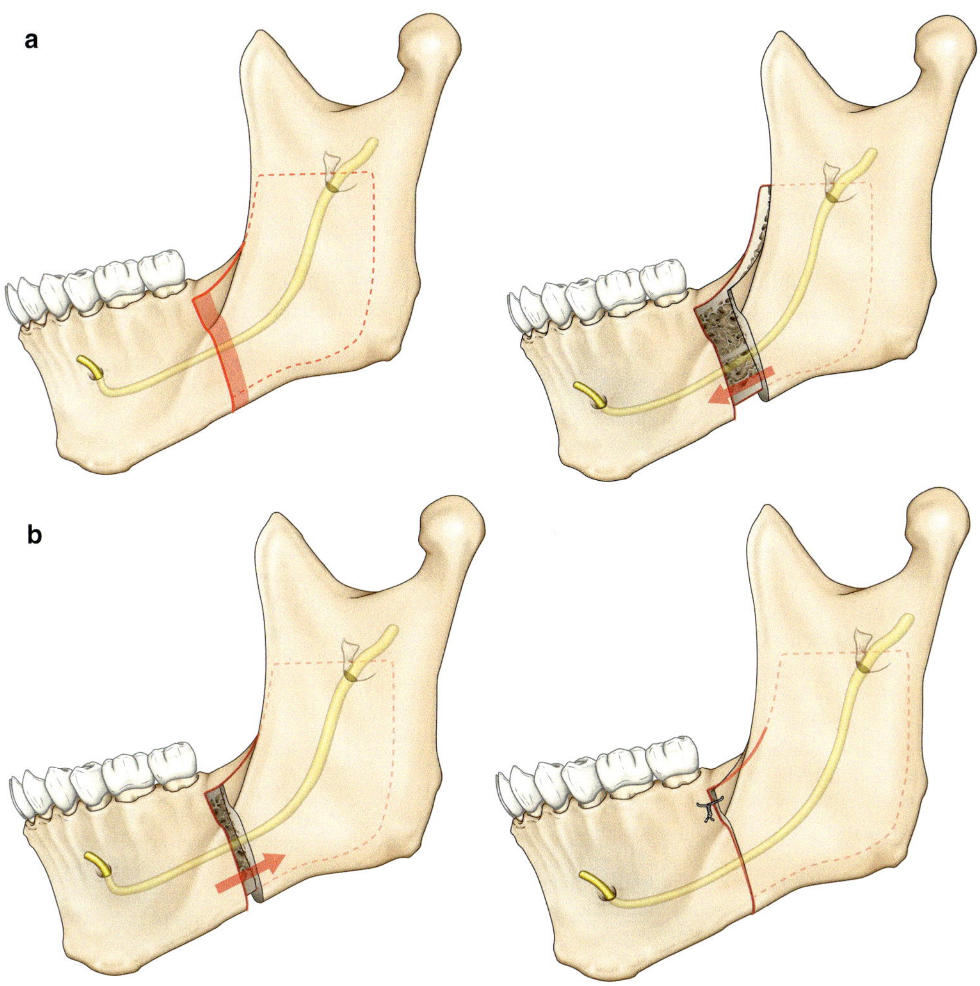

Fig. 1.18 Dal Pont–Hunsuck type of osteotomy which comes through the medial cortex above the lingula and anteriorly to the posterior border of the ramus—short lingual osteotomy—SLO (**a**) mandibular advancement (**b**) mandibular setback ©Copyright Keisuke Koyama 2020. All rights reserved

4 Conclusion

The sagittal split osteotomy, according to *Trauner-Obwegeser/Dal Pont*, has decisive advantages, a wide medullary bone contact as a prerequisite for uncomplicated bone healing and universal applicability in prognathic and retrognathic isolated and combined bimaxillary surgery. It is the most widely used technique today.

One of the most important innovations in the sagittal splitting process was the introduction of set and lag screw osteosynthesis by *Spiessl* [46, 47].

Broad experience has shown that the stable osteosynthetic fixation of the segments enabled uncomplicated, rapid bone healing, a significant reduction in the relapse frequency, a stable condyle position and improved patient comfort [4].

Since the first publication, the sagittal split osteotomy has been modified in various ways [48–50, 52]. The numerous surgical techniques and modifications reflect the collective but also the individual interest in this technique, as well as the individually different surgical experiences of the authors.

References

1. Bell HW, Proffit WR, White RP. Surgical correction of dentofacial deformities Vol. 1–3. Saunders; 1980.
2. Kashani H, Rasmusson L. Osteotomies in orthognathic surgery. In: Hosein M, Motamedi K, editors. A textbook of advanced oral and maxillofacial surgery–volume 3. IntechOpen; 2016.
3. Steinhäuser EW. Historical development of orthognathic surgery. J Craniomaxillofac Surg. 1996;24:195–204.
4. Steinhäuser EW. Rückblick auf die Entwicklung der Dysgnathiechirurgie und Ausblick. Mund-Kiefer- und Gesichtschirurgie. 2003;7:371–9.
5. Angle EH. Double resection for treatment of mandibular protrusion. Dent Cosmos. 1903;45:268–74.
6. von Eiselsberg J. Über Plastik bei Ektropium des Unterkiefers (Progenie). Wien Klin Wochenschr. 1906;19:1505–8.
7. Blair VP. Instances of operative correction of malrelation of the jaws. Int J Orthodont. 1915;1(8):395–432.
8. Dingman RO. Surgical correction of the mandibular prognathism. Am J Orthod. 1944;30(11):683–92.
9. Dingman RO. Surgical correction of development deformities of the mandible. Plastic Reconstr Surg. 1948;3(2):124–46.
10. Kazanjian V, Converse J. The surgical treatment of facial injuries. 2nd ed. Baltimore: Williams a. Wilkins; 1959.
11. Limberg A. Treatment of open-bite by means of plastic oblique osteotomy of the ascending rami of the mandible. Dent Cosmos. 1925;67:1191–200.
12. Berger P. Du traitement chirurgical du prognathisme. These: Lyon; 1892.
13. Dufourmentel M. Le Traitement chirurgical du prognathisme. Presse Méd. 1921:235–7.
14. Dufourmentel M, Darcissac M. Quelques cas de résections condyliennes unilatérales et bilatérales avec présentation d'anciens opérés. Revue de Stomat. 1932;34(6):340.
15. Kostecka F. A contribution to the surgical treatment of open bite. Int J Orthod. 1934;28:1082–92.
16. Fox GL, Tilson HB. Mandibular retrognathia: a review of the literature and selected cases. J Oral Surg. 1976;34:53–61.
17. Hebert JM, Kent JN, Hinds EC. Correction of prognathism by an intraoral vertical subcondylar osteotomy. J Oral Surg. 1970;33:384.
18. Hall HD, Chase DC, Payor LG. Evaluation and refinement of the intraoral vertical subcondylar osteotomy. J Oral Surg. 1975;33:333.
19. Robinson M. Micrognathism corrected by vertical osteotomy. Of ascending ramus and iliac bone graft: a new technique. Oral Surg Oral Med Oral Pathol. 1957;10:1125–30.
20. Caldwell JB, Amaral WJ. Mandibular micrognathism corrected by vertical osteotomy in the rami and iliac bone graft. J Oral Surg. 1960;18:3–15.
21. Robinson M, Lytle JJ. Micrognathism corrected by vertical osteotomies of the rami without bone grafts. Oral Surg Oral Med Oral Pathol. 1962;15:641–5.
22. Caldwell JB, Hayward JR, Lister RL. Correction of mandibular retrognathia by vertical-L osteotomy: a new technique. J Oral Surg. 1968;26:259–64.
23. Hawkinson RT. Retrognathia correction by means of an arcing osteotomy in the ascending ramus. J Prosthet Dent. 1968;20:77–86.
24. Hayes PA. Correction of retrognathia by modified "C" osteotomy of the ramus sagittal osteotomy of the mandibular body. J Oral Surg. 1973;31:682–6.
25. Schuchardt K. Ein Beitrag zur chirurgischen Kieferorthopädie unter Berücksichtigung ihrer Bedeutung für die Behandlung angeborener und erworbener Kieferdeformitäten bei Soldaten. Dtsch Zahn Mund Kieferheilkd. 1942;9:73.
26. Schuchardt K. Formen des offenen Bisses und ihre operativen Behandlungsmöglichkeiten. In: Fortschr Kiefer–Gesichtschir 1955; 1:222–230.

27. Schuchardt K. Experience with the surgical treatment of some deformities of the jaws: prognathia, microgenia and open bite. In: Wallace AB, editor. Transactions of the International Society of Plastic Surgeons. Second congress. Baltimore: Williams and Wilkins; 1961. p. 73–8.
28. Weinstein I. C-osteotomy for correction of mandibular retrognathia: report of cases. J Oral Surg. 1971;29:358.
29. Blair VP. Report of a case of double resection for the correction of protrusion of the mandible. Cosmos. 1906;48:817–20.
30. Blair VP. Operations of the jaw bone and face. Surg Gynecol Obstet. 1907;4:67–78.
31. Ernst F. Die Prognathie. In: Kirschner M, Nordmann O, editors. Die Chirurgie Bd. IV 1. Berlin: Urban u. Schwarzenberg; 1927. p. 803–11.
32. Ernst F. Über die chirurgische Beseitigung der Prognathie des Unterkiefers. Deutsche zahnärztl Wschr. 1934;37:949–53.
33. Ernst F. Über die chirurgische Beseitigung der Prognathie des Unterkiefers. Zentralbl Chir. 1938;65:179.
34. Perthes G. Die Kieferköpfchen und ihre operative Behandlung. Arch Klin Chir. 1924;1333:425.
35. Trauner R, Obwegeser HL. The surgical correction of mandibular prognathism and retrognathia with considerations of genioplasty. Surgical procedures to correct mandibular prognathism and reshaping the chin. Part I. Oral Surg Oral Med Oral Pathol. 1957;10:677–89.
36. Bloomquist DS. Principles of mandibular orthognathie surgery. In: Peterson LJ, Andresano AT, Marciani RD, Roser SM, editors. Principles of oral and maxillofacial surgery. Philadelphia: Lippincott; 1992. p. 1415–63.
37. Hoffmann-Axthelm W. Chirurgie der Zahnstellungs- und Kieferanomalien. In: Hoffmann-Axthelm W, Neumann HJ, Pfeifer G, Stiebitz R, editors. Die Geschichte der Mund-, Kiefer- und Gesichtschirurgie. Berlin: Quintessenz-Verlag; 1995.
38. Fonseca RJ, Marciani RD, Turvey TA. Oral and maxillofacial surgery. Orthognathic surgery, esthetic surgery, cleft and craniofacial surgery. Saunders; 2009.
39. Obwegeser HL, Trauner R. Zur Operationstechnik bei der Progenie und anderen Unterkieferanomalien. Dtsch Zahn Kieferheilkd. 1955;23:1.
40. Obwegeser HL. The surgical correction of mandibular prognathism with consideration of genioplasty. Oral Surg Oral Med Oral Path. 1957;10:677–89.
41. Dal Pont G. L'osteotomia retromolare par la converzione della progenia. Minerva Chir. 1959;14:1138.
42. Obwegeser HL. The indication for surgical correction of mandibular deformity by sagittal splitting technique. Br J Surg. 1963;1:157–60.
43. Wassmund M. Frakturen und Luxationen des Gesichtsschädels unter Berücksichtigung der Komplikationen des Hirnschädels. In: Klinik und Therapie. Praktisches Lehrbuch, Vol. 20. Meusser, Berlin 1927.
44. Dal Pont G. Retromolar osteotomy for the correction of prognathism. J Oral Surg. 1961;19:42–7.
45. Hunsuck EE. A modified intraoral sagittal splitting technic for correction of mandibular prognathism. J Oral Surg. 1968;26:250–3.
46. Spiessl B. The sagittal splitting osteotomy for correction of mandibular prognathism. Clin Plast Surg. 1982;9(4):491–507.
47. Tucker MR. Surgical correction of mandibular excess. Atlas Oral Maxillofac Surg Clin North Am. 1993;1:29–39.
48. Epker BN. Modification in the sagittal osteotomy of the mandible. J Oral Surg. 1977;35:157–9.
49. Spiessl B. Osteosynthese bei sagittaler Osteotomie nach Obwegeser-Dal Pont. Fortschr Kieferheilkd Gesichtschir. 1974;18:145–8.
50. Wolford LM, Davis WM. Mandibular inferior border split: a modification in the sagittal split osteotomy. J Oral Maxillofac Surg. 1990;48:92–4.
51. Bell B. A history of orthognathic surgery in North America. J Oral Maxillofac Surg. 2018;76(12):2466–81.
52. Obwegeser HL. Orthognathic surgery and a tale of how three procedures came to be: a letter to the next generations of surgeons. Clin Plast Surg. 2007;34:331–55.

Further Readings

Hoffmann-Axthelm W, Neumann HJ, Pfeifer G, Stiebitz R. Die Geschichte der Mund-, Kiefer- und Gesichtschirurgie. Quintessenz: Berlin, 1995.

Steinhäuser EW. Historical development of orthognathic surgery. J CranioMaxillofac Surg. 1996;24:195–204.

Classification and Facial Patterns

2

Peter Kessler and Nicolas Hardt

Contents

Abstract

The skeletal position of the jaws is genetically determined. Typical positional relationships of the jaws include classifiable occlusal forms and externally recognizable, almost typifying esthetic features of each face. Classification was essential for the development of systematic treatment concepts in order to enable structured treatments in the first place, which must also be communicated internationally (Becking et al., Ned Tijdschr Tandheelkd 2007; 114(1):34–40).

Keywords

Facial growth pattern · Classification of dysgnathias · Dentoalveolar dysgnathia · Skeletal dysgnathia

P. Kessler (✉)
Department of Cranio-Maxillofacial Surgery, Maastricht University Medical Center, Maastricht, The Netherlands
e-mail: peter.kessler@mumc.nl

N. Hardt (✉)
Kantonsspital Lucerne, Clinic and Policlinic of Cranio-Maxillofacial Surgery, Lucerne, Switzerland

P. Kessler et al. (eds.), *Illustrated Manual of Orthognathic Surgery*,
https://doi.org/10.1007/978-3-031-06978-9_2

1 Introduction

Dysgnathia refers to a disturbance of the regular jaw and tooth row relationship between the mandible and maxilla. The different forms of dysgnathias can be classified on the basis of clinical differences in the size and positional relationship of the jaws to each other and according to their radiological manifestation.

The positional anomalies can be classified according to the sagittal, vertical, and transversal orientation of the jaws into skeletal dysgnathias (dento-maxillofacial) and dentoalveolar dysgnathias. In addition, the third group are the cranio-maxillofacial disorders associated with dysgnathia [1].

2 Skeletal Dysgnathia

In skeletal dysgnathia, the positional relationship of the bases of the jaws to the skull and skull base is affected (neurocranium), whereby the positional relationship of the jaws to each other is usually also disturbed, e.g., through disproportional growth of the facial skeleton (viscerocranium).

The relationship of the mandible to the base of the skull is mediated by the temporomandibular joints, whereby dysgnathias can in turn result from condylar growth disorders. Condylar growth disorders represent a separate entity. Symmetric and asymmetric dysgnathias can be distinguished [1, 2].

2.1 Symmetric Dysgnathia

Symmetric dysgnathias where only *one vector* is affected:

- Sagittal dysgnathia—prognathism versus retrognathism.
- Vertical dysgnathia—vertical overgrowth including open bite and deep bite.
- Transversal dysgnathia—symmetric laterognathism/crossbite.

Dysgnathias, where mostly all *three vectors* are affected:

Mandible:

- Mandibular micrognathia.
- Mandibular macrognathia.
- Chin microgenia.
- Chin macrogenia.

Maxilla:

- Maxillary macrognathia.
- Maxillary micrognathia.

Often different forms of dysgnathia are combined with each other. If dysgnathias are present in both the lower jaw and the upper jaw, they are called bimaxillary dysgnathias.

Note

- Dysgnathias are often present in different directions in space.
- Combinations of the aforementioned malformations are common.
- Although, from a practical point of view, a skeletal anomaly can often be reduced to a vector (sagittal, transverse, vertical), in principle all dysgnathias include three-dimensional growth deficits.
- Occasionally, all three dimensions are affected to a similar, usually however, to a different extent.

2.2 Asymmetric Dysgnathia

Mandibular unilateral asymmetries.

- Laterognathism.
- Hemimandibular hyperplasia/elongation.
- Hemimandibular hypoplasia.
- Unilateral condylar hyperplasia.
- Unilateral condylar hypoplasia.
- Isolated unilateral dento-maxillofacial growth disorders.

Maxillary unilateral asymmetries.

- Unilateral maxillary hyperplasia.
- Unilateral maxillary hypoplasia.

3 Dentoalveolar Dysgnathia

Dentoalveolar dysgnathias are skeletal growth disorders that are restricted to one or both alveolar processes including the teeth, with the jaw base correctly positioned. Combinations of different dentoalveolar malocclusions are common.

Dentoalveolar occlusal anomalies—especially in the sagittal plane—are divided into three classes:

Class I—regular occlusion is defined by the position of the canines and the mesio-buccal cusp of the first molar in the maxilla which occludes in the buccal groove of the mandibular first molar. Overbite and overjet of the incisors must be regular, no midline deviation.

Class II—distal occlusion.

Class II/1—distal occlusion with extruded front.

Class II/2—distal occlusion with deep bite.

Class III—mesial occlusion.

Note

- The motivation of the patient is leading in the decision-making process for surgical orthognathic treatment.
- Complex combined orthodontic and surgical therapy should only be performed on patients who know the needs and risks of combined treatment and are able to meet the treatment requirements.
- The prerequisite is a clear agreement between patient and surgeon on the achievability of the treatment goals.

4 Surgical Classification of Dysgnathias

(Adapted from [3])

Sagittal-skeletal Dysgnathia	Dentoalveolar Dysgnathia
Overdeveloped lower face	
Skeletal mandibular prognathism	Dentoalveolar protrusion and dento-maxillofacial prognathism
Chin macrogenia	
Underdeveloped lower face	
Skeletal mandibular retrognathism	Dentoalveolar retrusion and dento-maxillofacial retrognathism
Skeletal mandibular micrognathia	
Chin microgenia	
High lower face	
Chin macrogenia	Dentoalveolar open bite
Low lower face	
Chin microgenia	Dentoalveolar deep/closed bite
Underdeveloped midface	
Maxillary hypoplasia	
Maxillary retrognathism	
Mandibular pseudo-prognathism	
Overdeveloped midface	
Maxillary hyperplasia	Dentoalveolar protrusion
Maxillary prognathism	
Transversal growth disorders	
Mandibular hypoplasia	
Mandibular hyperplasia	
Chin hypoplasia	
Chin hyperplasia	
Maxillary hypoplasia	
Maxillary hyperplasia	

5 Asymmetric Skeletal Growth Disorders

- Skeletal laterognathia.
- Hemimandibular hyperplasia/elongation.
- Unilateral condylar hyper-/hypoplasia.

6 Facial Patterns in Typical Forms of Dysgnathia

The three *basic facial growth patterns* are:

A. *Hyperdivergent* facial growth pattern.
B. *Neutral* facial growth pattern.
C. *Hypodivergent* facial growth pattern.

The *neutral growth pattern* is generally considered the ideal facial growth scheme because it makes a straight facial profile with good dental occlusion possible (Fig. 2.1b).

A *posterior growth rotation* is seen in the "long face" syndrome with an anterior open bite (Fig. 2.1a). These cases have short rami with steep mandibular plane angles.

The *anterior growth rotation* can be associated with prognathism when the mandibular growth far exceeds the maxillary growth in the horizontal direction. It can also lead to bimaxillary protrusion as represented in Fig. 2.1 on the right (Fig. 2.1c) [2, 5].

6.1 Mandibular Growth

The mandible is suspended from the cranial base and there are two separate growth centers. The anterior downward movement of the maxilla is matched by a vertical increase in the condylar region of the posterior mandible. As the teeth show a vertical growth pattern, this must be matched by vertical growth in the condylar region or the mandible will show a posterior inclination [2, 5].

6.2 Anterior Mandibular Rotational Growth Pattern

Growth of the orofacial region is quantitatively described by locating the center of mandibular rotation relative to the cranial base. The anterior rotational growth pattern is associated with an increase in vertical condylar growth and reduced dentoalveolar height [4, 5].

The center of mandibular rotation is defined by the ratio of vertical facial growth—anterior versus posterior facial height—and the direction of condyle growth. To achieve the occlusal level, the molars must show stronger vertical growth than the incisors. In class II patients with open bite, e.g., changes in growth pattern reduce or stop favorable anterior mandibular rotation and redirect the mean condylar growth vector more posteriorly.

In extreme cases, a reduced facial height may also reduce the volume of the elevating muscles that results in a wider maxillary buccal space. In

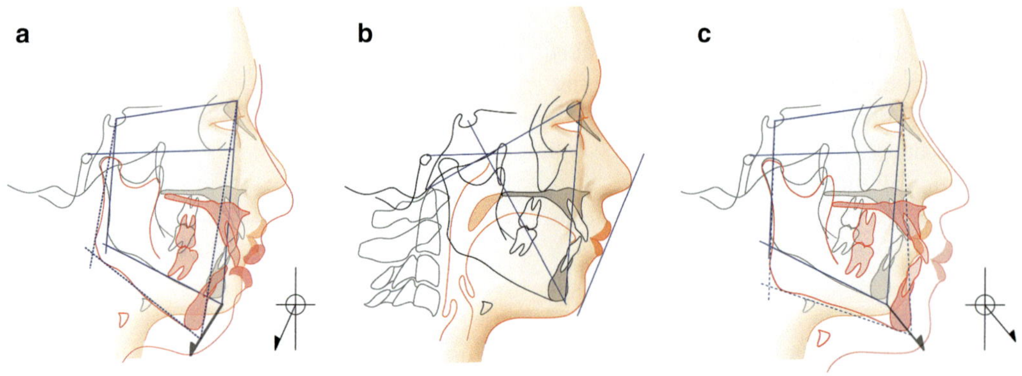

Fig. 2.1 Basic facial growth patterns [4] (**a**) Hyperdivergent (**b**) Neutral (**c**) Hypodivergent

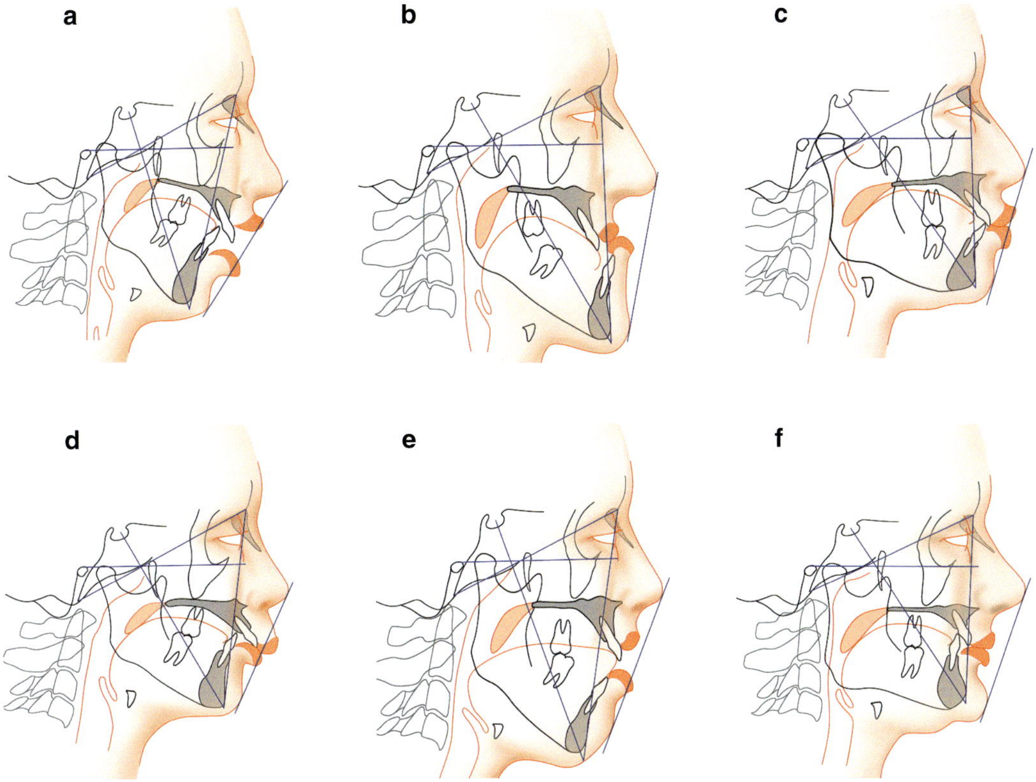

Fig. 2.2 Various types and typical forms of dysgnathias [6]. (**a**) Mandibular retrognathism. Retrognathism with steep mandibular angle. Pronounced overbite and overjet. Chronic breathing through the mouth. (**b**) Mandibular prognathism. Prognathism of the lower jaw with retrognathic maxilla and midface hypoplasia. (**c**) Underdeveloped face. Brachyfacial growth pattern with low facial height, dentoalveolar protrusion in both jaws. (**d**) Mandibular retrognathism. Moderate retrognathia with maxillary dentoalveolar protrusion and deep bite. (**e**) Overdeveloped face—long face. Long flat lower face with severe functional problems of the tongue, extreme open bite and insufficient lip closure. (**f**) Low lower face. Extremely deep bite with reduced lower facial height.

this situation, the transversal growth will result in a buccal overjet. A lingual crossbite is almost never present in anterior mandibular rotation or short face growth patterns.

The reduction in facial height is found almost exclusively in the lower face and is associated with a reduction in vertical alveolar development.

Figure 2.2 illustrates typical facial pattern variations in pronounced growth-related isolated or combined dysgnathias of the maxillo-mandibular complex.

7 Conclusion

No planning and no therapy without classification. Classification of dysgnathia is essential for functional and esthetic treatment. Furthermore, the classification defines the cooperation between orthodontists and surgeons. Both must speak this common language, which is based on a generally accepted classification. It also gives the patient certainty and the possibility of comparison when a therapeutic alternative is presented.

References

1. Becking AG, Hoppenreijs TJM, Tuinzing DB. Disturbances of growth and development of the maxillofacial skeleton. Ned Tijdschr Tandheelkd. 2007;114(1):34–40.
2. Hultgren BW, Isaacson RJ, Erdman AG, Worms FW, Rekow ED. Growth contributions to class II corrections based on models of mandibular morphology. Am J Orthod. 1980;78(3):310–20.
3. Spiessl B. Osteosynthese bei sagittaler Osteotomie nach Obwegeser-Dal Pont. Fortschr Kieferheilkd Gesichtschir. 1974;18:145–8.
4. Isaacson RJ, Erdman AG, Hultgren BW. Facial and dental effects of mandibular rotation craniofacial biology, monograph no. 10, Craniofacial growth series. University of Michigan; 1981.
5. Berkowitz S. Orthodontic analysis and treatment planning in patients with craniofacial anomalies. In: Wolfe SA, Berkowitz S, editors. Plastic surgery of the facial skeleton. Boston, Toronto: Little, Brown; 1989.
6. Ricketts ARE. The biology of occlusion and the temporomandibular joint. In: Modern man, 1972.

Types of Osteotomies in the Mandible

3

Peter Kessler and Nicolas Hardt

Contents

Abstract

Corrections of the bite position in skeletal malformations or esthetic corrections with the aid of the skeleton can only be achieved by osteotomies and relocation of bone and soft tissue components. The nomenclature of common osteotomies must be clearly understood. They can be applied individually, in combination, and in both jaws.

Keywords

Classification of dysgnathias · Development of orthognathic surgery · Basic osteotomy procedures · Ramus osteotomies · Sagittal mandibular split · Bilateral sagittal split osteotomy · BSSO · Segment osteotomies · Chin osteotomies · Genioplasty · Chin osteotomy

P. Kessler (✉)
Department of Cranio-Maxillofacial Surgery, Maastricht University Medical Center, Maastricht, The Netherlands
e-mail: peter.kessler@mumc.nl

N. Hardt (✉)
Kantonsspital Lucerne, Clinic and Policlinic of Cranio-Maxillofacial Surgery, Lucerne, Switzerland

1 Introduction

Orthognathic surgery includes surgical interventions on the facial skeleton to restore normal anatomical and functional intermaxillary relationships in patients with maxillo-mandibular anomalies affecting the face.

P. Kessler et al. (eds.), *Illustrated Manual of Orthognathic Surgery*,
https://doi.org/10.1007/978-3-031-06978-9_3

The compartments of the facial skeleton can be surgically repositioned through a variety of established osteotomies, redefining facial contours such as the facial profile.

Most mandibular deformities can essentially be treated with four basic osteotomy procedures, which in turn can be combined with each other.

2 Surgical Corrections in the Lower Jaw

1. Ramus osteotomies.
2. Mandibular body osteotomies.
3. Segmental osteotomies.
4. Chin osteotomies.

2.1 Ramus Osteotomies

are differentiated into.

- Sagittal split ramus osteotomy.
- Vertical ramus osteotomy.
- Inverted L- and C-ramus osteotomy.

2.2 Mandibular Body Osteotomies

Mandibular body osteotomies are differentiated into.

- Anterior mandibular body step osteotomy-ostectomy.
- Posterior mandibular body step osteotomy-ostectomy.
- Inter- or retromolar vertical osteotomy combined with distraction osteogenesis - DOG.

2.3 Segmental Osteotomies

Segmental osteotomies are differentiated into

- Anterior segmental osteotomies.
- Posterior segmental osteotomies.

2.4 Chin Osteotomies

Chin osteotomies are differentiated into.

- Augmentation/advancement genioplasty.
- Reduction genioplasty.
- Straightening genioplasty.
- Lengthening genioplasty.

3 Classification of Surgical Corrections

See Table 3.1

Table 3.1 Classification of orthognathic procedures in the mandible

Classification of surgical correction possibilities in the lower jaw through transoral accesses		
Ramus osteotomies	Body osteotomies	Segmental osteotomies
Sagittal split ramus osteotomy	Anterior mandibular body step osteotomy-ostectomy	Anterior segmental osteotomies
Vertical ramus osteotomy	Posterior mandibular body step osteotomy-ostectomy	Posterior segmental osteotomies
Inverted L- and C-ramus osteotomy	Inter-or retromolar osteotomy for distraction osteogenesis - DOG	–
–	Augmentation/advancement genioplasty	–
–	Reduction genioplasty	–
–	Straightening genioplasty	–
–	Lengthening genioplasty	–

4 Conclusion

Brief and concise listing of possible mandibular osteotomy techniques including genioplasties. The planning and technical procedure and the appropriate indications are described in the following parts.

Further Reading

Bell HW, Proffit WR, White RP. Surgical correction of dentofacial deformities. Saunders. 1980;1-3

Fonseca RJ, Marciani RD, Turvey TA. Oral and maxillofacial surgery. Orthognathic surgery, esthetic surgery, cleft and craniofacial surgery. Saunders. 2009;

Reyneke JP. Essentials of orthognathic surgery. Quintessence Publishing Co Inc; 2019.

Steinhäuser EW. Rückblick auf die Entwicklung der Dysgnathiechirurgie und Ausblick. Mund-Kiefer- und Gesichtschirurgie. 2003;7:371–9.

Definition of Standard Procedures

4

Peter Kessler and Nicolas Hardt

Contents

P. Kessler (✉)
Department of Cranio-Maxillofacial Surgery,
Maastricht University Medical Center,
Maastricht, The Netherlands
e-mail: peter.kessler@mumc.nl

N. Hardt (✉)
Kantonsspital Lucerne, Clinic and Policlinic of
Cranio-Maxillofacial Surgery, Lucerne, Switzerland

P. Kessler et al. (eds.), *Illustrated Manual of Orthognathic Surgery*,
https://doi.org/10.1007/978-3-031-06978-9_4

Abstract

The surgical standard interventions are differentiated between procedures in the region of the mandibular angle and ascending ramus—concerning the sagittal and vertical osteotomy to perform the typical sagittal split—and stepped or oblique osteotomies in the tooth-bearing mandibular body for horizontal shifts. In addition, segmental anterior and posterior partial osteotomies of the horizontal branch and chin osteotomies are distinguished. Combinations of these procedures are possible.

Keywords

Classification of dysgnathias · Orthognathic surgery · Basic osteotomy procedures · Classification of surgical corrections · Ramus osteotomies · Sagittal mandibular split · Bilateral sagittal split osteotomy · BSSO · Mandibular advancement · Mandibular setback · Segment osteotomies · Distraction osteogenesis · Chin osteotomies · Genioplasty

1 Bilateral Sagittal Split Osteotomy - BSSO/ Osteotomies in the Mandible

The transoral approach to the sagittal splitting of the mandible in the region of the jaw angle as described by *Trauner* and *Obwegeser* [1] and modified by *Dal Pont* in [2] ensures a maximum overlap of the proximal and distal bone surfaces. This allows an extensive displacement of the bone segments in both posterior and anterior directions (mandibular setback or advancement).

Advantages:

- Possibility of a functionally stable fixation of the fragments.
- Due to stable fixation reduced risk of recurrence and pseudarthrosis.
- No visible scars.

1.1 Indications—Standard Sagittal Split Osteotomy

The versatility of the BSSO allows the lower jaw to be shifted into a functionally ideal position:

1. Anterior displacement to correct a skeletal class II malocclusion or a large overjet.
2. Posterior repositioning (setback surgery) to correct a class III malocclusion with reversed overjet.
3. Horizontal and vertical rotation to correct a mandibular asymmetry or an open or crossbite.

1.2 Surgical Principle—BSSO

A successful split will result in the split region in a lateral monocortical segment with little cancellous bone and a medial monocortical segment with much more cancellous bone.

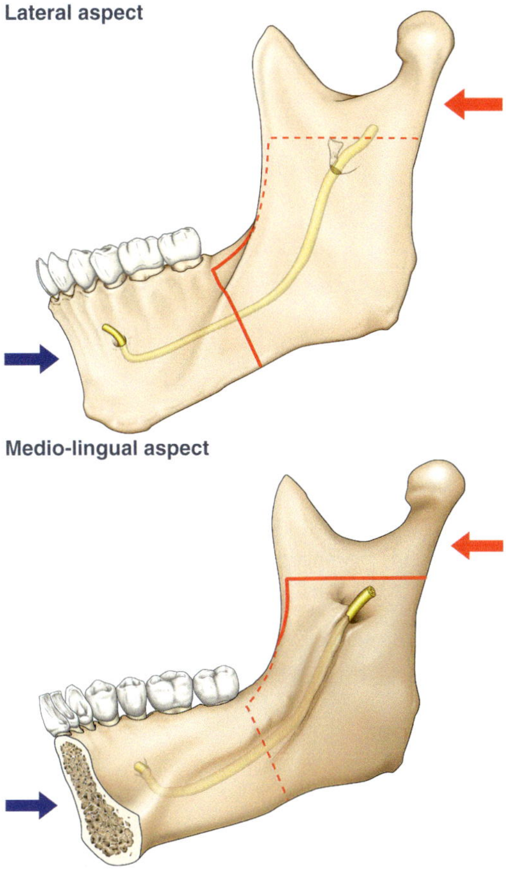

Fig. 4.1 Course of the osteotomy lines in a typical BSSO according to Obwegeser-Dal Pont: Bucco-lateral and medio-lingual osteotomy lines (——) and sagittal connecting osteotomy (-------). Red arrow = proximal segment, blue arrow = distal segment [3]

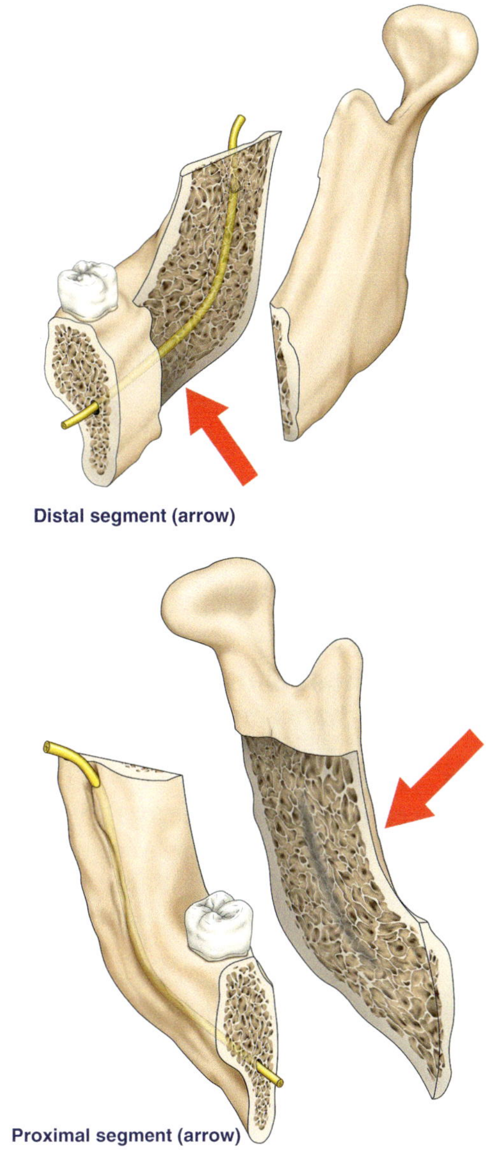

Fig. 4.2 Split mandibular segments after sagittal osteotomy. The inferior alveolar nerve is ideally fully embedded in the medio-distal mandibular segment. Only a thin layer of cancellous bone remains on the lateral-proximal segment [3]

The division is performed by three bone cuts (osteotomies), which are applied vertically-laterally and horizontally-medially; both are connected by a sagittal osteotomy line (Fig. 4.1).

The principle of the sagittal splitting is the division of the ascending ramus into a proximal-lateral and a distal-medial segment in a sagittal plane (Fig. 4.2).

In the sagittal splitting osteotomy (SSO), the buccal vertical osteotomy lies directly behind the second molar. The linguo-medial osteotomy runs about 8–10 mm below the semilunar notch and the sagittal connecting osteotomy runs medially along the anterior edge (external oblique line) of the ascending ramus.

1.3 Sagittal Splitting as Setback Surgery

1.3.1 Principle

In mandibular prognathism, after SSO and repositioning of the mandible, the proximal segment is shortened according to the distance by which the mandible has been setback (Fig. 4.3).

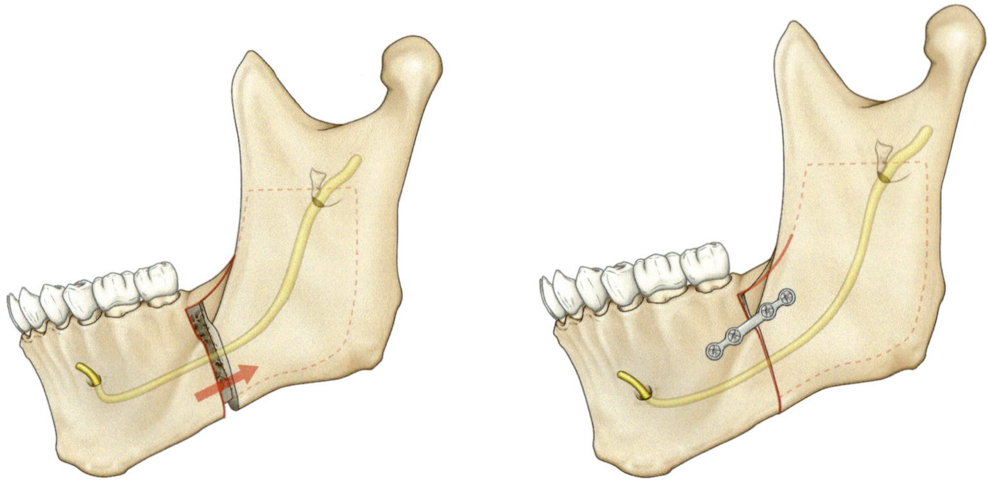

Fig. 4.3 Mandibular Excess—Prognathism. Situation after sagittal split and mandibular setback. The red arrow marks the posterior repositioning (backward displacement). The overlapping buccal bone lamella is removed [3].

1.4 Sagittal Splitting as Advancement Surgery

1.4.1 Principle

In mandibular retrognathism the SSO is the same as in mandibular prognathism. After sufficient mobilization the mandible will be advanced. There is no need to shorten the segments (Fig. 4.4).

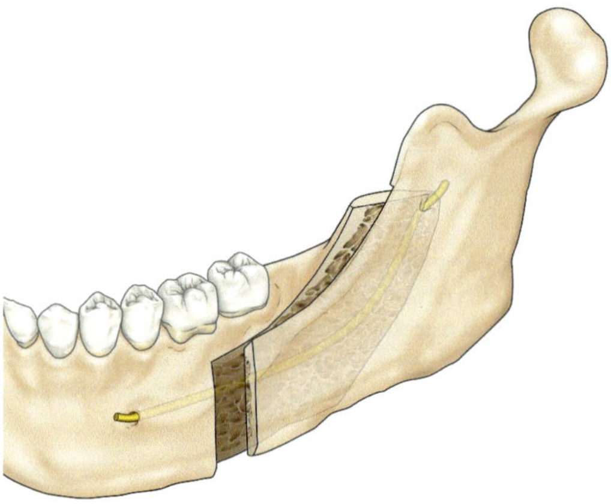

Fig. 4.4 Mandibular Deficiency—Retrognathism, SSO with horizontal mandibular advancement. Note bone overlap

1.5 Mandibular Body Osteotomy

Osteotomies in the tooth-bearing body of the mandible are now only performed for very selective indications, such as the anterior mandibulotomy, anterior ostectomy, and the stepwise osteotomy.

1.6 Stepwise Osteotomy

This type of osteotomy is preferred for very selected cases of prognathism with anterior open bite, excessive mandibular growth in the anterior dentoalveolar block, a negative overjet, and asymmetries of the mandibular arch, especially if the first or second premolars are missing or need to be extracted (Figs. 4.5 and 4.6) [4].

1.6.1 Principle

Methodically, this type of osteotomy can be used as a segmental or total osteotomy to reposition the anterior section of the mandible in any desired direction, e.g., into a posterior position with/without a cranial tilt.

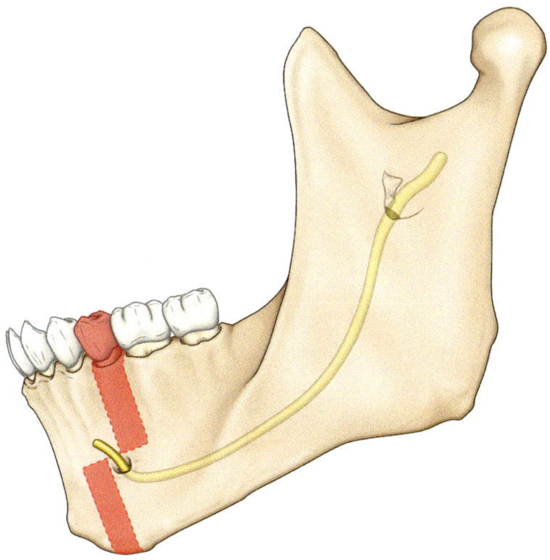

Fig. 4.5 The stepwise body osteotomy can be used for a segmental alveolar osteotomy or total osteotomy of the mandible

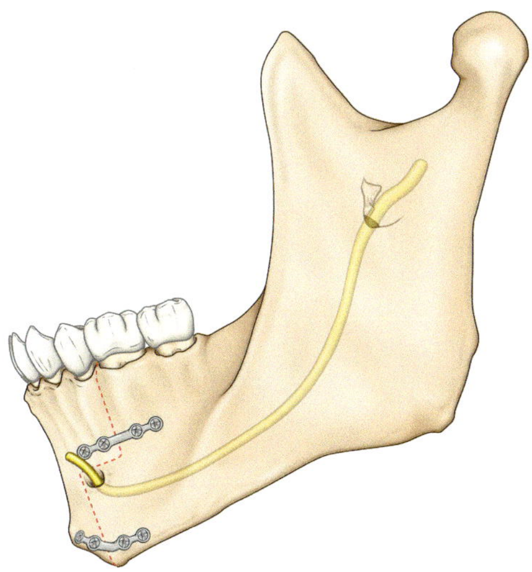

Fig. 4.6 Rigid internal fixation after lateral body osteotomy is performed with miniplates [4]

1.7 Horizontal Mandibular Distraction Osteogenesis

Retromolar and intermolar mandibular distraction osteogenesis are forms of bone distraction surgery. The decisive advantage of distraction osteogenesis is the combined, simultaneous growth of soft tissue together with the growth of bone tissue. Both guarantee postoperative stability using a dynamic technique (Figs. 4.7 and 4.8).

1.7.1 Indication

Only class II dysgnathias can be treated by distraction. Horizontal distraction to lengthen the mandible applying retromolar distractors is rarely indicated. This concerns, e.g., pronounced cases of mandibular retrognathia, such as mandibular hypoplasia (unilateral or bilateral hypoplasia of the mandible) and micrognathia, severe cleft facial malformations and congenital craniofacial anomalies/malformations such as hemifacial microsomia as well as retrognathia with TMJ-ankylosis and facial asymmetries. Intermolar osteotomies, on the other hand, can be used primarily in younger class II patients to avoid standard treatment with BSSO at the end of growth. Above all, this can save treatment time.

1.7.2 Principle

Three-dimensional increase of bone volume by horizontal distraction of the lower jaw. The distraction is carried out with bone—less frequently combined bone and tooth-anchored—unidirectional or bi-multidirectional distractors. The distraction rate is usually 1 mm/day divided into two fractions of 0.5 mm [6].

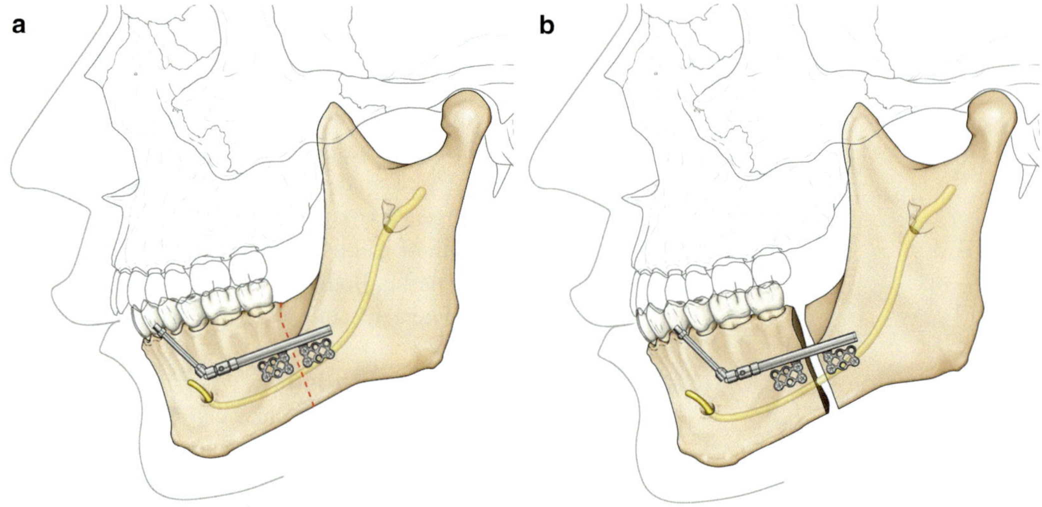

Fig. 4.7 Horizontal mandibular distraction [5] (**a**) Vertical osteotomy and placement of distractor on the buccal side. (**b**) Distraction distal of the last molar tooth ©Copyright Keisuke Koyama 2020. All rights reserved

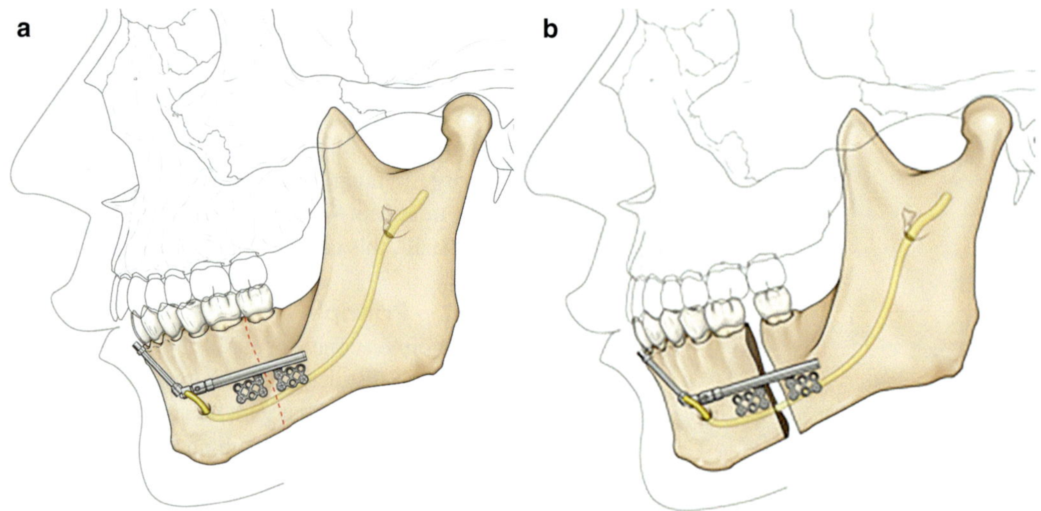

Fig. 4.8 (**a**) Intermolar vertical osteotomy as special form of horizontal mandibular distraction (**b**) Vertical mandibular osteotomy between first and second molar, activation of distractor ©Copyright Keisuke Koyama 2020. All rights reserved

1.8 The Anterior Mandibulotomy

1.8.1 Indications

Occasionally, in patients with a short lower face, there is very little bone between the root tips of the incisors and the lower edge of the mandible. In such cases adequate vertical segment relocation cannot be achieved without damaging the tips or leaving a precariously thin strut of cortical bone (Fig. 4.9).

1.8.2 Technique

This problem can be overcome in two ways:

1. Two vertical osteotomy lines mostly distal to the canines lead to a three-piece mandible, whereby the middle segment can be shifted vertically (Fig. 4.9a).
2. Combination of the abovementioned technique with a horizontal osteotomy in the chin area (genioplasty), resulting in a four-piece mandible (Fig. 4.9b).

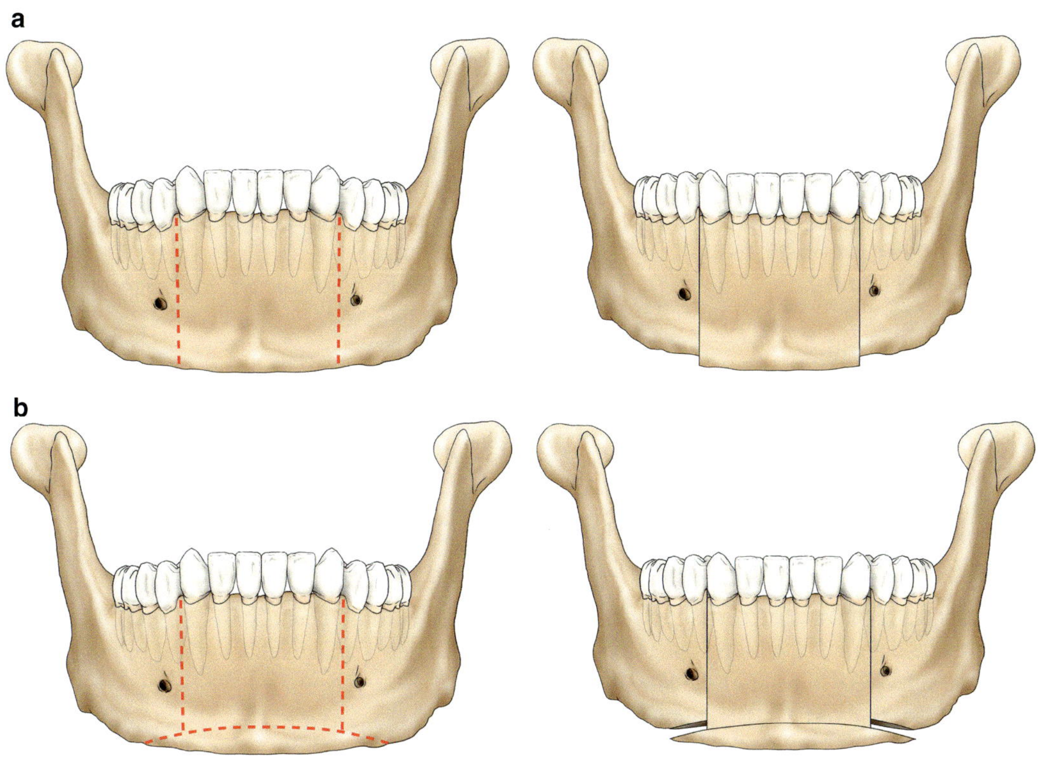

Fig. 4.9 Representation of the vertical (**a**), or vertical and horizontal osteotomy lines (**b**) for displacement of the mandibular middle segment.

The mandibular front segment is then set down and fixed as planned, and shifts the chin bone downward, thus avoiding any bone loss. The anterior inferior dentoalveolar height is increased and improves the lower facial proportions. Bone plates must be used for stable fixation [7].

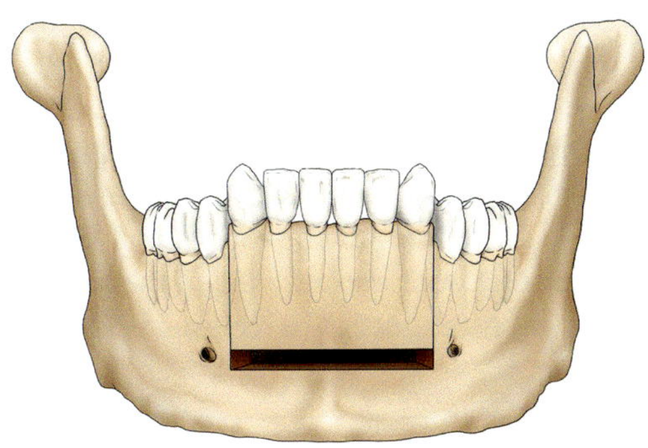

Fig. 4.10 The subapical area can be clearly exposed and provides sufficient access for the subapical osteotomy

2 Segmental Alveolar Osteotomies

2.1 Anterior Subapical Osteotomy

An anterior subapical osteotomy is indicated when there is a skeletal class I relationship, but a vertical frontal bone excess or deficiency cannot be corrected by orthodontic treatment.

2.1.1 Principle

The anterior subapical osteotomy allows the mandibular alveolar segment to be repositioned in any desired direction. Even a slight tilting of the segment is possible. Surgically, the subapical area provides sufficient access for the osteotomy under the root tips (Fig. 4.10). The subapical area is reached through an intraoral, vestibular incision.

The horizontal osteotomy is performed subapically approx. 5 mm below the root tips and is then connected with two interdental vertical osteotomies between the canines and the first premolars, the segment is then carefully mobilized and adjusted to the preoperatively predetermined position (Fig. 4.10).

2.2 Posterior Subapical Osteotomy

2.2.1 Indication

Correction of super-erupted molars in the mandible or ankylosis of posterior teeth.

2.2.2 Principle

The transoral incision starts at the anterior edge of the vertical ramus and continues into the canine area.

In the area of the intended osteotomy, the incision is made marginally, starting one tooth width behind, respectively in front of the intended posterior and anterior vertical osteotomies. The two vertical oblique incisions are made and connected with the horizontal subapical osteotomy.

The periosteal attachment of the segment is removed only in the area of the osteotomy lines. This ensures the soft tissue contour and perfusion of the segment.

The horizontal osteotomy is performed subapically about 5 mm below the root tips. The horizontal osteotomy is then connected to the two vertical osteotomies between the first molar and the second premolar. After mobilization of the segment, the posterior segment can be repositioned.

3 Chin Osteotomies

Various craniofacial skeletal deficiencies such as the deep bite of class II or class III and the open bite can be simultaneously associated with morphological changes of the chin, which vary greatly from one individual to another. Class II mandibles might be associated with microgenia or retrognathia, whereas in a class III relation (prognathism) is often related with progenia.

The correction of chin disharmonies can be performed surgically by three-dimensional reduction, advancement, or augmentation of the chin segment, namely vertically, transversely, and sagittally.

The determination of the chin anomaly types is objectified at the jaw position to the orthograde profile line.

The following basic types of shape deviations are distinguished (Fig. 4.11):

Microgenia

Small chin is present with an overall deficiency of bone, generally in all three dimensions.

Retrogenia

Chin is not necessarily small but is positioned posterior to its desired position. Pure retrogenia exists when the occlusion is normal. If there is mandibular retrognathia, the retrogenia is secondary.

Macrogenia

Chin is large in size. As with microgenia, macrogenia can exist with normal occlusion or be associated with mandibular prognathism.

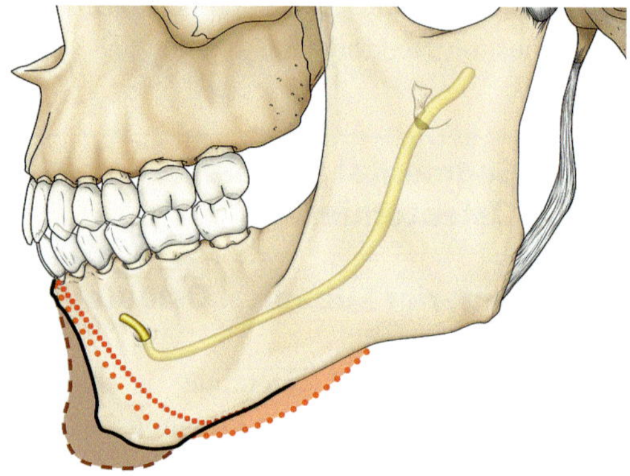

Fig. 4.11 Disharmonic chin shapes objectified at the chin position to the mandible and the orthograde profile line.

4 Principal Surgical Techniques in Chin Osteotomies

Chin reshaping can provide a more pronounced facial appearance in patients undergoing orthognathic surgery. The "sliding" genioplasty has the most potential for reshaping the chin.

The following surgical variants (sliding osteotomies and ostectomies) are distinguished:

4.1 Horizontal Sliding Genioplasty

Indications:
The sliding genioplasty serves:

- To build up a chin prominence.
- For chin elongation in cases with too short vertical lower faces.
- For horizontal reduction of a prominent chin.
- For rotation and straightening of an asymmetric chin.
- Advancement of a receded chin.
- For vertical reduction of a chin with excess height.
- For vertical augmentation and lengthening of a shortened chin.

A transoral approach is obligatory. The anterior mandibular base—if necessary also the lateral base up to the mandibular angle—is osteotomized and repositioned in the desired position.

A distinction is made between the following genioplasties:

4.2 Horizontal Sliding Osteotomy

Chin Augmentation Genioplasty
After horizontal osteotomy, the lower fragment can be pushed directly forward, similar to a drawer that is opened, until its posterior cortex is in contact with the anterior cortex of the symphysis. A vertical dislocation to lengthen the chin is possible. In addition, bone-graft material can be used for vertical augmentation (Fig. 4.12) [8].

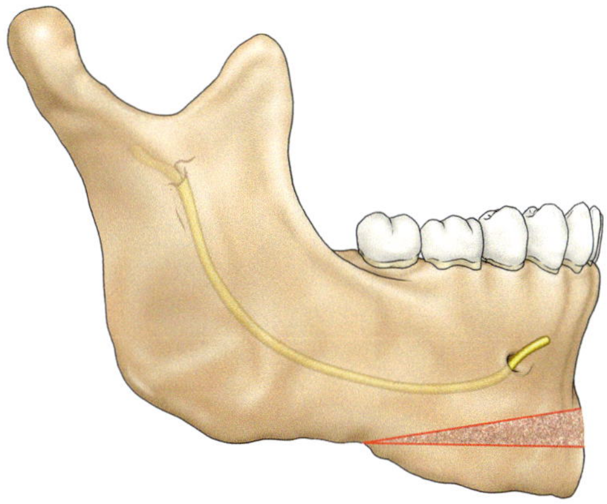

Fig. 4.12 Horizontal osteotomy—horizontal sliding osteotomy with vertical augmentation—augmentation genioplasty.

Chin Reduction Genioplasty
During reduction, a piece of bone is removed, the chin is pulled backward and sometimes moved upward. To achieve this a bone disc under the root tips is osteotomized and removed, but the shape of the chin prominence itself is not changed. The chin prominence is shifted dorsally. The chin can also be reduced by grinding away the caudal edge of the chin. This measure inevitably and irreversibly leads to the loss of the original shape of the chin apex [8].

4.3 Oblique Osteotomy for Chin Advancement

Osteotomy for chin advancement and elevation of the chin apex.

Chin forward displacement with simultaneous rotation of the chin upward [9]. The advantage of this technique is that it allows maximum forward and upward displacement of the chin apex (Fig. 4.13). It is very important that the muscles remain attached to the bony chin. As a result, the muscle attachments are also shifted upward and forward, thus relaxing the entire perioral region.

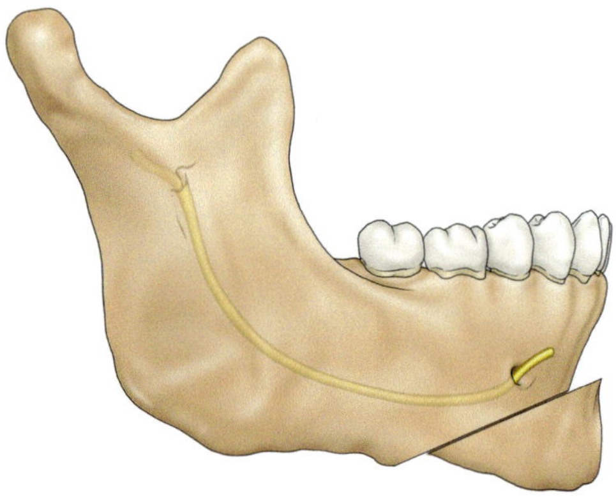

Fig. 4.13 Oblique osteotomy for chin advancement

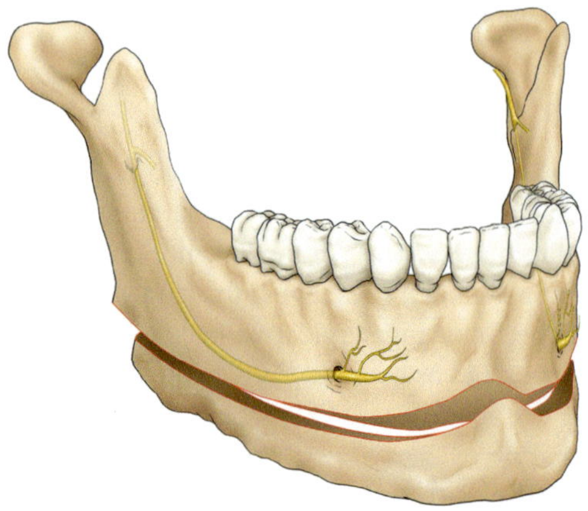

Fig. 4.14 Chin wing osteotomy

4.4 Jumping Genioplasty

The lower border fragment is lifted so it rests on the main mandibular segment, thereby shortening the chin vertically as well as giving more anteroposterior projection than can be obtained by the sliding genioplasty.

4.5 Centering Genioplasty

The lower fragment is moved horizontally to correct a transversal asymmetric deformity.

4.6 Two-Tiered or Tandem Genioplasty

A double horizontal osteotomy is performed. Whereas simple genioplasty can be easily performed by sliding or jumping osteotomies, extreme chin advancement, i.e., an advancement greater than 10 mm, requires the use of the double-step sliding technique [10].

4.7 Chin Wing Osteotomy

The chin wing osteotomy is performed as an aesthetic correction not only of the chin but also of the mandibular lower margin, either only in the front part of the lower margin or it covers the entire lower mandibular base (Fig. 4.14) [11].

The monocortical osteotomy line runs in a descending direction from above the mandibular angle to inferior below the mandibular canal and the mental foramen and then bi-cortically to the middle of the chin.

4.8 Less Common Variants and Alternatives

However, depending on the individual situation, double horizontal osteotomies, reduction osteotomies, wedge osteotomies, propeller genioplasties, triple and quadruple osteotomies, and genioplasties with interposition grafts of various materials are also performed.

Chin corrections can be performed as isolated or combined intervention with any orthognathic surgery of the maxilla and/or the mandible.

Besides the procedures mentioned here, the chin region can also be corrected with augmentation materials up to individualized implants.

5 Conclusions

In this part, the common surgical techniques for replacement of the mandible are presented [1, 2, 12]. Whenever possible, an osteotomy in the retromolar region (BSSO) will always be preferred over segmental osteotomies because they carry more risks and offer significantly fewer correction options. Special forms of osteotomies in the region of the ascending mandibular ramus, the inverted L osteotomy and the inverted vertical ramus osteotomy (IVRO) are discussed in detail in part VII. The chin osteotomy is a procedure often used to correct asymmetries in the frontal but lateral view on the patient. Genioplasties can be used alone or in combination.

Knowledge of the long evolution of osteotomy techniques in the context of orthognathic surgery in the mandible facilitates understanding of the BSSO as the standard and basic technique for all orthognathic correction procedures. Classification and definition of diagnosis-related treatment options creates systematics in patient handling, but also in training as well as comparability of results.

On this basis, complementary and alternative treatments can be understood. Also, the combination with other technical procedures, but also the limitations of monomaxillary treatments, become clear.

References

1. Trauner R, Obwegeser HL. The surgical correction of mandibular prognathism and retrognathia with considerations of genioplasty. Surgical procedures to correct mandibular prognathism and reshaping the chin. Part I. Oral Surg Oral Med Oral Pathol. 1957;10:677–89.
2. Dal Pont G. L'osteotomia retromolare par la converzione della progenia. Minerva Chir. 1959;14:1138.
3. Wolfe SA, Berkowitz S. Plastic surgery of the facial skeleton. Little Brown; 1989.
4. Kashani H, Rasmusson L. Osteotomies in orthognathic surgery. In: Hosein M, Motamedi K, editors. A textbook of advanced Oral and maxillofacial surgery, vol. 3. IntechOpen; 2016.
5. Michel C, Reuther J. Orthopädische Chirurgie. In: Hausamen E, Machtens E, Reuther J, editors. Mund-, Kiefer- und Gesichtschirurgie. Operationslehre und Atlas. Springer; 1995.
6. Karun V, Agarwal N, Singh V. Distraction osteogenesis for correction of mandibular abnormalities. Nat l J Maxillofac Surg. 2013;4(2):206–13.
7. Harris M, Reynolds IR. Fundamentals of orthognathic surgery. Saunders; 1991.
8. Hoenig JF. Sliding osteotomy genioplasty for facial aesthetic balance: 10 years of experience. Aesthet Plast Surg. 2007;31(4):384–91.
9. Joos U, Delaire J, Scheibe B, Schilli W. Funktionelle Aspekte der Kinnplastik. Fortschr Kiefer Gesichtschir. 1981;26:86.
10. Wiese KG. Extreme chin advancement with tandem genioplasty. Mund Kiefer Gesichts Chir. 1997;1(1):105–7.
11. Triaca A, Brusco D, Guijarro-Martínez R. Chin wing osteotomy for the correction of hyperdivergent skeletal calss III deformity: technical modification. Br J Oral Maxillofac Surg. 2015;53(8):775–7.
12. Dal Pont G. Retromolar osteotomy for the correction of prognathism. J Oral Surg. 1961;19:42–7.

Part II

Ramus Split Osteotomies / Bilateral Sagittal Split Osteotomies (BSSO) - General Planning

The Patient

5

Veronique C. M. L. Timmer, Peter Kessler, and Nicolas Hardt

Contents

Abstract

An accurate orthognathic planning is based on a combination of clinical examination, imaging, and facial analysis. Röntgen imaging commonly used for orthognathic diagnosis and planning includes conventional X-rays or cone-beam computerized tomography (CBCT).

Especially CBCT can reproduce an accurate visualization of the bone structures of the face but are less accurate in depicting soft tissues. However, soft tissue evaluation and prediction of soft tissue changes after surgery are essential to obtain a satisfying end result for the patient as well as for the surgeon.

Therefore, physical examination and analysis of the facial soft tissues remain a fundamental step in orthognathic planning. This chapter will discuss the chronological steps of planning in orthognathic surgery. The frequently used radiologic imaging modalities and their technical background and clinical indications will be briefly evaluated.

Keywords

Patient · Intake · Clinical examination · Photo documentation · Radiology · Basic measurements · Panoramic radiograph · Lateral

V. C. M. L. Timmer (✉) · P. Kessler (✉)
Department of Cranio-Maxillofacial Surgery, Maastricht University Medical Center, Maastricht, The Netherlands
e-mail: v.timmer@mumc.nl; peter.kessler@mumc.nl

N. Hardt (✉)
Kantonsspital Lucerne, Clinic and Policlinic of Cranio-Maxillofacial Surgery, Lucerne, Switzerland

P. Kessler et al. (eds.), *Illustrated Manual of Orthognathic Surgery*,
https://doi.org/10.1007/978-3-031-06978-9_5

cephalogram · Cone-beam computerized tomography (CBCT) · Cephalometric analysis · Facial analysis · Soft tissue analysis · Computer-based planning · General planning · 2D-Planning · 3D-Planning · Simulation surgery · Preoperative assessment · Preparations for the surgical procedure

1 Intake

The first step of the planning process already starts with the intake of a new patient. For every surgeon, it is essential to discover the motivation of the patient to undergo invasive surgery. Few question examples to ask the patient and yourself:

- Any functional problems involving speaking or eating?
- Problems with breathing or apnea?
- Complaints about joint pain?
- Is the motivation for surgery more related to the esthetics of the face?
- Are the wishes of the patient realistic and can we meet their expectations?

The motivation of the patient needs to be taken into account to achieve a good end result where the patient is satisfied and happy with.

2 Clinical Examination and Photo Documentation

Close observation of the face and profile provides a prediction of which jaw movements need to be made during surgery. It is preferable that the orthognathic planner has seen the patient himself rather than relying solely on photo documentation. The photographer's ability to obtain standardized and reproducible photographs is critical to planning accurate surgical jaw repositioning.

An experienced photographer can provide reliable photographs suitable for planning, but a less experienced photographer can produce photographs that lead to critical planning errors.

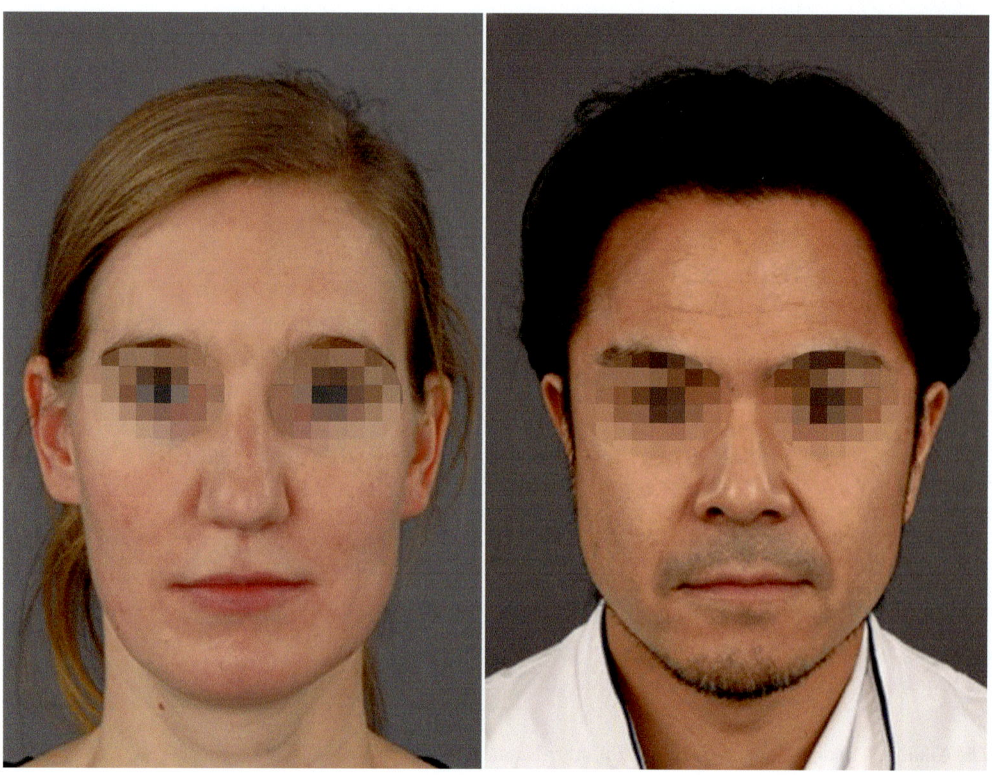

Fig. 5.1 Natural head position, frontal view

Photo documentation and evaluation of the face should always be done in a standardized way with the patient in natural head position, ears visible, and the patient should not wear jewelry during the photo shoot.

- The natural head position is a position of the head with the patient standing straight and looking straight to a point in the distance or to him/herself in the mirror (Fig. 5.1).

2.1 Examination of the Face from Top to Bottom

Frontal (portrait) position with closed lips, both ears visible:

- Assess the overall harmony of the face.
  - Do the proportions of the face look natural?
  - What is the shape of the face? (long, short, broad)
  - Are there any severe asymmetries present that may suggest craniofacial deformities?
- The rule of thirds

Horizontal lines divide the face into three sections which are ideally equal in vertical height (Fig. 5.2).

- The upper border of the face is indicated by the hair line.
- The second horizontal line is indicated by the eyebrows/glabella.
- The third horizontal line is indicated by the alar base of the nose and subnasal point.
- The lower border of the face is indicated by the edge of the chin (menton point).

The lower facial third can be divided by a horizontal line through the lips. The height of the upper lip to the subnasal point should ideally be 50% of the lower lip height to the menton point (Fig. 5.3).

- Facial midline

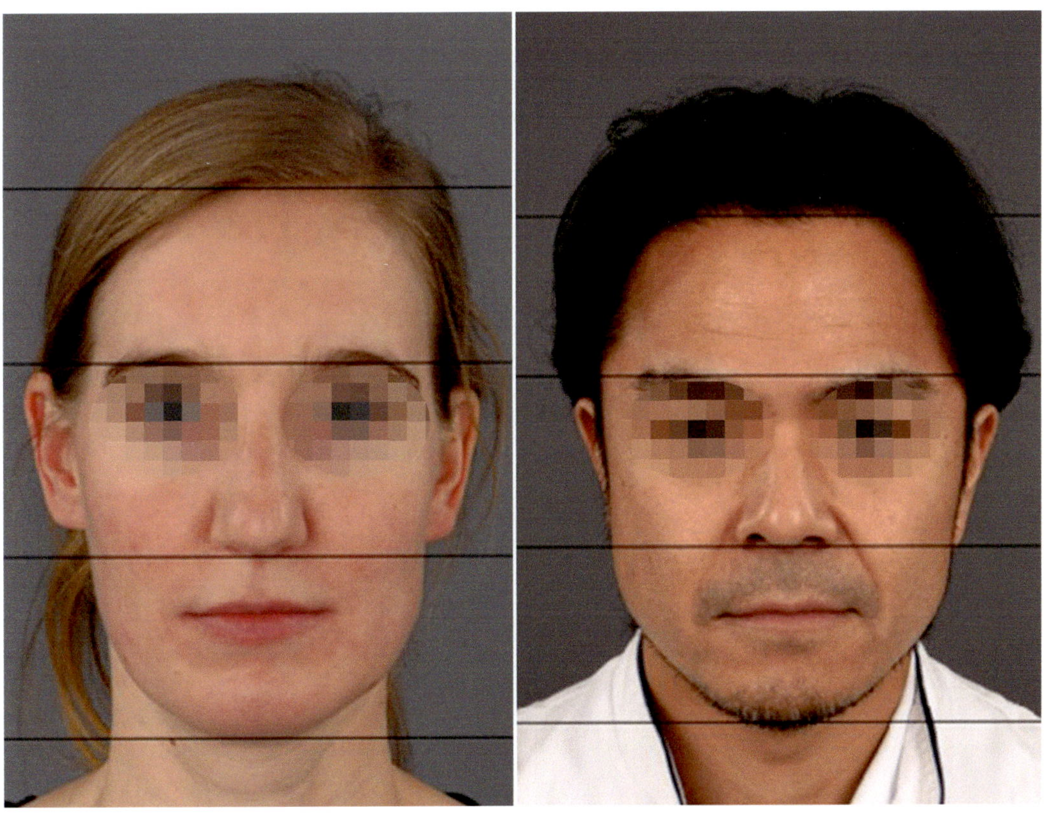

Fig. 5.2 Rule of thirds

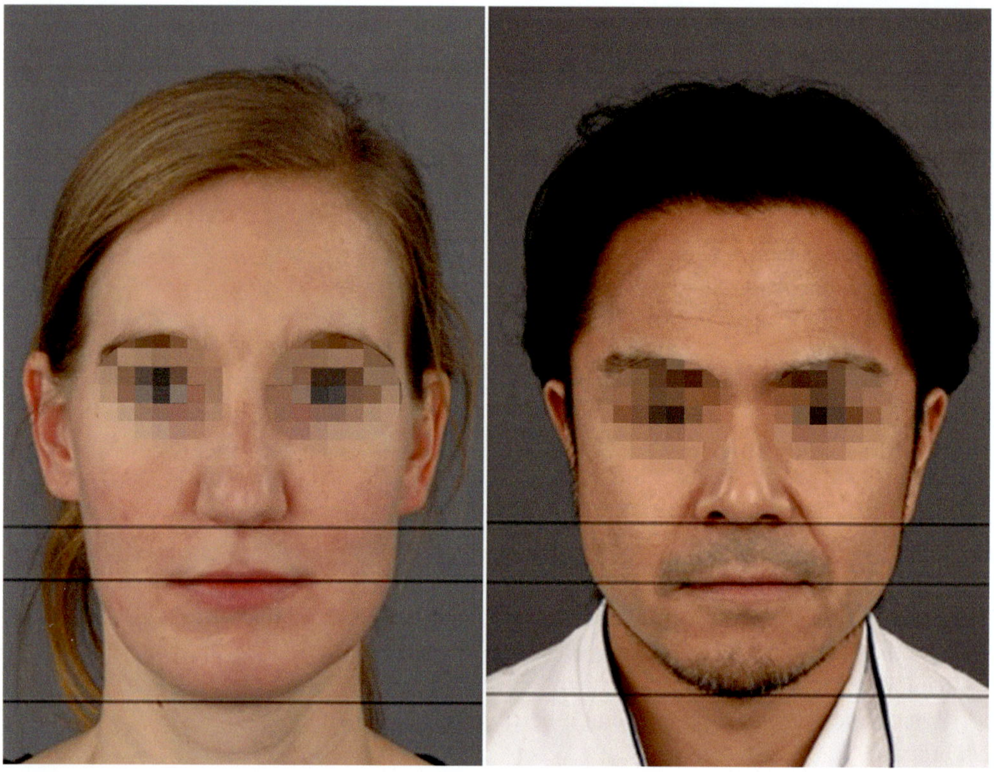

Fig. 5.3 Analysis of the lower facial third

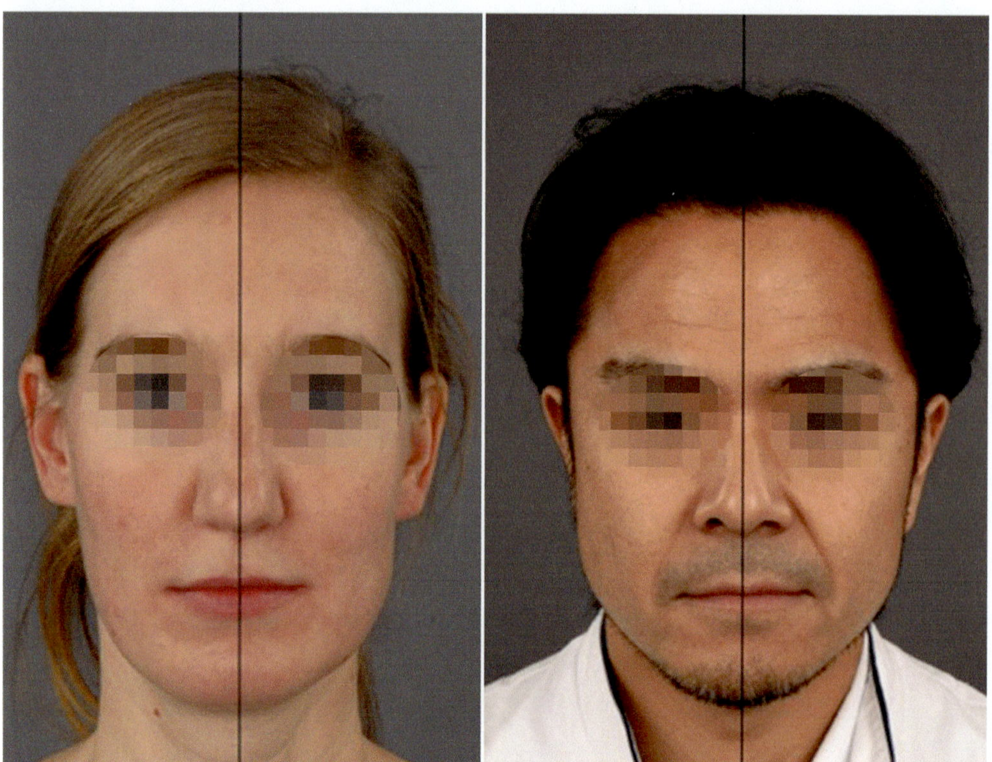

Fig. 5.4 Facial midline

The facial midline is a vertical center line through the glabella/nasion and subnasal point. The philtrum can be used as an anatomical landmark when there is no asymmetry as in cleft lips, e.g. (Fig. 5.4).

Assess the following anatomical landmarks:

Deviation of the tip of the nose (pronasale).

Deviation of the chin point (pogonion).

Compare left and right orbito-zygomatic complex.

Position of the eyebrows, eyes, ears, nose, and mouth.

> **Note**
>
> Be aware that every individual face has slight asymmetries.

The rule of five

The face can be divided vertically into five equal sections (Fig. 5.5).

In a well-proportioned face:

- The intercanthal width should be even to the width of the eyes (medial to lateral canthus).
- The nose and chin should be positioned in the center section of the five.
- The width of the alar base is ideally as wide as or a bit wider than 1/5 of the face.
- The mouth is positioned in the center section.
- The width of the mouth should equal the interpupillary distance.

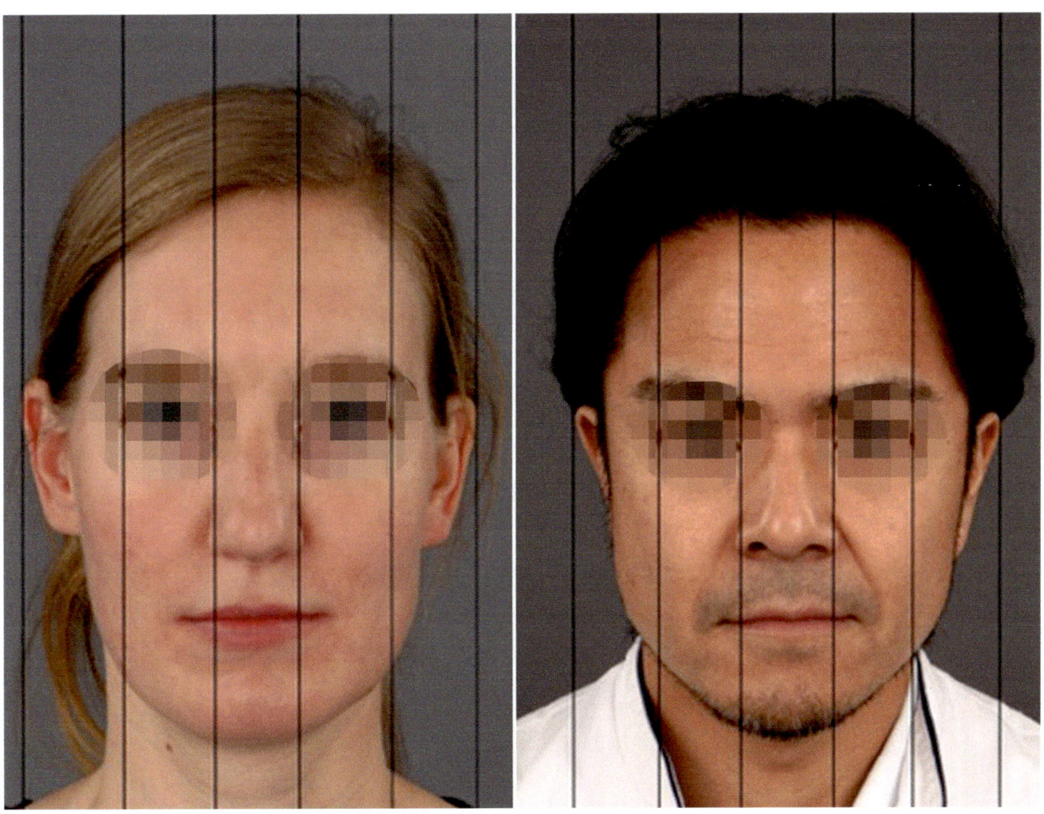

Fig. 5.5 Rule of five

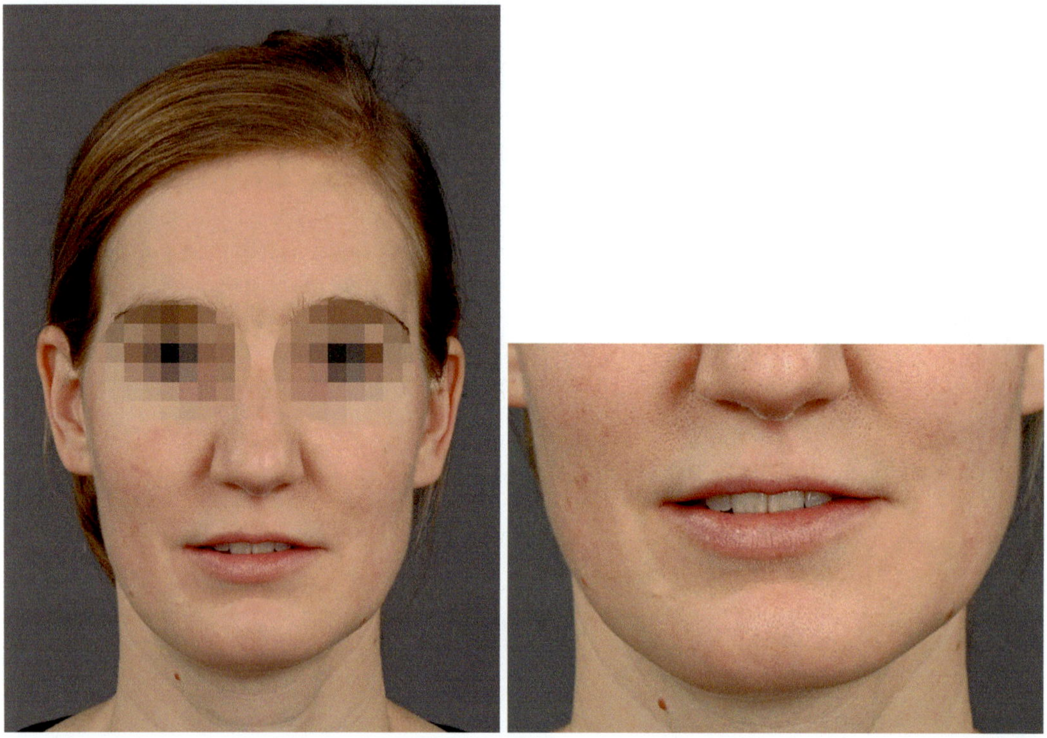

Fig. 5.6 Photo relaxed upper lip position with close-up

- Frontal position with relaxed soft tissues where the lips are slightly parted:
- Assess the relation of the upper lip to the front teeth. The dental show with relaxed facial tissue should be around 1–2 mm (Fig. 5.6).
- Assess the dental midline of the upper teeth.

Frontal position when smiling and showing teeth:

Assess the relation of the upper lip to the upper front teeth: The dental show when smiling should ideally be 9–10 mm, but is dependent on the length of the crowns (Fig. 5.7).

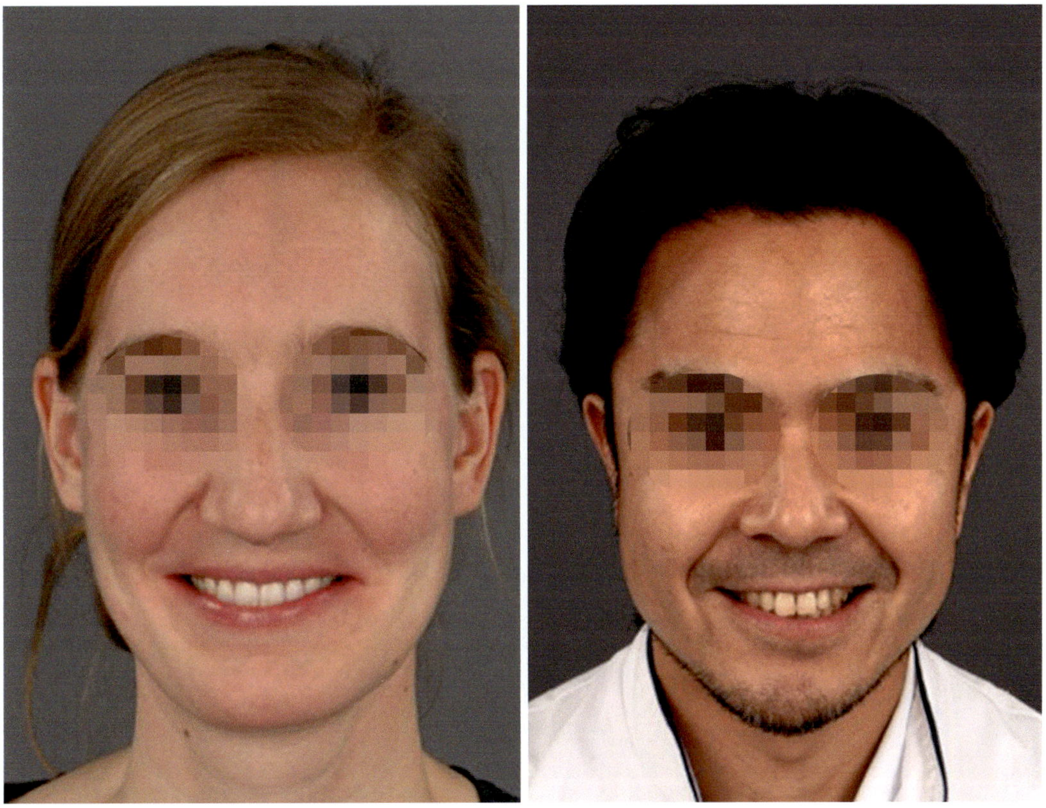

Fig. 5.7 Frontal portrait with a smile

Gummy smile.
Dental midlines of upper and lower teeth.
Occlusal canting.

Tip

Occlusal canting can be evaluated using a wooden spatula. The spatula is placed horizontally in occlusion at the height of the premolars. Check the cervical region of the cuspids and premolars besides the tips of the teeth; the tips of the cuspids can be worn down and may affect the accuracy of your observation.

- Profile position in 90° with relaxed soft tissues (Fig. 5.8).
  (45° profile pictures can be added as well):
  Evaluate the following structures:

- Profile shape: convex, concave, straight.
- Skeletal relation of the mandible and maxilla.
- Mandibular angle.
- Projection of infraorbital rim.
- Projection and shape of the nose.
- Projection of the lips, competence and support.
- Projection of the chin.
- Soft tissues, muscle tension.

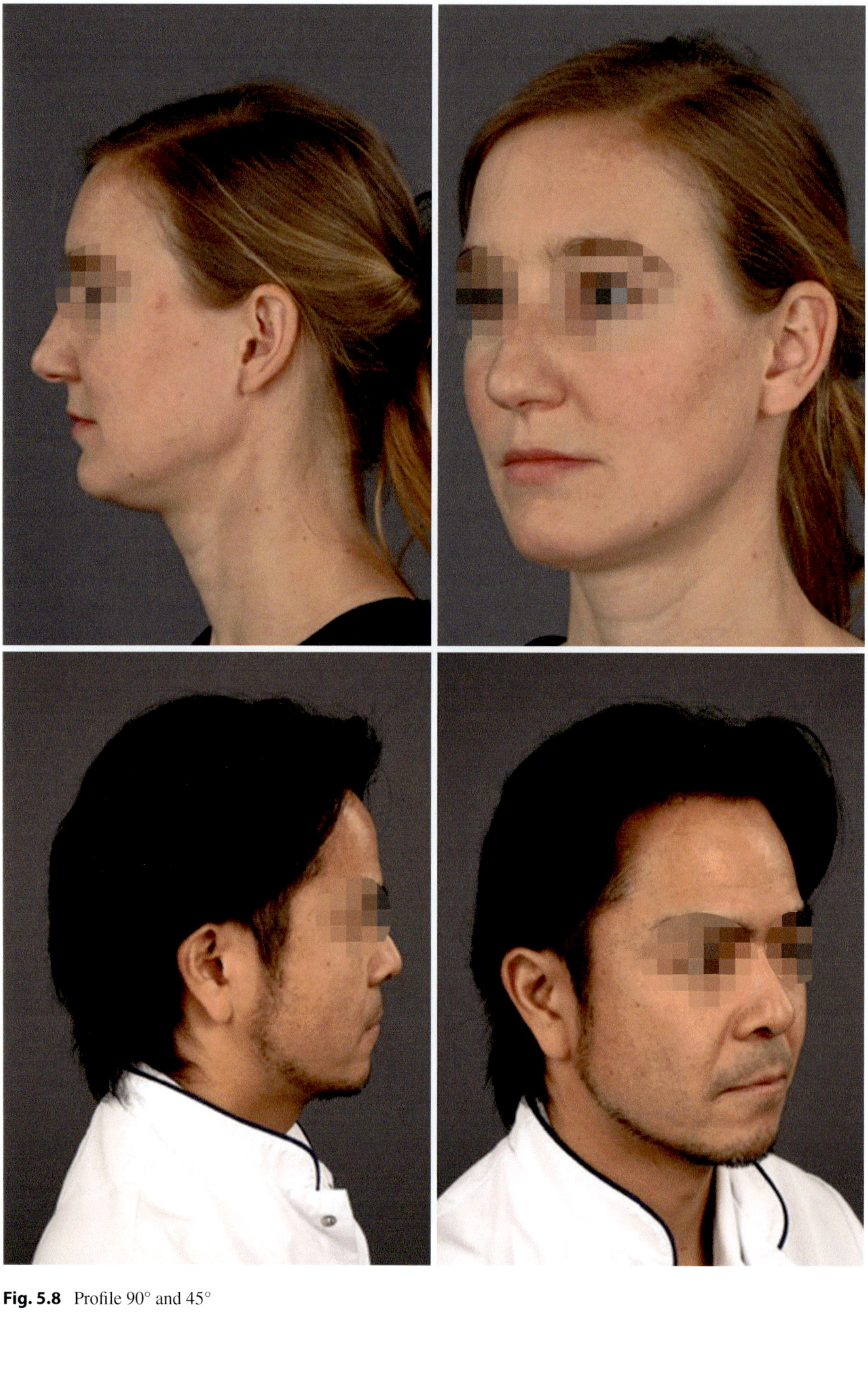

Fig. 5.8 Profile 90° and 45°

> **Note**
> Be aware of a "Sunday-bite": a habitual forward posturing of the mandible to compensate the sagittal deficit in overjet.

3 Dental Examination (Fig. 5.9)

- Dental hygiene and general condition of the gum and teeth.
- Number of teeth present.
- Occlusion: angle classification.
- Deep bite/palate bite, traumatic bite, open bite.
- Cross bite.
- Midline shift.
- Dental compensation.

3.1 Additional Clinical Examination

- Dental impressions or intraoral scans of the upper and lower teeth.
- Bite registration in centric relation with a thick wax bite. The bite registration can also be taken with the intraoral scanner. The centric relation is a reproducible mandibular position with the condyles in the most superior-posterior position in the fossa and the teeth in occlusion.

3.2 How to Proceed

- No assistance of the patient when trying to find the right occlusion.
- Guide the chin with one hand on the chin point and the other hand on the head of the patient (chin point guidance technique).
- The patient needs to be in an upright seated position.

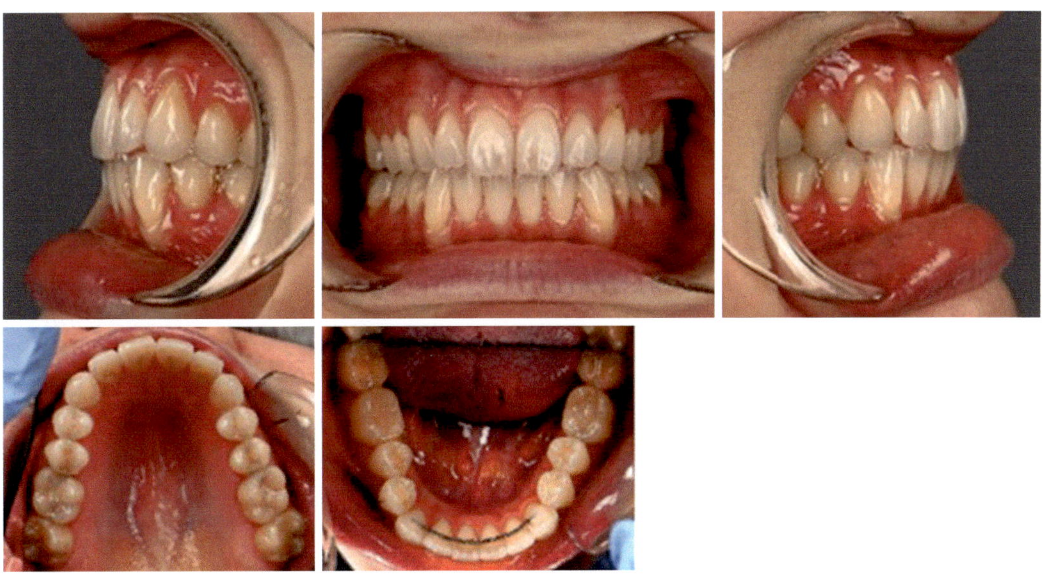

Fig. 5.9 Occlusion and dental arches

3.3 Facebow

With a single jaw mandibular osteotomy, precise model surgery planning using a facebow and anatomical articulator is not required.

4 Conclusion

The quality of the preoperative preparation determines the success of the treatment. The surgeon must be familiar with the individual planning steps in order to be able to implement them intraoperatively. An essential part of the planning is the cephalometric analysis.

Further Reading

Meneghini F, Biondi P. Clinical facial analysis. Springer-Verlag Berlin Heidelberg; 2021.

Proffit WR, Raymond P, White RP, Sarver DM. Contemporary treatment of dentofacial deformity. India: Elsevier; 2012.

Steinhäuser EW, Janson I. Kieferorthopädische Chirurgie, Eine interdisziplinäre Aufgabe, Band I. Quintessenz-Verlag GmbH. 1988;

Radiology and Basic Measurements

6

Veronique C. M. L. Timmer, Peter Kessler, and Nicolas Hardt

Contents

Abstract

Radiological imaging is an adjunct to the clinical examination. Imaging is needed to obtain a complete picture of the patient, to provide precise and individualized planning, and to detect hidden pathologies.

The standard preoperative radiological examination and assessment before a planned surgical treatment in the orthognathic surgery includes:

- The panoramic radiograph (panoramic X-ray).
- The lateral cephalometric X-ray of the skull.
- The cone-beam computed tomography (CBCT).

Occasionally the multi-slice computed tomography (MSCT).

Keywords

Radiology · Basic measurements · Panoramic radiograph · Lateral cephalogram · Cone-beam computerized tomography (CBCT) · Cephalometric analysis · Facial analysis · Soft tissue analysis · Computer-based planning · General planning · 2D Planning · 3D Planning · Simulation surgery · Preoperative assessment · Preparations for the surgical procedure

V. C. M. L. Timmer (✉) · P. Kessler (✉)
Department of Cranio-Maxillofacial Surgery, Maastricht University Medical Center, Maastricht, The Netherlands
e-mail: v.timmer@mumc.nl; peter.kessler@mumc.nl

N. Hardt (✉)
Kantonsspital Lucerne, Clinic and Policlinic of Cranio-Maxillofacial Surgery, Lucerne, Switzerland

P. Kessler et al. (eds.), *Illustrated Manual of Orthognathic Surgery*,
https://doi.org/10.1007/978-3-031-06978-9_6

1 Radiological Imaging

1.1 Panoramic X-Ray

The panoramic X-ray is a standardized diagnostic tool in preoperative screening of maxillofacial patients. It gives a general overview of the development of the teeth, the presence of third molars, and dental pathology, such as root resorption or periapical lesions. Furthermore, it shows basic information about the mandibular shape, TMJ morphology, and the mandibular canal (Figs. 6.1, 6.2, 6.3, 6.4).

Radiological findings can alter the course of the original surgery planning. For example, existing M3s in the mandible are preferred to be removed before BSSO to decrease the risk of a bad split during surgery. Any other hidden pathology revealed on panoramic X-ray, like mandibular cysts or periapical granuloma, should be properly treated before undergoing elective orthognathic surgery.

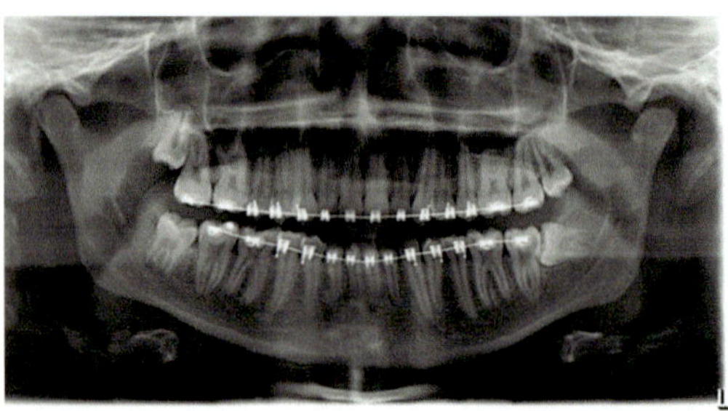

Fig. 6.1 A preoperative panoramic X-ray of an orthognathic patient with partially impacted third molars. Ideally the wisdom teeth need to be removed before the BSSO is performed to reduce the risk of a bad split during surgery

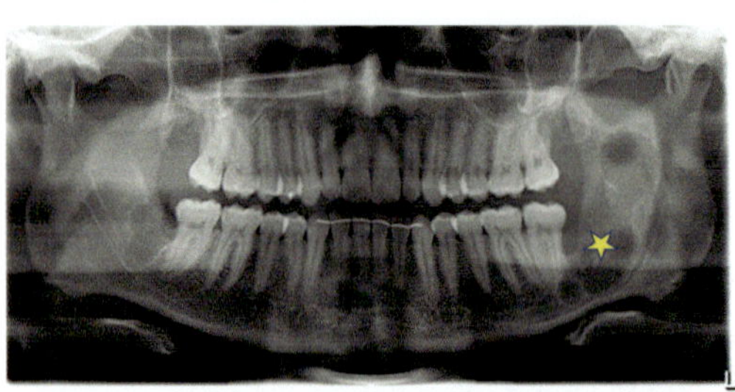

Fig. 6.2 A preoperative panoramic X-ray of an orthognathic patient showing an accidental finding [1] (should be further investigated before any orthognathic surgery will be performed)

The panoramic X-ray is not used in the actual orthognathic planning process concerning the positioning of the jaws, but it can easily be used for postoperative follow-up imaging (Fig. 6.4).

1.2 Lateral Cephalometric X-Ray

The lateral cephalometric X-ray represents a lateral view of the whole skull (Fig. 6.5). The X-ray is taken with the patient in a standardized reproducible position, perpendicular to the X-ray beam: in natural head position with the patient looking straight forward to a point in the far distance with relaxed facial soft tissues.

The lateral cephalometric images are used in orthodontics for cephalometric analysis, tracing, and follow-up of the development of the jaws and teeth during orthodontic treatment.

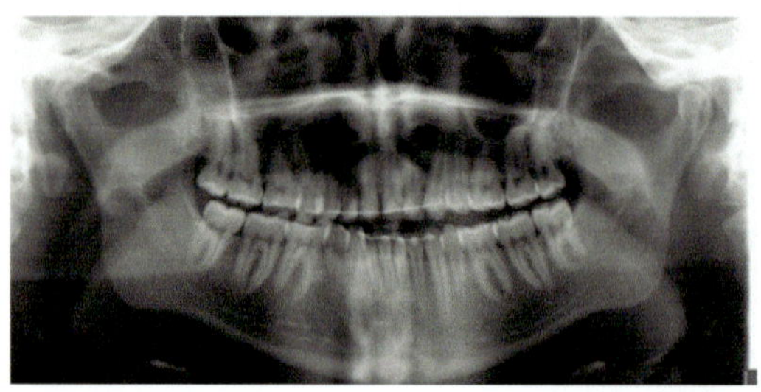

Fig. 6.3 A preoperative panoramic X-ray of a patient with an evident left midline-shift of the mandible. Note the changes in the bone structure of the right condylar head. A possible unilateral condylar hyperplasia or other (TMJ) pathology should be excluded before orthognathic correction of the mandibular asymmetry can be planned

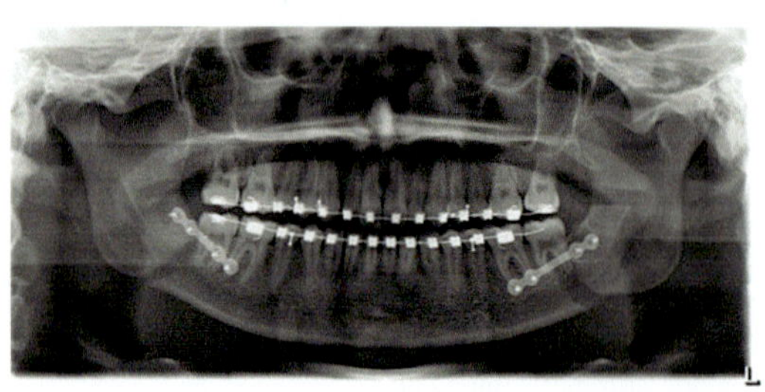

Fig. 6.4 A postoperative panoramic X-ray of a patient after BSSO treatment with advancement of the mandible. The osteotomy lines on both sides of the mandible are clearly visible and the osteosynthesis material can be evaluated. The condyles are both positioned in the mandibular fossa

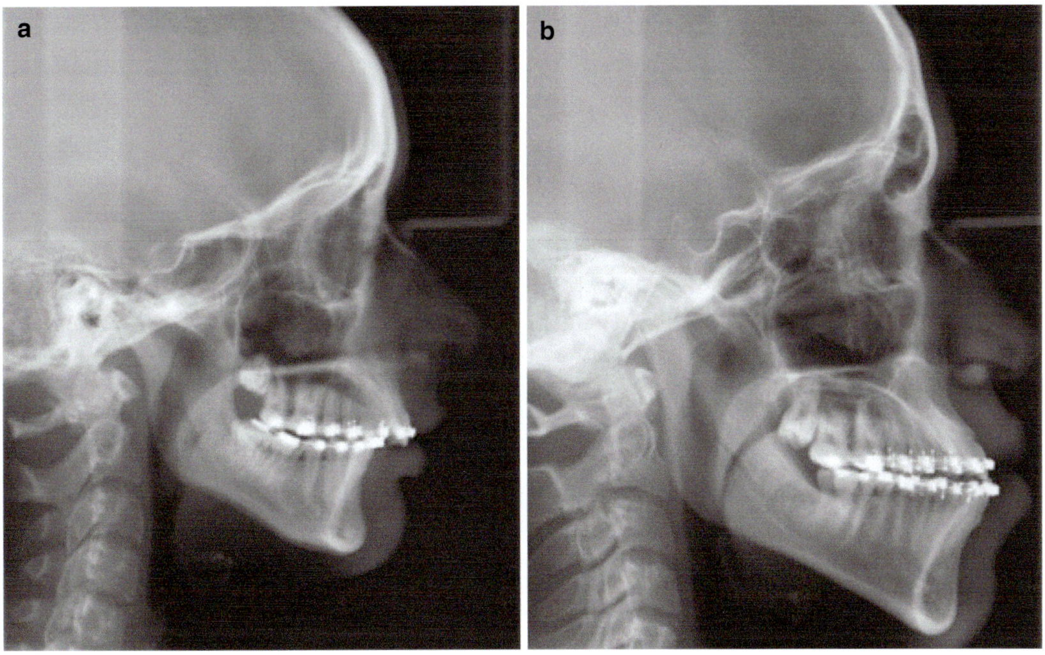

Fig. 6.5 Two examples of preoperative lateral cephalometric X-rays: (**a**) Patient with a skeletal class II and deep bite based on mandibular hypoplasia (**b**) Patient with a skeletal class III based on a mandibular hyperplasia

Important items to evaluate on a lateral cephalometric X-ray for the orthognathic surgeon:

- The sagittal relationship of the maxilla and mandible to the skull base before and after surgery.
- The angulation of the maxilla and mandible to each other and to the skull base.
- The angulation of the mandibular angle.
- The angulation of the incisors according to the base of upper and lower jaw.
- Soft tissue analysis with the focus on the projection of the nose, lip position, and chin.

1.3 Cone-Beam Computed Tomography (CBCT)

The CBCT is widely used for the tomographic and three-dimensional evaluation of possible norm deviations of osseous dento-maxillofacial structures and for the closer differentiation of pathological findings such as the three-dimensional position of the wisdom teeth. Other dental and skeletal anomalies can be visualized such as supernumerary teeth or the determination of the position and course of the mandibular canal. The data set is a prerequisite for three-dimensional planning in any planning program.

Furthermore, the CBCT images allow the assessment of skeletal anomalies and asymmetries in a coronal, transversal, and sagittal plane, which cannot be achieved with conventional X-rays (Fig. 6.6). Cone-beam data sets also allow for the evaluation of the soft tissue structures of the face so that the gain of information by the CBCT is invaluable. From this and medicolegal point of view, a three-dimensional skull or jaw X-ray should be considered obligatory.

Note

The CBCT-based preoperative visualization of the prospective osteotomy area allows the surgeon an individual risk assessment and risk management with regard to technique and procedure of the osteotomy.

It also facilitates the preoperative information of the patient about possible difficulties and complications during the intervention.

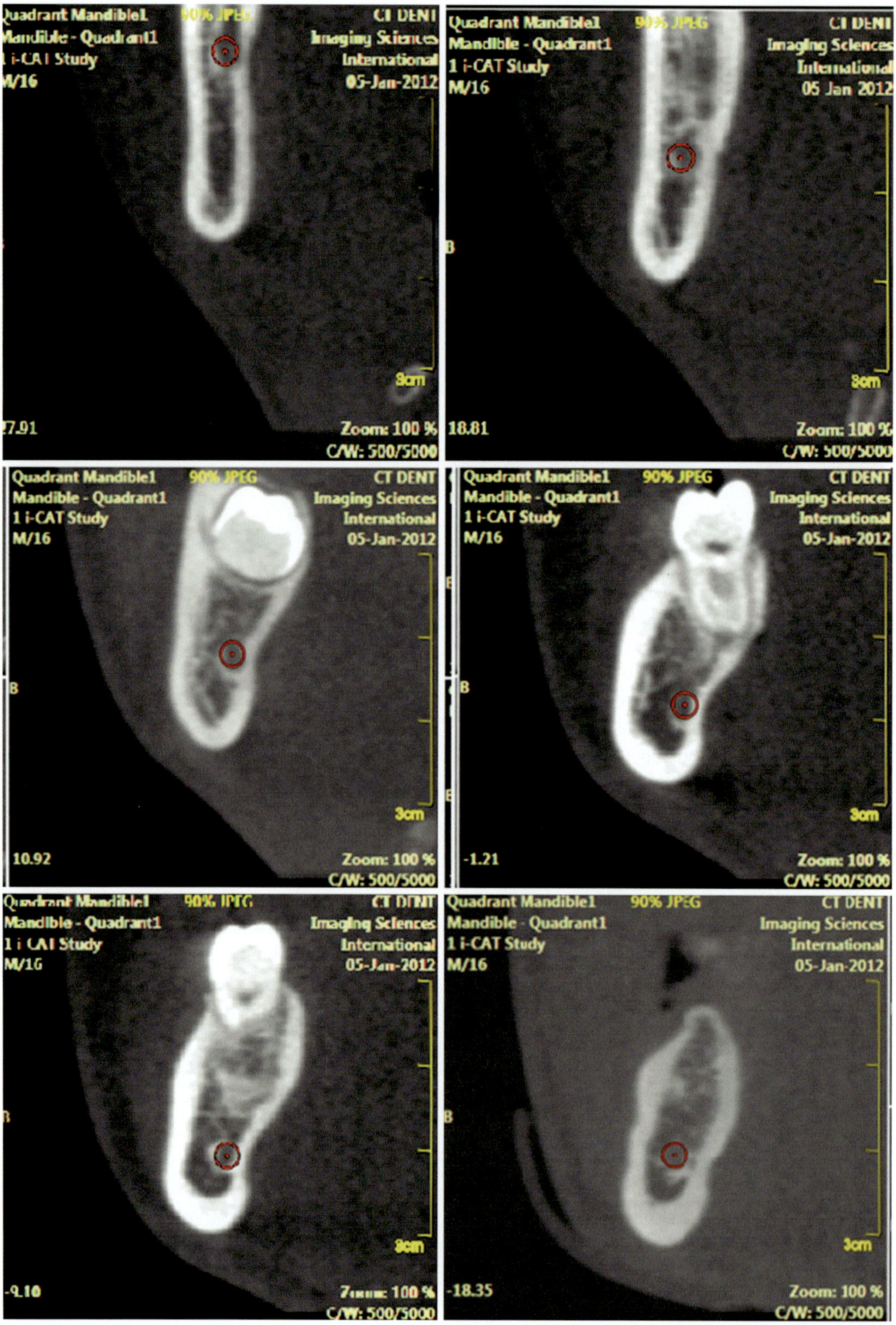

Fig. 6.6 Determination of the mandibular canal from the post molar region to the first molar on the right mandibular side

1.4 Multi-Slice Computed Tomography (MSCT)

In some rare cases of complex dysgnathias, severe facial asymmetries, and patients suffering from soft or hard tissue deficits, a MSCT scan can be indicated. For intraoperative navigation thin-slice MSCT's deliver the best quality data. In asymmetric cases and cases with hard tissue deficits, MSCT data can be used to analyze changes in the shape, size, and volume of osseous, but also soft tissue structures.

MSCT delivers the best quality data in the evaluation and measurement of the prospective mandibular osteotomy region, with regard to the bone quality, transverse extension of the mandibular body, the width of the buccal and lingual mandibular cortico-cancellous bone, and the position and intrabony course of the inferior alveolar nerve (IAN). With standard X-rays, statements or measurements in the transverse plane are impossible.

The use of computerized tomographic X-ray techniques in the jaws allows the exact definition and marking of position and course of the mandibular canal, as well as the distance between the mandibular canal and the buccal cortex.

The width of cancellous bone between the mandibular canal and the buccal cortex is essential for the exact planning of the buccal vertical osteotomy (Fig. 6.6).

This precise control of the individual nerve course on the one hand and the relationship of the IAN to the surrounding cortico-cancellous structures on the other hand allows an individual risk assessment of possible nerve injuries caused by surgical splitting. This and the fact that CBCT or MSCT's in particular are required as the basis for computer-based planning make three-dimensional X-rays indispensable today.

1.5 CT-Based Distance Measurements in the Pre-Masseteric Region (Buccal Osteotomy)

At the caudal end of the buccal vertical osteotomy, the metric distances between the buccal cortex and the mandibular canal vary between 7.0 and 1.5 mm and correspond to the existing cancellous bone thickness between the two structures (Figs. 6.7, 6.8) [2].

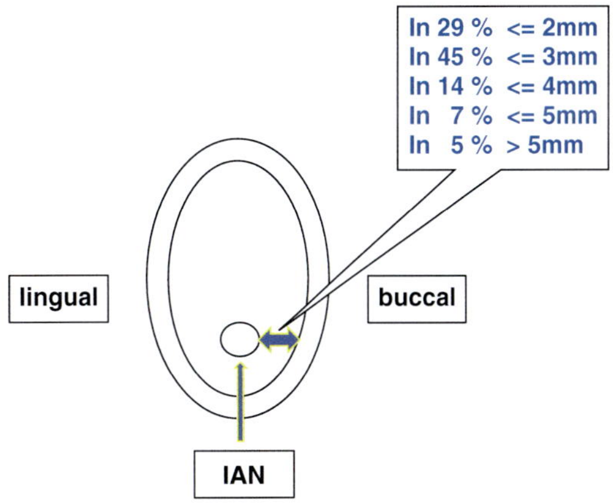

Fig. 6.7 Distance measurement of cancellous bone thickness between the mandibular canal and the buccal cortex in the inferior region of the buccal vertical osteotomy (*IAN* = inferior alveolar nerve)

The mean distance is 2.9 mm with a standard deviation of ±1.2 mm. In detail, the distance-maintaining cancellous bone layer between the mandibular canal and buccal cortex is:

- In 29% ≤ 2 mm.
- In 45% ≤ 3 mm.
- In 14% ≤ 4 mm.
- In 7% ≤ 5 mm.
- 5 mm.

Note

The distances between the mandibular canal and the buccal cortex are small and variable in the pre-angular and angular region of the mandible [2, 3].

In the inferior region of the buccal vertical osteotomy there is on average only a narrow cancellous bone zone between the nerve canal and the buccal cortex.

The average mean value of the cancellous bone layer is 2.9 mm +/−1.2 mm. In 58%, the thickness of the cancellous bone layer is between 2 and < 4 mm and in 45% it is < 3 mm.

1.6 CT-Based Distance Measurements in the Region of the Mandibular Angle

Serial preoperative horizontal CT-based measurements of the distance between the mandibular canal and the external buccal cortex in the area of the cranial osteotomy zone on the lingual side of the ascending ramus starting at the lowest point of the mandibular foramen in 2 mm intervals down to 22 mm inferior to the foramen led to the following result:

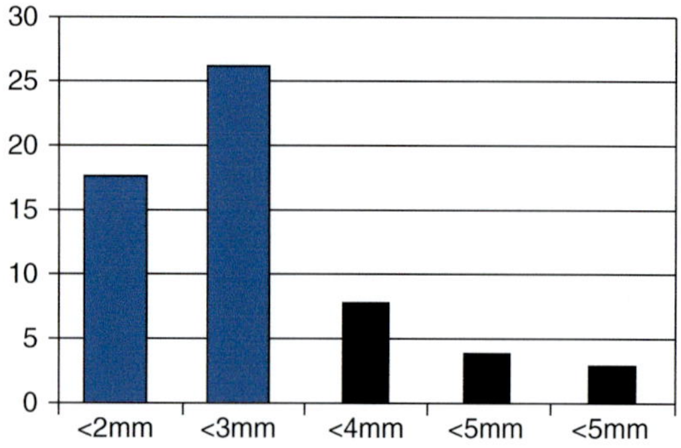

Fig. 6.8 Distance measurement between mandibular canal and buccal cortex in mm in the inferior region of the buccal vertical osteotomy ($n = 58$) [2]

- In 25% of the cases the mandibular canal was in direct contact with the lateral cortical bone.
- In 75% there was no direct contact between the mandibular canal and the lateral buccal cortex ($p < 0.05$).

The vertical contact area between the lateral, external cortex and the canal varied between 2 and 18 mm (average 10.6 ± 4.9 mm) (Fig. 6.9).

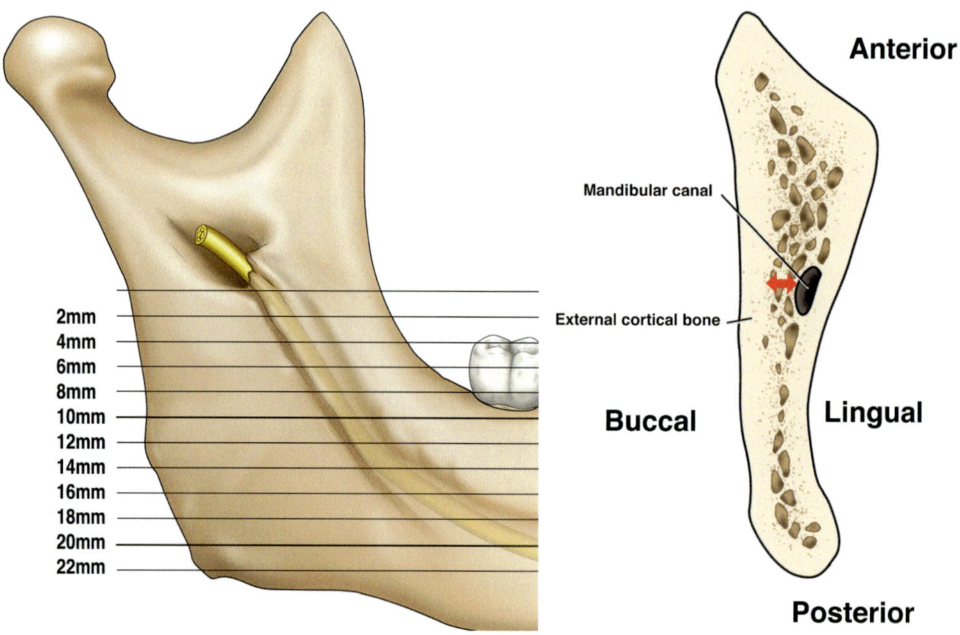

Fig. 6.9 Relationship of the mandibular canal to the lateral cortex of the mandibular ramus [1, 4–6]. ©Copyright Keisuke Koyama 2020. All rights reserved

2 Conclusion

Radiographic analysis is a condition sine qua non for surgery in general and orthognathic surgery in particular. The basis and standard of careful planning are three-dimensional imaging procedures. Two-dimensional X-ray photos are taken for overview and rough orientation.

References

1. Yamamoto R, Nakamura A, Ohno K, Michi K. Relationship of the mandibular canal to the lateral cortex of the mandibular ramus as a factor in the development of neurosensory disturbance after bilateral sagittal split osteotomy. Oral Maxillofac Surg. 2002;60(5):490–5.
2. Pilling E, Schneider M, Mai R, Eckelt U. Präoperative Lagebestimmung des Canalis Mandibulae vor sagittaler Ramusosteotomie des Unterkiefers. Mund Kiefer Gesichtschir. 2004;8(1):18–23.
3. Bell HW, Proffit WR, White RP. Surgical correction of dentofacial deformities, vol. 1–3. Saunders; 1980.
4. Huang CY, Yu-Fang L. Anatomical position of the mandibular canal in relation to the buccal cortical bone in Chinese patients with different dentofacial relationships. J Formos Med Assoc. 2016;115(11):981–90.
5. Rich J, Golden BA, Phillips C. Systematic review of preoperative mandibular canal position as it relates to postoperative neurosensory disturbance following the sagittal split ramus osteotomy. Int J Oral Maxillofac Surg. 2014;43(9):1076–1081. Thieme, Stuttgart.
6. Yoshioka I, Tanaka T, Khanal A, Habu M, Kito S, Kodama M, Oda M, Wakasugi-Sato N, Matsumoto-Takeda S, Fukai Y, Tokitsu T, Tomikawa M, Seta Y, Tominaga K, Morimoto YJ. Relationship between inferior alveolar nerve canal position at mandibular second molar in patients with prognathism and possible occurrence of neurosensory disturbance after sagittal split ramus osteotomy. Oral Maxillofac Surg. 2010;68(12):3022–7.

General Planning and Preoperative Assessment

7

Veronique C. M. L. Timmer, Peter Kessler, and Nicolas Hardt

Contents

V. C. M. L. Timmer (✉) · P. Kessler (✉)
Department of Cranio-Maxillofacial Surgery, Maastricht University Medical Center, Maastricht, The Netherlands
e-mail: v.timmer@mumc.nl; peter.kessler@mumc.nl

N. Hardt (✉)
Kantonsspital Lucerne, Clinic and Policlinic of Cranio-Maxillofacial Surgery, Lucerne, Switzerland

Abstract

After clinical diagnosis and evaluation of the current situation of the patient's face, profile, and dentition, the surgeon must decide which treatment procedure will be necessary. Will one-jaw surgery be sufficient to achieve the desired final result, or is it better to perform corrective surgery in both jaws? And if correction in one jaw is sufficient, should the surgery be performed in the upper or lower jaw? The surgical plan, which includes the actual movements of the jaw, provides guidance during surgery and a prediction of the final result. A 2D cephalomet-

P. Kessler et al. (eds.), *Illustrated Manual of Orthognathic Surgery*,
https://doi.org/10.1007/978-3-031-06978-9_7

ric analysis on the lateral cephalogram is performed to predict the sagittal transposition of the bony structures. Three-dimensional analysis is used to prepare for surgery.

Keywords

Clinical examination · Diagnosis · Photo documentation · Radiology · Basic measurements · Panoramic radiograph · Lateral cephalogram · Cone beam computerized tomography (CBCT) · Cephalometric analysis · Facial analysis · Soft tissue analysis · Computer-based planning · General planning · 2D Planning · 3D Planning · Simulation surgery · Preoperative assessment · Preparations for the surgical procedure

1 2D Cephalometric Analysis

1.1 Tracing

The analysis starts with a tracing of the anatomical structures on the lateral cephalometric X-ray:

- Bone structures including sella turcica, nasal bone, orbit, maxilla, and mandible.
- Soft tissue structures including forehead, nose, lips, chin, and anterior neck.
- Teeth: First molar and central incisor in upper and lower jaw.

1.2 Marking of Anatomical Landmarks and Planes

The cephalometric analysis in orthognathic surgery includes a reduced number of reference points and lines for surgical necessities compared to the orthodontic analysis [1, 2].

Evaluation of the lateral cephalometric X-ray of the skull of a patient in central/habitual occlusion (eugnathia, Angle Class I). The essential dentoalveolar and skeletal reference points and lines as well as the ratio of upper and lower osseous facial height show standard values.

Most important cephalometric landmarks:

- Nasion (N): Most anterior point of the nasofrontal suture.
- Sella (S): Center of Sella turcica.
- Basion: Most caudal point of the clivus.
- Articulare (Ar): Intersection point of the skull base with the dorsal contour of the mandibular ascending ramus.
- A-point (A): Deepest point in the anterior contour of the superior alveolar process.
- B-point (B): Deepest point in the anterior contour of the inferior alveolar process.
- Pogonion (Pg): Most anterior point of the chin bone.
- Gnathion (Gn): Most caudal point of the mandibular symphysis.
- Gonion angle (tgo): Intersection point of ramus line and mandibular line.
- Anterior nasal spine (ANS): Most anterior point of the maxilla.
- Posterior nasal spine (PNS): Most posterior point of the posterior nasal spine/maxilla.
- Infraorbitale (Io): Most caudal point of the infraorbital rim.
- Is: Most anterior point of the upper central incisor.
- Isa: Apex of the upper central incisor.
- Ii: Most anterior point of the lower central incisor.
- Iia: Apex of the lower central incisor.
- Axis through Is and Isa.
- Axis through Ii and Iia.

Most important planes for cephalometric analysis:

- NSL: Nasion-Sella Line: Horizontal line connecting Sella with Nasion.
- NL: Nasal line: Horizontal line connecting ANS (Sp) with PNS (Pm).
- ML: Mandibular line: Horizontal line connecting Gonion with Gnathion.

1.3 Analysis

The Segner-Hasund analysis (1991) has proven itself for planning in orthognathic surgery:

1.3.1 Important Angles Used for Measuring Skeletal Relations

- SNA: Sagittal relation of the maxilla related to the skull base. Evaluates the amount of pro–/retrognathism of the maxilla.
- SNB: Sagittal relation of the mandible related to the skull base. Evaluates the amount of pro–/retrognathism of the mandible.
- ANB: Angulation between the sagittal position of the maxilla and mandible.
- SNPg: Sagittal relation of the chin related to the skull base.
- Mandibular angle: Angulation of the ascending mandibular ramus related to the lower mandibular border. Evaluates the vertical growth of the mandible: long face/short face.
- ML-NL: Angulation between the mandibular and maxillary bases: a large angle is related to open bite, a small angulation is related to deep bite.
- ML-SNL: Angulation between the mandibular base and the skull base.
- NL-SNL: Angulation between the maxillary base and the skull base.

1.3.2 Important Angles Used for Measuring Dental Relations

- NL–Is: Angulation of upper incisor to maxillary base, proclination/retroclination of the upper incisors.
- ML–Ii: Angulation of the lower incisor to mandibular base, proclination/retroclination of the lower incisors.
- Is–Ii: Vertical angulation between the axis of upper and lower incisor.

2 Soft Tissue Analysis

In contrast to the analysis of the bony base, which is based on internationally recognized landmarks and analysis procedures, soft tissue analysis is subject to sociocultural and genetic-ethnic influences. Various concepts are applied, which cannot be said to be universally valid.

Several recognized analytical methods are used: S-line according to Steiner, E-line—esthetic line according to Ricketts [3], H-line—harmony line according to Holdaway [4, 5], or the soft tissue analysis according to Schwarz [6]. These soft tissue analyses are based on the Frankfurt horizontal plane or the cranial base, which can differ evidently among patients.

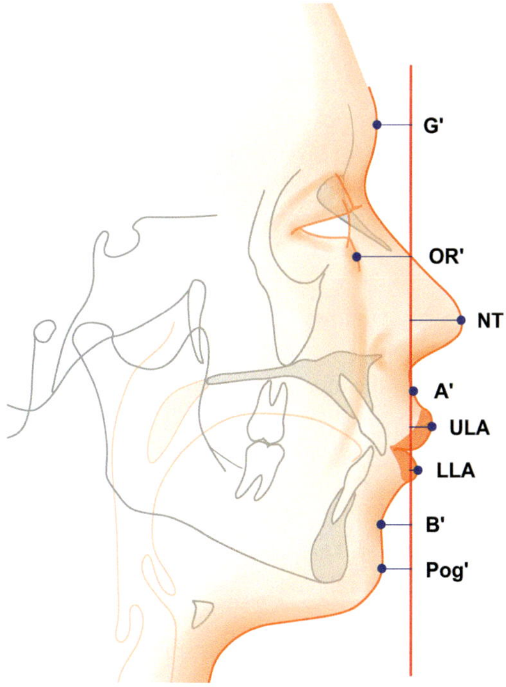

Fig. 7.1 The projection of soft tissue landmarks to the true vertical line (TVL). The distance between the landmarks and TVL is measured horizontally and compared to standardized mean values. Soft tissue landmarks named are glabella (G'), soft tissue orbital rim (OR'), nasal tip (NT), soft tissue A' point (A'), upper lip anterior (ULA), lower lip anterior (LLA), soft tissue B′ point (B′), and soft tissue pogonion (Pg') ©Copyright Keisuke Koyama 2020. All rights reserved

The more recently developed true vertical line (TVL) analysis is based on the use of the natural head position and a true vertical through the subnasal soft tissue point perpendicular to the natural head position (Fig. 7.1).

The projection of the soft tissue landmarks to the TVL are measured horizontally. The individual values should be compared to the standardized values of the socio-ethnic group the patient belongs to.

Independent of which soft tissue analysis is used, it should always be taken into account that the bone movement of the jaws does not result in a 1:1 ratio soft tissue movement. Furthermore, soft tissue thickness and dentoskeletal factors such as the orthodontic positioning of the upper and lower incisors also play an important factor in the outcome of facial profile and esthetics. Soft tissue analysis should always be combined with clinical examination and cephalometric analysis.

2.1 Planning

The size of the aforementioned angles and additional vertical and horizontal relational determinations are compared to standardized reference measurements based on mean values, which must be consistent with the age, gender, and ethnicity of the patients. The Asian population has different facial morphology than the European or African population (Fig. 7.2).

Men and women also differ in facial proportions. This should be taken into account in planning. Based on this information, the new—in the best case ideal—position of the lower and/or upper jaw can be calculated and planned by means of a surgical simulation using plaster models of the teeth rows. By measuring the difference in distance between the old and the new position of the jaws, the surgeon can check the new position of the jaws pre- and later intraoperatively before osteosynthetic fixation.

During planning, the surgeon must always have the esthetic aspects of the patient in mind in order to transfer the skeletal movements to the face.

Examples of cephalometric analyses with regard to the planning of surgery:

1. Mandibular retrognathism—Fig. 7.3.
2. Mandibular prognathism with maxillary retrognathism—Fig. 7.4.
3. Mandibular retrognathism and maxillary prognathism—Fig. 7.5.

2.1.1 Mandibular Retrognathism.

Figure 7.3 As a consequence of the cephalometric analysis, for later surgical planning skeletal harmonization will prospectively be achieved by correction of the mandibular base. This is achieved by anterior displacement of the lower

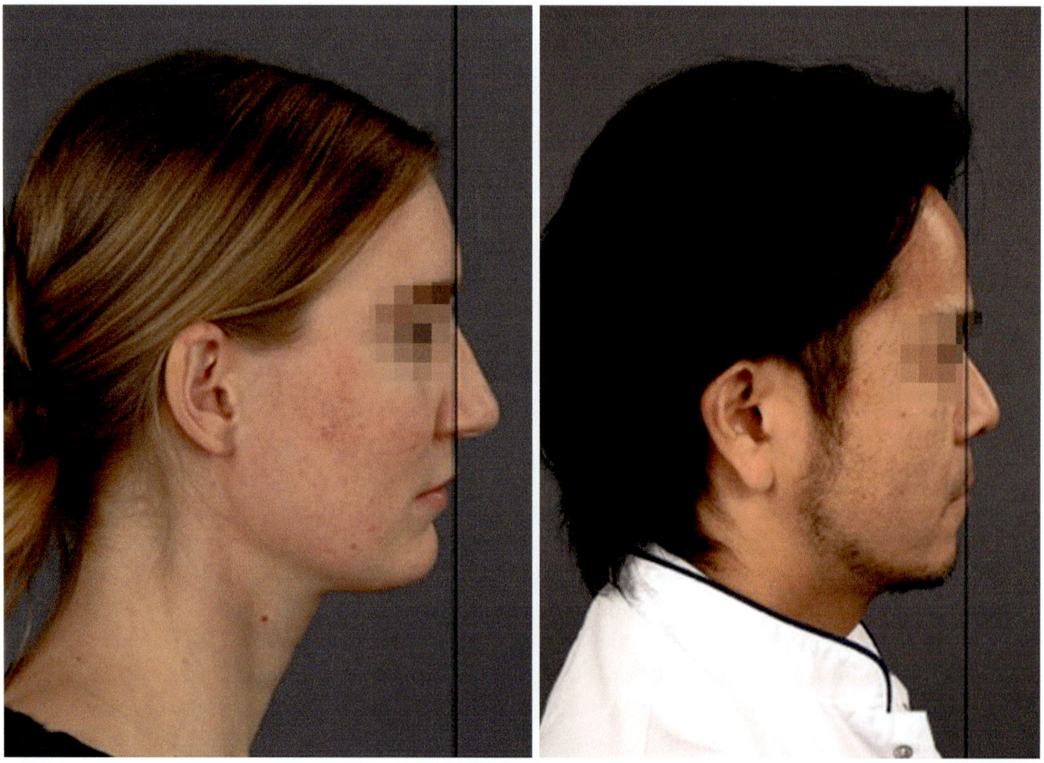

Fig. 7.2 The TVL in the individual patient's profile photodocumentation in a European and Asian face

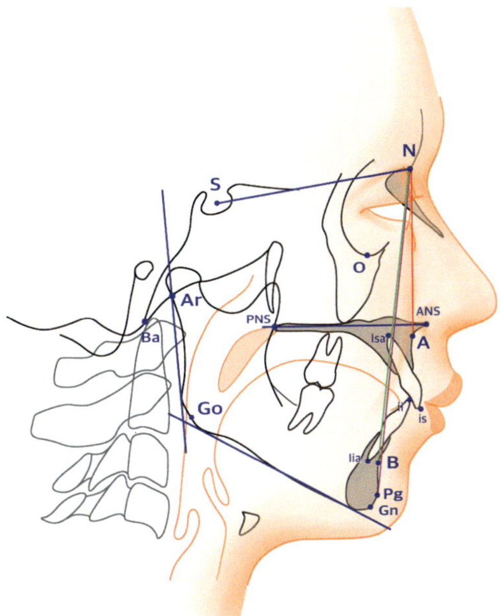

Fig. 7.3 Mandibular retrognathism with Angle Class II occlusion with a retrusive jaw base relation and relatively harmonious vertical jaw base relation: distal occlusion, retrusive occlusion, increased vertical overbite

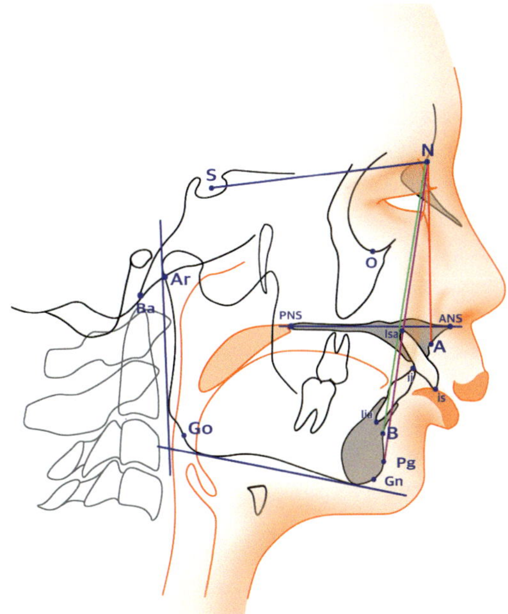

Fig. 7.5 Mandibular retrognathia and maxillary protrusion in a patient with Angle Class II malocclusion with a wide sagittal step (overjet) and a deep bite vertically and a sagittal-distal, vertically slightly open jaw base relation

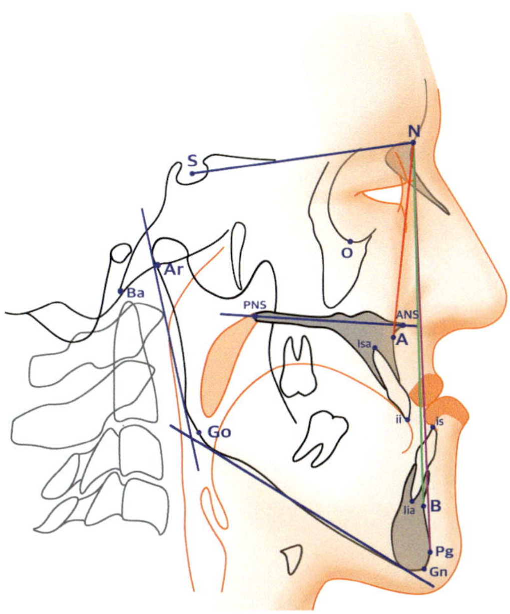

Fig. 7.4 Cephalometric tracing of a patient with mandibular prognathism and maxillary retrognathia in a patient with an Angle Class III occlusion and anterior open bite and a more horizontally directed sagittal-mesial growth pattern with vertically open jaw base relation (vertical malocclusion)

jaw, combined with a simultaneous correction of the pogonion, if necessary.

2.1.2 Mandibular Prognathism and Maxillary Retrognathism.

Figure 7.4 As consequence of the cephalometric analysis, the necessity of a bimaxillary skeletal jaw base harmonization can be derived for treatment planning. This should be achieved by ventral (anterior) repositioning of the upper jaw and a dorsal (posterior) displacement of the lower jaw simultaneously combined with a reduction of the pogonion, if necessary.

2.1.3 Mandibular Retrognathism and Maxillary Prognathism.

Figure 7.5 As a consequence of the cephalometric analysis, the necessity of skeletal harmonization in the maxillary and mandibular base area arises for treatment planning. In the upper jaw, however, only a dorsal and cranial displacement in the anterior region may be necessary (segment). At the same time, the lower jaw should be shifted ventrally by means of a BSSO. The vertical changes can be insignificant in terms of interbasal relation and of upper and lower facial height ratio

3 3D Imaging and 3D Planning

Performing orthognathic surgery on a patient means movement of the maxilla or mandible in three dimensions:

- Translation in the sagittal, vertical, and transvers plane.
- Rotational movements around the sagittal, vertical, and transverse axis, described as pitch, roll, and yaw.

If you use two-dimensional imaging as a basis for planning, you will never get a true representation of a real three-dimensional object like the skull and not all three-dimensional movements can be realistically planned and predicted.

Within the spectrum of 3D imaging modalities, MSCT and magnetic resonance imaging (MRI) have been available for years. Both modalities are used in cranio-maxillofacial surgery to assess certain facial deformities or craniofacial syndromes. However, due to difficult accessibility and high costs, these imaging modalities are not suitable for routine imaging in orthognathic surgery planning.

The CBCT is the most accessible 3D imaging tool for the general OMF surgeon and available in private dental and orthognathic practices. By combining CBCT data with intraoral scanning tools, the entire orthognathic planning process can be performed in a virtual 3D environment without the need for dental models and articulators. The analysis of the preoperatively planned movements of the osteotomized bone segments of the maxilla and mandible, the simulation of the operation, increases the intraoperative accuracy and the predictability of the results [7–9].

3.1 Using Virtual Surgery Planning

- The desired osteotomy lines can be visualized on a virtual 3D skull model (Fig. 7.6).
- The bone segments of the upper and lower jaw can be brought into the desired position and the effect of this positioning on the treatment

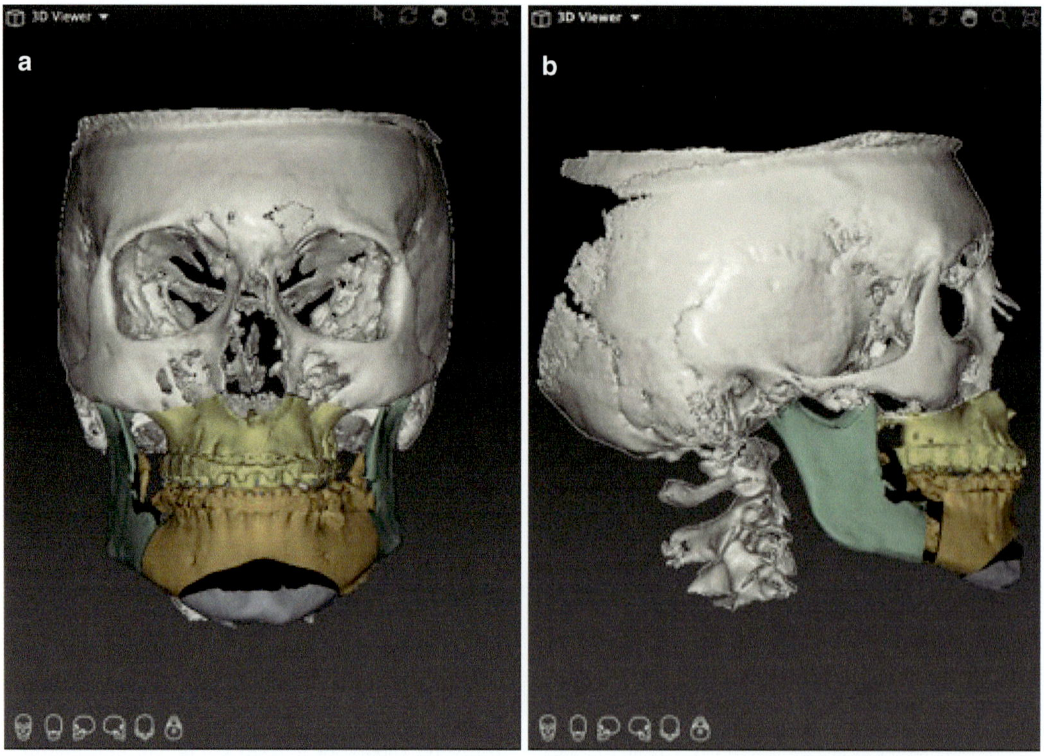

Fig. 7.6 An example of a 3D virtual planning of a bimaxillary osteotomy with genioplasty (**a**) frontal view (**b**) lateral view

goal can be examined and if necessary corrected.
- In rotational movements of the mandible the impact of flaring on the proximal segments and the TMJ can be visualized (Fig. 7.7).
- Cephalometric analysis can be generated from the 3D data set (Fig. 7.8).
- The virtual planning can be used for the production of CAD/CAM interocclusal wafers.
- Patient-specific implants (fixation plates) with individualized cutting and drill guides can be made.
- 3D photographs of the face can be added to the planning software to visualize facial soft tissue changes before and after surgery.

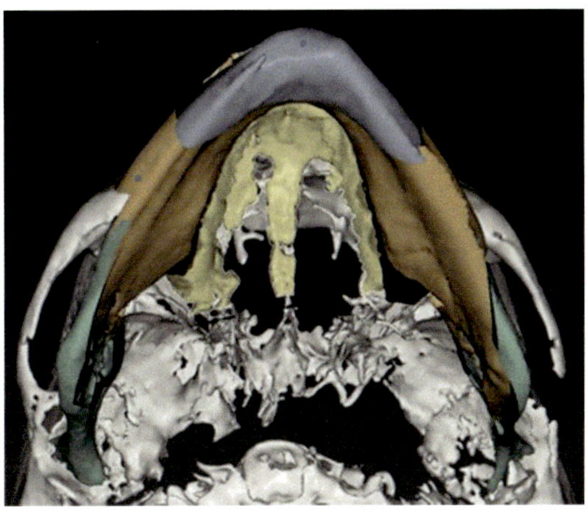

Fig. 7.7 The rotation of the mandible will cause some flaring on the right sight: Note the overlap of the lingual side of the mandibular segment with the distal mandibular segment

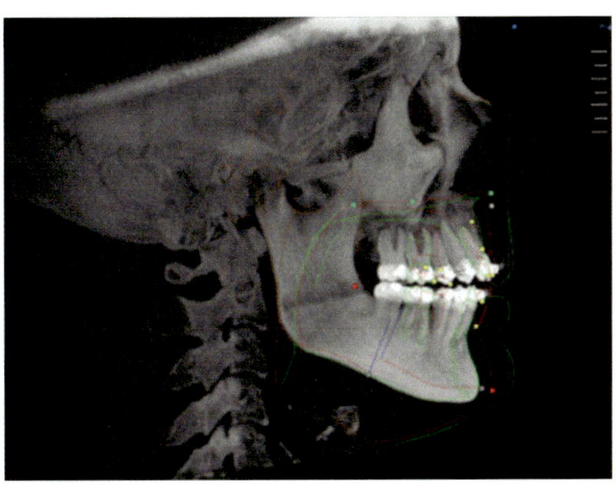

Fig. 7.8 3D cephalometric analysis

In addition, the CBCT enables quality control in postoperative imaging by comparing preoperative virtual planning with actual results. The actual fracture patterns of the osteotomy lines and the position of the condyles can be accurately assessed. The final result is compared with the preoperatively planned positioning of the jaws. This allows the accuracy of translational and rotational movements of the bone and soft tissue structures to be controlled and planning improved. This improves the performance and results of combined orthognathic planning and surgery. In addition, the use of virtual planning software and three-dimensional imaging allows us to easily exchange data and improve communication between the multiple involved practitioners including the surgeon, orthodontist, and technician and to evaluate the teaching success of educational programs.

3.2 Summary of the Advantages of 3D Imaging and 3D Planning

- A realistic three-dimensional representation of the anatomical structures of the face can be obtained.
- A precise planning of all jaw movements in the three-dimensional space of translation (sagittal, transverse, and vertical) and rotation (pitch, yaw, roll) is possible.
- Precision in planning leads to more precision during surgery and to more predictable end results.
- A virtual 3D procedure can be performed without dental casts.
- Interocclusal wafers or waferless surgery with drilling templates and patient-specific osteosynthesis plates can be generated using CAD/CAM technology.
- 3D allows more accurate postoperative imaging for the evaluation of osteotomy lines.
- The patient can be informed more adequately about the surgical procedure. A pre- and postoperative simulation can be shown to give the patient a better idea of the procedure and the final result.

- A comparison of the pre- and post-operative situation can lead to new insights in planning and surgical techniques.
- Teaching and communication are improved by 3D technology.

4 Conclusion

The two-dimensional X-ray analysis is used for preparation and initial orientation. If the treating team and the patient decide to correct a dysgnathia for functional and esthetic reasons, three-dimensional surgical planning is inevitable in order to keep the surgical risks of the procedure as small as possible and achieve the treatment goal as good as possible.

References

1. Hardt N, Paulus GW. Kephalometrische Aspekte bei der Korrektur von Gesichtsdeformitäten. In: Mühlbauer W, Anderl H, editors. Kraniofaziale Fehlbildungen. Stuttgart, New York: Thieme; 1983.
2. Steinhäuser EW, Janson I. Kieferorthopädische Chirurgie Bd. I. Berlin, Chicago, London, Sao Paulo, Tokyo: Quintessenz; 1988.
3. Ricketts RM. New persepectives on orientation and their benefits to clinical orthodontics–part I. Angle Orthod. 1975;45(4):238–48.
4. Holdaway RA. A soft-tissue cephalometric analysis and its use in orthognathic treatment planning. Part I Am J Orthod 1983;84(1):1–28.
5. Holdaway RA. A soft-tissue cephalometric analysis and its use in orthognathic treatment planning. Part II Am J Orthod 1984;85(4):279–293.
6. Schwarz AM. Wie der angehende Kieferorthopäde Gesicht und Schädel verstehen lernt. I. Auflage. Wien/Innsbruck: Urban&Schwarzenberg; 1955.
7. Ackerman L, Proffit WL, Sarver DM, Ackerman MB, Martin RK. Pitch, roll, and yaw: describing the spatial orientation of dentofacial traits. J Orthod Dentofacial Orthop. 2007;131(3):305–10.
8. Segner D, Hasund A. Individualisierte Kephalometrie. 3. Auflage. Hamburg: Segner; 1988.
9. Swennen GR, Schutyser J, Filip AC, Hausamen JE. Three-Dimensional Cephalometry. A Color Atlas and Manual. Springer; 2006.

Preparations for the Surgical Procedure

8

Veronique C. M. L. Timmer, Peter Kessler, and Nicolas Hardt

Contents

Abstract

Orthognathic surgery is considered to be one of the elective forms of treatment in most cases. In order to ensure the safety of the extensive interventions as well as possible, solid planning and problem analysis is required. Only in this way can trust between patient and surgeon develop and lead to a successful result. The necessary patient contacts must be well structured in order to be able to work effectively and in a targeted manner. The presence of an orthodontist may be desirable in the initial phase.

Keywords

Patient · Patient contacts · Guidelines · Radiology · Computer-based planning · General planning · 2D-Planning · 3D-Planning · Simulation surgery ·

V. C. M. L. Timmer (✉) · P. Kessler (✉)
Department of Cranio-Maxillofacial Surgery, Maastricht University Medical Center, Maastricht, The Netherlands
e-mail: v.timmer@mumc.nl; peter.kessler@mumc.nl

N. Hardt (✉)
Kantonsspital Lucerne, Clinic and Policlinic of Cranio-Maxillofacial Surgery, Lucerne, Switzerland

P. Kessler et al. (eds.), *Illustrated Manual of Orthognathic Surgery*, https://doi.org/10.1007/978-3-031-06978-9_8

Preoperative assessment · Preparations for the surgical procedure · Medication · Patient journey · Postoperative Instructions

1 A Short Guideline for the Patient Journey in Orthognathic Surgery

1.1 The First Contact—Basic Analysis

- Always be friendly and empathic! Most patients are a little scared.
- Look at the patient and the patient's face from all sides to get a first impression: at rest and while smiling.
- Is the patient in orthodontic treatment?
- Is the patient sent for surgical preparation or just seeking for information?
- Place a wooden spatula between the rows of teeth and compare the occlusal plane with the bipupillary line: parallel? Cant?
- Check the centerline of the jaws in relation to the face.
- Dental show: sufficient, too little, too much: 2–3 mm crown length should be visible with relaxed upper lip.
- Dental show when smiling: Does the patient have a gummy smile?
- For sagittal displacement: Assess rotational components in lateral view.
- Think of flaring in case of transversal shifting—yaw?
- Remember: With mandibular misalignment, a sagittal component is often connected to a transverse one.
- Is a chin osteotomy necessary for aesthetic reasons?

2 Take a Thorough Medical History and Deliver Appropriate Information

2.1 The Second Contact

Collection of all clinical parameters for orthognathic surgery (Fig. 8.1):

- Clinical facial analysis and measurements in detail—anthropometry.
- Photo documentation.
- Impressions or intraoral scan, wax bite in a relaxed head position.
- Evaluation of orthodontic pretreatment.
- Radiological imaging.

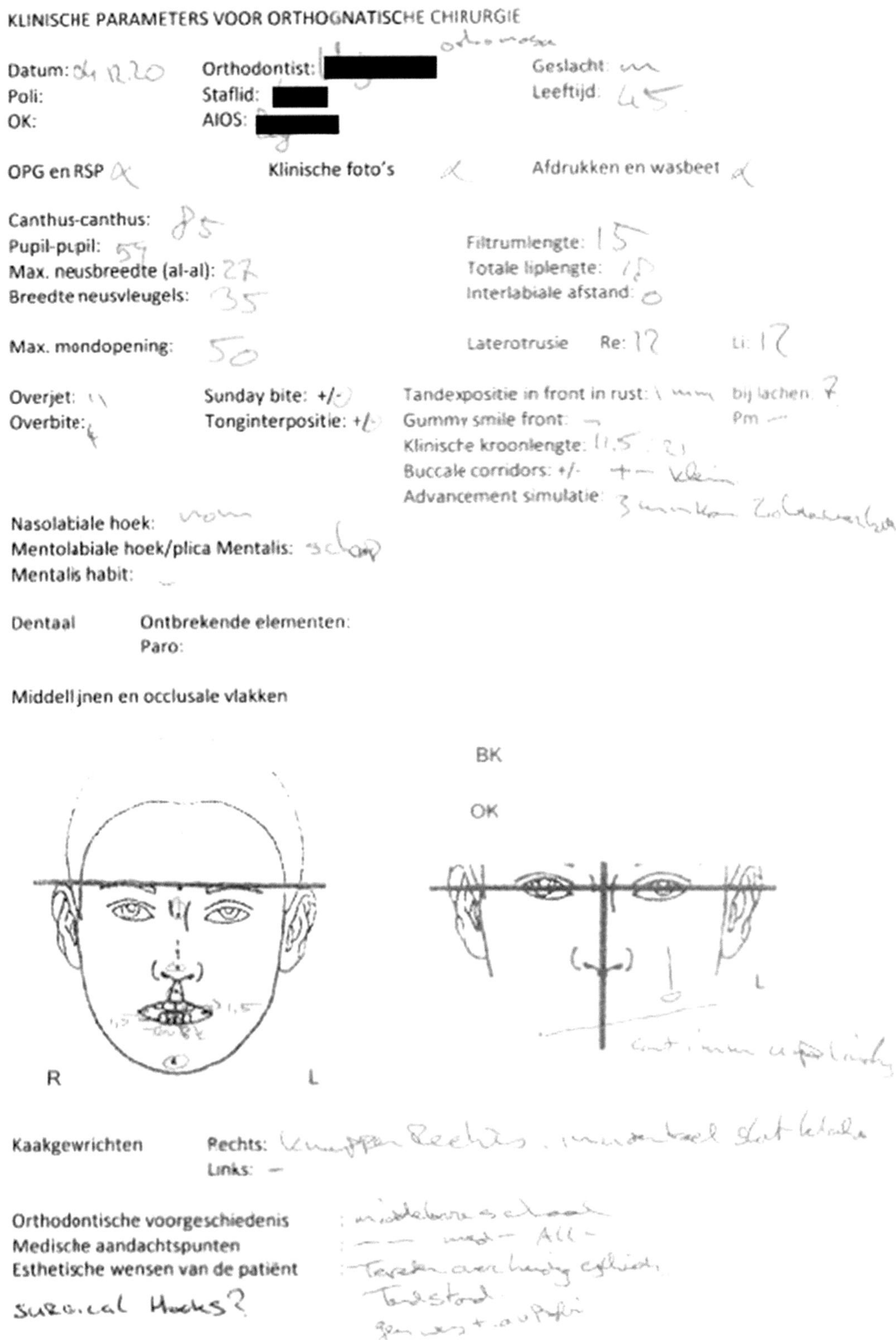

KLINISCHE PARAMETERS VOOR ORTHOGNATISCHE CHIRURGIE

Datum: 04 12.20 Orthodontist: Geslacht: m
Poli: Staflid: Leeftijd: 45
OK: AIOS:

OPG en RSP Klinische foto's Afdrukken en wasbeet

Canthus-canthus: 85
Pupil-pupil: 59
Max. neusbreedte (al-al): 27
Breedte neusvleugels: 35
Filtrumlengte: 15
Totale liplengte: 18
Interlabiale afstand: 0

Max. mondopening: 50
Laterotrusie Re: 12 Li: 12

Overjet: Sunday bite: +/-
Overbite: Tonginterpositie: +/-
Tandexpositie in front in rust: 1 mm bij lachen: 7
Gummy smile front: — Pm —
Klinische kroonlengte: 11.5
Buccale corridors: +/-
Advancement simulatie:

Nasolabiale hoek:
Mentolabiale hoek/plica Mentalis:
Mentalis habit:

Dentaal Ontbrekende elementen:
Paro:

Middellijnen en occlusale vlakken

BK
OK
R L
L

Kaakgewrichten Rechts:
Links: —

Orthodontische voorgeschiedenis
Medische aandachtspunten
Esthetische wensen van de patiënt

SURGICAL HOOKS?

Fig. 8.1 Personal remarks as a reminder (in Dutch language)

2.2 The Third Contact

- Inform the patient and, if necessary, the patient's family and relatives about the treatment plan. Explain the procedure and show the treatment simulation.
- Mention all relevant risks of a surgical intervention and also name alternatives or consequences of not having the treatment.
- Explain the patient management—admission, ward, transport, etc.—all around the surgical treatment.
- Send the patient to the preoperative anesthesiologic consultation.
- Check your records for completeness and assign an operation date after the patient has documented his informed consent in an appropriate form.

3 Specific Advice

- Advise the patient to ensure healthy sleep for a few days before the procedure, not to consume alcohol or tobacco. This lifestyle should be maintained for at least 2 weeks after the surgery.
- Advise the patient that the intake of food will be more difficult after surgery. The patient will lose weight.
- Liquid and soft or softly cooked food should be prepared for the first 2 weeks.
- After 2 weeks the patient can build up his or her diet: Pasta, rice, boiled vegetables, potatoes, bread without hard edges, soft meat.
- Dairy products are suitable but should only be recommended if good oral hygiene is maintained. The patient should be able to enjoy normal diet after 6 weeks.

3.1 The Week before Surgery

- Is the planning complete? Cephalometry done? Photos of good quality available? Does planning and patient match?
- Patient's written consent to the procedure documented? If underage: do the parents agree with the operation?
- Patient is informed, hospital and *OR* know about the planned procedure?
- Patient-labeled implants, if necessary individually manufactured, have been delivered and sterilized?
- Is the model surgery available digitally or on a plaster model?
- Are splints required and manufactured?
- Have splints been checked for accuracy?

3.2 The Operation Day

- Is the patient present?
- Is the patient fasting and ready to undergo the surgery?
- Is the surgical team present?
- The *OR* should be prepared, everyone in the medical supply chain must be informed: ward, transport, *OR* preparation, *OR* nurses, the anesthesia team, the staff in the operating room.
- The technical equipment must be prepared: Instruments and implants available.
- The planning material needed to perform the operation must be in the operating room and should be labeled to the patient—case specific.
- Briefing and time-out procedure with all relevant professionals involved.
- The surgery begins with the induction of anesthesia.

3.3 Pre- and Perioperative Medication

After anesthetic induction, a suitable, weight-adapted antibiotic is given and a single dose of 16 mg dexamethasone.

- Nasal intubation.
- Positioning of the patient, usually in supine position with head in the body axis, head not hanging in extension/flexion.
- Disinfection of the surgical area and sterile covering.
- Local anesthesia for BSSO: Para mandibular and lingual with a suitable dental local anes-

thetic with vasoconstrictor, e.g., Ultracain-forte, 4 ampoules, two per side.
- Documentation of the incision.

Note
A possible antibiotic regimen can be as follows: cefazolin and metronidazole at the initiation, continuing postoperatively with amoxicillin-clavulanic acid.

Usually the patient will be extubated on the *OR*. After ensuring safe spontaneous breathing, the patient is transferred to the recovery ward for further postoperative observation. The patient usually remains there for 3 h. Afterwards, the patient is transferred to the normal ward. See the patient there and tell the patient how the surgery went. If necessary, inform his family.

4 Instructions at the End of Operation

- If necessary, wafers and intermaxillary fixation elastics remain intraorally. Inform the anesthesiologist or recovery staff to cut the elastics in occurrence of an emergency situation.
- Continue antibiotic therapy for at least 24 h.
- Pain medication is based on acetaminophen (paracetamol) and NSAIDs.
- Repeat dexamethasone doses of 8 mg 10 and 20 h after the procedure.
- Position head and upper body at least 30° high.
- Cool wound area: cool packs and individual cooling masks are suitable.
- Start feeding with water and tea.

5 Conclusion

Careful preparation of orthognathic treatment reduces adverse events during the surgical procedure. This increases the probability of success, patient satisfaction, and strengthens the confidence of the treating team in its capabilities. Confidential guidance of the patient through the entire treatment protocol is essential, and the technical possibilities help in this.

Further Reading

Hardt N, Paulus GW. Kephalometrische Aspekte bei der Korrektur von Gesichtsdeformitäten. In: Mühlbauer W, Anderl H, editors. Kraniofaziale Fehlbildungen. Stuttgart, New York: Thieme; 1983.

Proffit WR, Raymond P, White RP, Sarver DM. Contemporary Treatment of Dentofacial Deformity. India: Elsevier; 2012.

Schwarz AM. In: Auflage I, editor. Wie der angehende Kieferorthopäde Gesicht und Schädel verstehen lernt. Wien/Innsbruck: Urban& Schwarzenberg; 1955.

Segner D, Hasund A. Individualisierte Kephalometrie. Hamburg: Auflage, Signer; 1988.

Steinhäuser EW, Janson I. Kieferorthopädische Chirurgie Bd. I. Chicago, London, Sao Paulo, Tokyo: Quintessenz–Berlin; 1988.

Swennen GR, Schutyser J, Filip AC, Hausamen JE Three-Dimensional Cephalometry. A Color Atlas and Manual Springer 2006.

9 Osteosynthesis for Sagittal Splitting

Peter Kessler and Nicolas Hardt

Contents

P. Kessler (✉)
Department of Cranio-Maxillofacial Surgery, Maastricht University Medical Center, Maastricht, The Netherlands
e-mail: peter.kessler@mumc.nl

N. Hardt (✉)
Kantonsspital Lucerne, Clinic and Policlinic of Cranio-Maxillofacial Surgery, Lucerne, Switzerland

P. Kessler et al. (eds.), *Illustrated Manual of Orthognathic Surgery*,
https://doi.org/10.1007/978-3-031-06978-9_9

Abstract

All osteosynthesis techniques evolved from traumatology. There, the anatomically correct and stable positioning of fracture ends is the goal of treatment. In orthognathic surgery, however, the displacement of bone segments is the goal of treatment, which places different demands on osteosynthesis techniques. Under aspects of stability, functional adaptation, and masticatory function, the functionally stable osteosynthesis, originally developed by Champy for traumatology, has gained acceptance.

Keywords

3D Planning in orthognathic surgery · Simulation surgery · Preoperative assessment · Preparations for the surgical procedure · Wire osteosynthesis · Screw osteosynthesis · Bicortical screw fixation · Plate osteosynthesis · Monocortical plate osteosynthesis · Rigid fixation · Plates and screws · Intermaxillary fixation (IMF) · Condylar head · TMJ · Plate removal

1 Wire Osteosynthesis/ Intermaxillary Fixation

Prior to the introduction of stable osteosynthesis, long-term mandibulo-maxillary fixation for at least 6–8 weeks with alloyed splints and wire ligatures was necessary to secure the occlusion of the osteotomized mandible or mandibular segments [1].

The positionally stable adaptation osteosynthesis of the early days was able to prevent unintentional fragment displacement, but immobilization of the segments under functional loading was not guaranteed.

2 Rigid Internal Segment Fixation

With the development of less invasive and less morbid osteotomy designs, questions about general osteotomy stability arose. The transition from extended intermaxillary fixation and wire osteosynthesis to rigid internal fixation has raised questions about the most effective fixation technique. These questions represent a still ongoing debate and discussion as measures have been taken to optimize patient outcomes and minimize patient morbidity.

Instead of the conventional non-rigid wire fixation or circum-mandibular cerclages with mandibulo-maxillary fixation, the rigid internal segment fixation with screw osteosynthesis according to *Spiessl* [2–4] was introduced and replaced the wire osteosynthesis and long-term intermaxillary fixation.

The principle of "functionally stable osteosynthesis" requires prerequisites for success:

- A direct interfragmentary contact of the split segment surfaces for undisturbed bone healing.
- A long-term secure positioning of the proximal and distal bone segments.
- A reliable possibility to position the condyles.

Depending on the interfragmentary osteosynthesis used—lag screw or positional screw osteosynthesis—bone healing proceeds either as primary or secondary bone healing [2, 4–8].

2.1 Advantages of Rigid Internal Fixation (RIF)

- RIF by screw fixation.
- RIF by plate fixation.

The many advantages of internal fixation make RIF an effective and predictable method in the surgical treatment of mandibular osteotomies [9].

The outstanding advantages of RIF are:

- Fast and uncomplicated bone healing due to a broad bone contact of the split segments.
- Secure segment stability and predictable surgical results.
- Stable results in mandibular advancement, setback and correction of asymmetry.
- Minor positional changes of the masticatory muscles—prevention of a relapse through muscular traction.
- Early restoration of functions, without a long-lasting mandibulo-maxillary fixation (MMF).
- Controlled positioning of the temporomandibular joints, which preventively reduces TMJ dysfunctions and TMJ long-term consequences.

2.2 Long-Term Versus Short-Term MMF

The comparison between long-term immobility with MMF prior to the introduction of stable osteosynthesis and short-term MMF immobilization was shown to significantly reduce the risk of secondary TMJ long-term problems, as functional stability allows the patient to undergo early physiotherapy with opening exercises as well as a rapid onset of the preoperative jaw function [10].

3 Osteosynthesis Techniques

Interfragmentary, stable fixation is achieved either by a:

Screw fixation as

- Lag screw osteosynthesis—bicortical compression screw osteosynthesis or
- Adjustable screw osteosynthesis—bicortical positioning screw osteosynthesis.

or by:

Plate and screw osteosynthesis as

- Monocortical miniplate osteosynthesis.

4 Rigid Screw Osteosynthesis

The use of osteosynthesis screws was the first form of stable and rigid osteosynthesis:

- Rigid bicortical compression screw osteosynthesis with 2.7/2.0 mm screws.
- Rigid bicortical positioning screw osteosynthesis with 2.0 mm screws.

4.1 Rigid Bicortical Compression Screw Osteosynthesis

The principle of lag or compression screw osteosynthesis consists in the creation of a threaded and gliding hole so that when the screw is tightened, an approximation/compression of the osteotomized segments is achieved (Fig. 9.1). The positioning of the fragments is not easy due to the application of tension and compression and is not always successful [4, 7, 11–14].

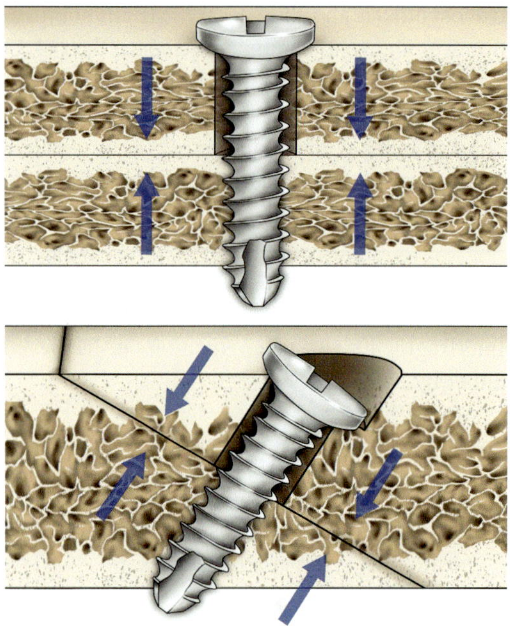

Fig. 9.1 Principles of compression screw osteosynthesis: By creating a threaded and sliding hole segment fixation is achieved during tightening the screw by compression of the segments [11]

- Drill a sliding hole on the lateral side of the split (proximal segment) in the *diameter of the screw* to be used.
- Drill a screw channel through the sliding hole in the diameter of the *screw core*. One must pay attention to the direction. Measure the total length of the drill channel for perfect screw fit.

4.1.1 Application

Bicortical screw osteosynthesis is usually performed transbuccally under instrumentation with a transbuccal trocar that can hold the drill, depth gauge, tap, screwdriver, and screw.

The system of interfragmentary compression using lag screws (2.7 mm diameter/alternatively 2.0 mm) consists of a buccal cortical gliding hole and a lingual cortical screw thread. The screw head causes compression of the lateral segment, and the lingual screw thread causes screw fixation [15].

Usually three compression screws are used. The localization for the compression screw application is carried out in the classical way, taking into account the course of the IAN and the position of the second molars.

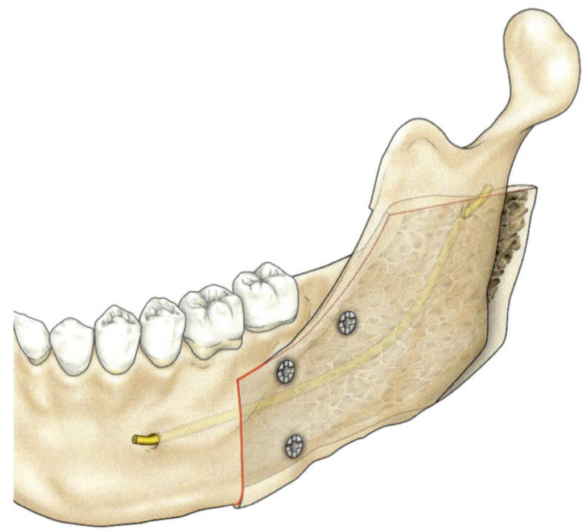

Fig. 9.2 Position scheme for compression screw application in equidistant position according to [3]

Position of the two anteriorly positioned screws: external oblique line ("oblique screw") and mandibular base ("base screw"). The position of the oblique and base screws are anatomically clearly defined in recognizable regions. Ensure that the osteosynthesis screws are evenly spaced (Fig. 9.2).

In addition to the classic screw application there are several variants (Fig. 9.3).

The triangular configuration of the screw position across the mandibular nerve canal presented less stress loading than the linear configuration, and hence provided better stability. When the screws were aligned in a linear setting, the stress values were four times higher, implying a less stable fixation. Neither two nor three screws applied at the superior border appeared to be better at exploiting the increased thickness of the cortical bone encountered in this region (external oblique line).

4.2 Rigid Bicortical Positioning Screw Osteosynthesis

As a functionally stable alternative to compression screw osteosynthesis, the distance- and angle-maintaining, non-compressive position screw osteosynthesis was developed, which clinically offers a rigidity equivalent to compression osteosynthesis.

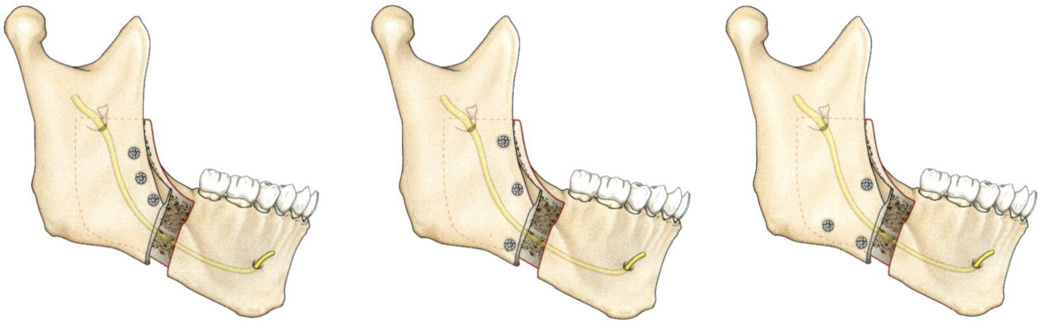

Fig. 9.3 Variants of compression screw application after mandibular split [16]

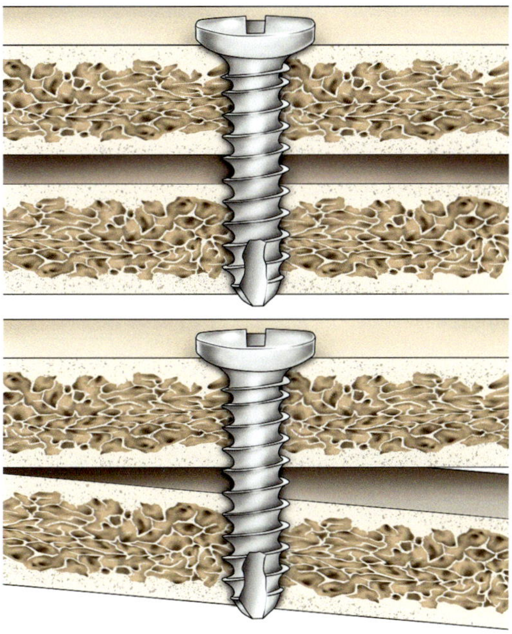

Fig. 9.4 Principle of bicortical position screw osteosynthesis: By creating two threaded holes, the intersegmental gap is preserved when tightening the screw according to [11]

In contrast to compression screw osteosynthesis, the interfragmentary gap between the segments remains intact when the position screws are tightened (Fig. 9.4) [17].

In addition, this form of osteosynthesis avoids the possible dislocation of the condyle during compression osteosynthesis (lateral/medial torqueing of the condyle) (Fig. 9.4) [8, 17–19].

4.2.1 Application

The segments are fixed on both sides by two self-tapping titanium screws each above and one screw below the mandibular canal, which are screwed in over the sleeve of the cheek trocar after pressure less pre-drilling with a twist drill.

A depth gauge inserted in the drill hole is used to determine the correct screw length, whereby the screw should protrude beyond the lingual cortex by a maximum of two thread turns.

To ensure a stable connection of the osteotomized bone segments for practice, the positioning screws must be able to grip the buccal and lingual segments bicortically [17–19].

The intersegmental gap existing when both threads are applied remains when the screws are tightened (Figs. 9.5 and 9.6).

In positioning screw osteosynthesis the bony gap will be bridged by secondary bone healing processes [8, 17].

Due to the anatomical conditions, however, in some cases only one screw can be implanted cranial to the mandibular canal, so that in these cases two screws must be inserted caudally of the canal to render sufficient stability for early mobilization in functionally stable osteosynthesis [17–19].

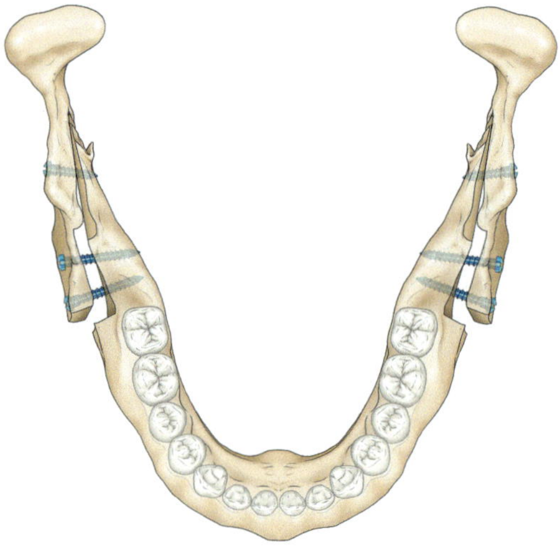

Fig. 9.5 Stable fixation of the segments by adjusted positioning screws. Note: No bone contact, no bone compression at the level of the osteosynthesis screws [20]

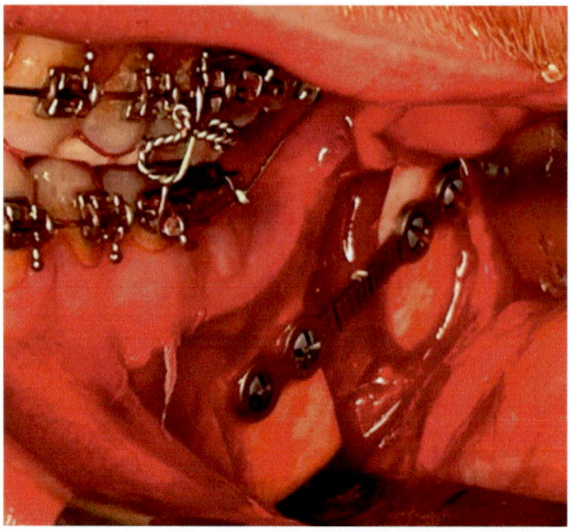

Fig. 9.7 Conventional miniplate osteosynthesis for stable internal fixation

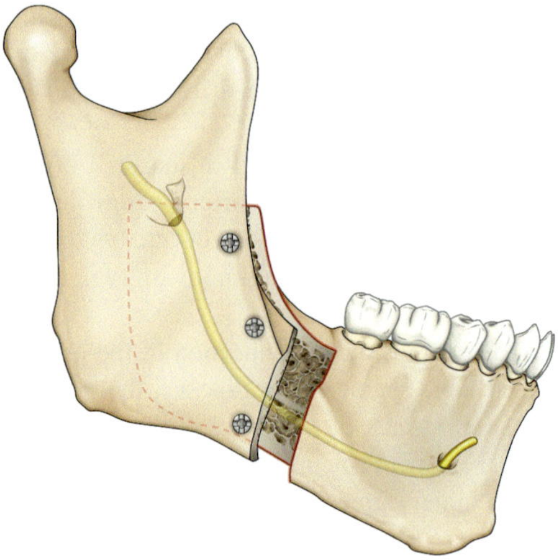

Fig. 9.6 Standard positioning of screws in bicortical positioning screw osteosynthesis

5 Rigid Internal Fixation: Osteosynthesis Plates

5.1 Rigid Monocortical Miniplate Osteosynthesis

The miniplate has also proven to be a reliable fixation device for mandibular osteotomies as well as for maxillary and segmental osteotomies [21–23].

A distinction is made between different plate types:

- Conventional osteosynthesis plates.
- Open sagittal split plates with sliders.
- Closed sagittal split plates with sliders.

5.2 Conventional Osteosynthesis Plates

As a standard, variably shaped fixation plates of the system size 2.0 mm and monocortical screws of 2.0 mm diameter are used for stable internal fixation after sagittal split osteotomies of the mandible (Fig. 9.7). The mandible is subject to greater chewing forces and has a thicker bone structure than the maxilla [16, 24].

The shape and thickness of the plate and screw system depends on the selected osteotomy line, the desired degree of stability, and the extent of bone displacement. The rigidity of the osteosynthesis plates can also be influenced by the choice of different titanium gradings (Fig. 9.8).

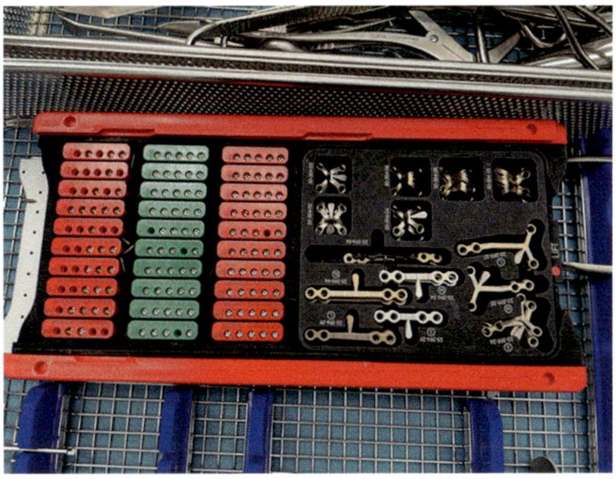

Fig. 9.8 Standard osteosynthesis set 2.0 mm plates and screws in routine use in the operation theater

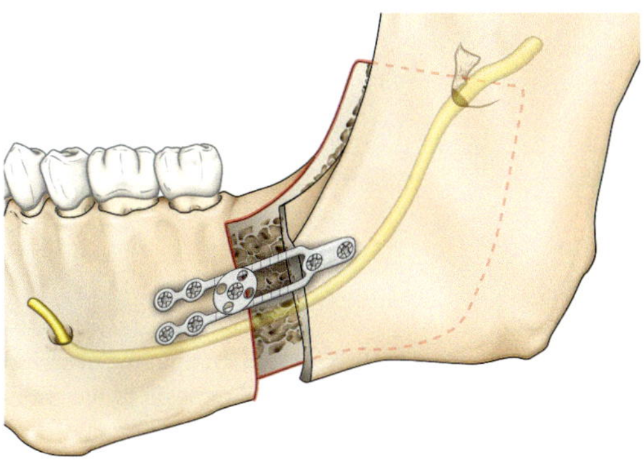

Fig. 9.9 Open sagittal split plate with sliding function ©Copyright Keisuke Koyama 2020. All rights reserved

5.3 Open Sagittal Split Osteosynthesis Plate

5.3.1 Application

After ideal positioning of the proximal segment (joint), the osteosynthesis plate with the slider is fixed to the proximal segment (2 screws) and a temporary osteosynthesis is performed through the sliding element: sliding screw in the distal segment close to the osteotomy (Fig. 9.9).

After checking the pre-planned occlusal position, the final completion of the osteosynthesis is achieved on the distal mandibular segment with four additional screws. The slider is an aid for intraoperative occlusion adjustment and will be removed when the osteosynthesis is completed [11].

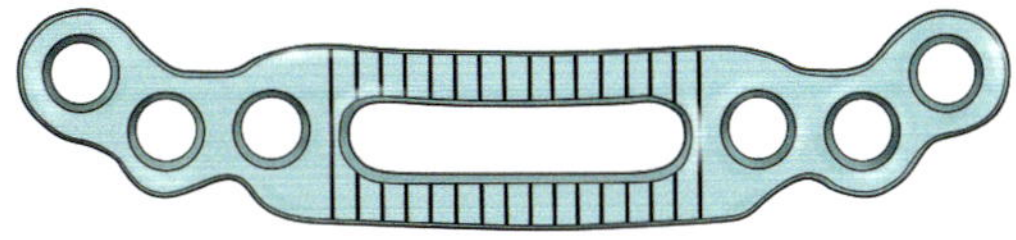

Fig. 9.10 Closed sagittal split sliding plates ©Copyright Keisuke Koyama 2020. All rights reserved

5.4 Closed Sagittal Split Plates with Sliding Function

Fixation of a sagittal split in the horizontal mandibular ramus with a closed, semirigid sagittal split plate with slider option (Figs. 9.10 and 9.11).

5.5 Monocortical Miniplate-Osteosynthesis Versus Bicortical Compression and Positioning Screw Osteosynthesis

In follow-up examinations, no significant differences were found in terms of rigidity and relapse behavior in mandibular advancement between miniplate osteosynthesis with monocortical screws and bicortical screw osteosynthesis [22].

However, excessive postoperative shear stress caused by strong traction from the masseteric and medial pterygoid muscle can—in exceptional cases—lead to bending of the monocortical osteosynthesis plate, with the distal segment rotating clockwise and the proximal segment rotating counterclockwise. An open bite can develop [25].

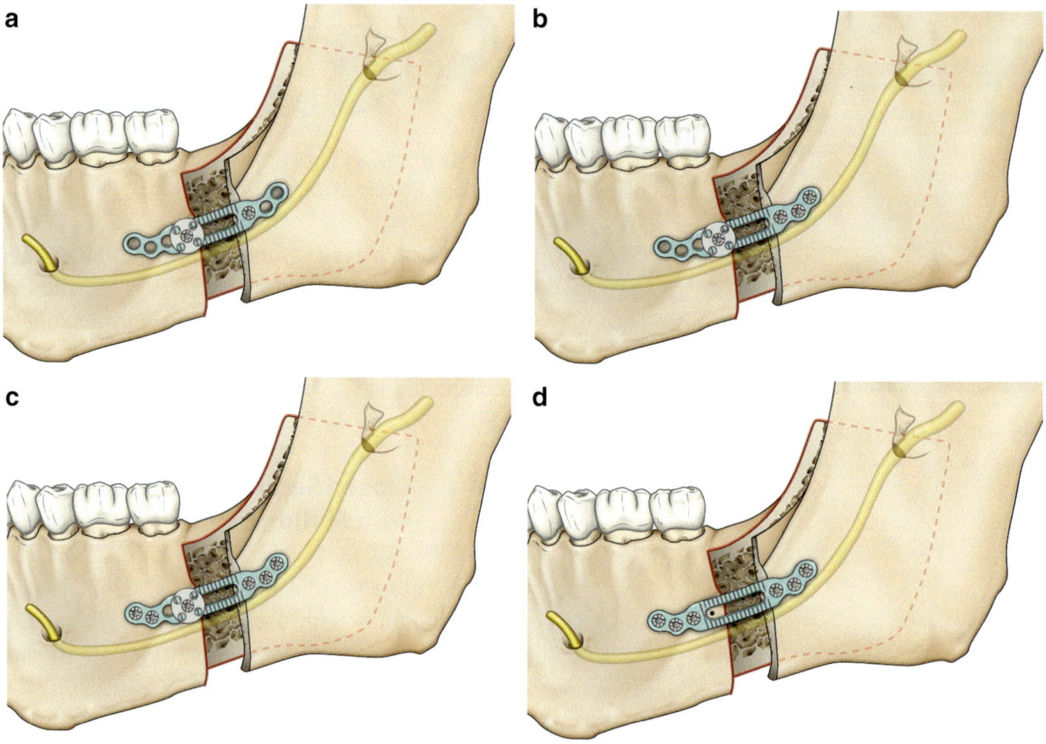

Fig. 9.11 Closed sagittal split plates with sliding function: Stepwise approach to stable fixation: (**a**) One screw proximal segment, check occlusion, IMF, fixation of the slider (**b**) Completion of screw fixation proximal segment (**c**) Check occlusion, IMF. If correct, completion of screws distal segment (**d**) Check occlusion, removal of the slider, if occlusion is correct

6 Osteosynthesis and Segment Positioning

6.1 Osteosynthesis with Intersegmental Distance

Intersegment interferences between the proximal and distal segments after BSSO is not always avoidable. Positioning of the proximal segment (TMJ) in a central condylar position in combination with bicortical screw osteosynthesis is sometimes associated with a wide osteotomy gap and a corresponding reduction of the bony attachment surface, especially when a horizontal dislocation of the mandible is indicated to correct a midline deviation.

Straight anterior and posterior repositioning of the mandible as well as small rotational or lateral movements lead to only small gaps in the osteotomy area, which are spontaneously bridged after 6 months by secondary bone healing even without osteoplasty.

For diastases of more than 5 mm in width, it is recommended to fill up the gap/split with autogenous cancellous or cortico-cancellous bone or a suitable bone replacement material [26].

Even if a wider intersegmental bone gap persists, rigid screw or plate fixation together with a gap filling cortico-cancellous bone graft ensures sufficient stability, since the bone graft can be rigidly fixed in position by osteosynthesis.

6.2 Condylar Position after BSSO and Bicortical Screw Fixation

A rigid, forced screw fixation disregarding intersegmental bone gaps can causally lead to a change of the condylar head and condylar disc position. This may lead to condylar resorption, damages to the articular disc, and relapse.

By placing the osteosynthesis in the region of the distal segment posterior to the last molar with interposition of a bone graft in the area of the segment gap, changes in the joint position can be avoided even with compression screw osteosynthesis. Positioning screw osteosynthesis or miniplate osteosynthesis have an even more favorable effect on a functionally correct condyle position and avoidance of a relapse [26, 27].

6.3 Osteosynthesis with Temporomandibular Dysfunction and Intersegmental Gaps

In patients with manifest temporomandibular joint dysfunction, a BSSO with mandibular repositioning can be performed. However, the following principles should be observed when planning the operation [26, 27].

- All bony interference between proximal and distal segment should be removed.
- The condylar head should be passively guided into the glenoid fossa during surgery.
- Not too rigid fixation with monocortical miniplate osteosynthesis is recommended for segment fixation. The use of compression or positioning screws should be avoided.

7 Rigid Osteosynthesis and Condylar Head Position

Unlike in traumatology, in orthognathic surgery the split jaw segments enter into a completely new positional relationship with each other after surgical correction caused by changes in the occlusion. Due to the parabolic, distally diverging lower jaw body and the individually different shape variants of the jaw angle, variable interfragmentary relationships, such as diastasis, compression, rotational or lateral dislocation, can occur depending on the three-dimensional jaw repositioning: sagittal, vertical, horizontal-rotational.

Under the given circumstances of the anatomical shape of the mandibular body, a forced, gap-free adaptation of the fragments can lead to a more or less large change in position of the proximal segment and the temporomandibular joint. The design of the mandibular split—long or short, vertical or more horizontal—also plays a decisive role. The position of the tooth-bearing distal mandibular body is determined by the occlusion and intermaxillary fixation and cannot be changed.

There is a consensus that rigid screw osteosynthesis can lead to unfavorable and unphysiological changes in the transverse intercondylar distance, the axial inclination of the condylar heads, and the horizontal and vertical positioning of the condyles affecting the condylar-fossa relation negatively [26, 28, 29].

Changes in the positional relationships between condylar head and fossa forced by rigid osteosynthesis can generally have long-term effects on the form and function of the TMJ and cause degenerative changes such as osteoarthritis/osteoarthrosis or condylar head resorption. However, in most patients, the condyle undergoes remodeling, resorption, and other adaptive changes with little or no temporomandibular joint symptoms.

7.1 Postoperative Changes in Condylar Position

Reasons for condylar position changes:

- Rotation of the proximal segment.
- Condylar sag.
- Torque on the proximal segment.

Condylar positioning changes can lead to:

- Skeletal mandibular relapse.
- Malocclusion.
- Hypomobility.
- Remodeling of the condyle.
- Pain.

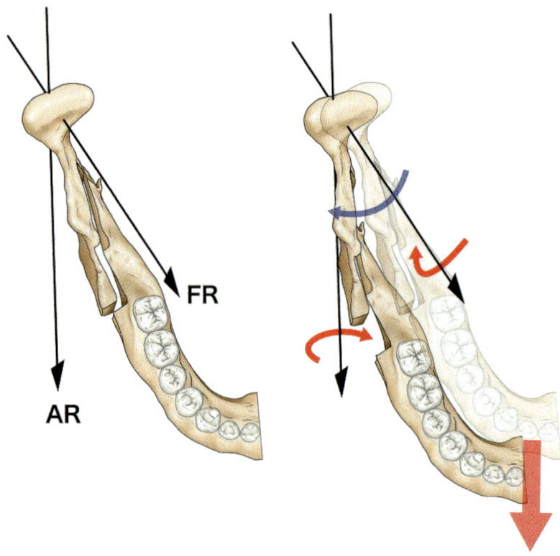

Fig. 9.12 Interference of the proximal bone segments supporting the TMJ with axial (AR) and frontal (FR) rotation of the condylar segment after pronounced mandibular advancement after a sagittal split ©Copyright Keisuke Koyama 2020. All rights reserved

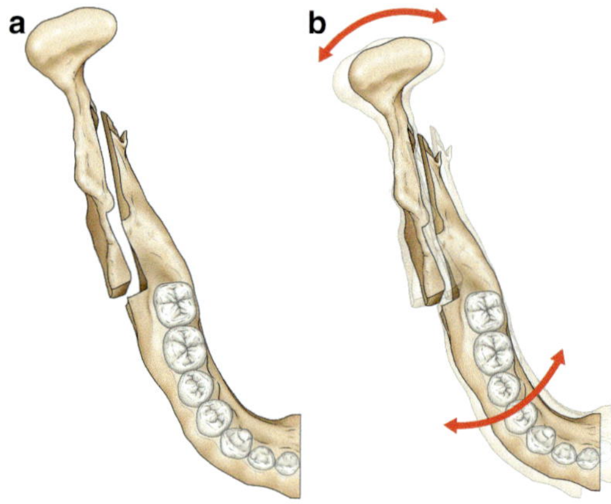

Fig. 9.13 Condylar torque (**a**) Position of split mandibular segments before repositioning (**b**) Medial/lateral torque on the condyle due to proximal segment interference ©Copyright Keisuke Koyama 2020. All rights reserved

7.2 Rotation of the Condyle

Axial (AR) and frontal (FR) rotations of the condylar segment can occur if the proximal bone segment interferes with the distal segment after significant mandibular advancement (Fig. 9.12).

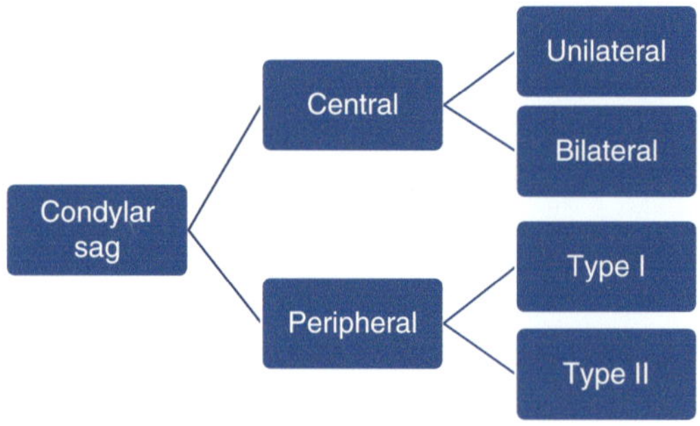

Fig. 9.14 Types of condylar sag (Condyle displacement) according to [31]

7.3 Change of the Intercondylar Distance

The intercondylar width can change when compression screws are used. In a mandibular setback procedure, medial condylar torque of the proximal mandibular segment may occur, narrowing the intercondylar distance.

In the mandibular advancement procedure, lateral condylar torque can occur with an increase in intercondylar distance (Fig. 9.13) [30].

The consequences of torque or displacement of the condyle can be an immediate or later change in position of the condyle in the glenoidal fossa, the so-called central or peripheral condylar sag (condyle displacement) with edema in and around the joint and intermediate occlusal discrepancies (Fig. 9.14). After splitting the mandible, the position of the temporomandibular joint can be unfavorably influenced by disturbing influences [31–33].

Interfering factors are:

- Active displacement of the temporomandibular joint head during osteosynthesis due to pressure.
- Displacement due to bony interference (flaring).
- Incomplete split.
- Muscular traction (especially horizontal pterygoid muscle.
- Traction by ligament.
- Intra- or periarticular edema or hematoma.

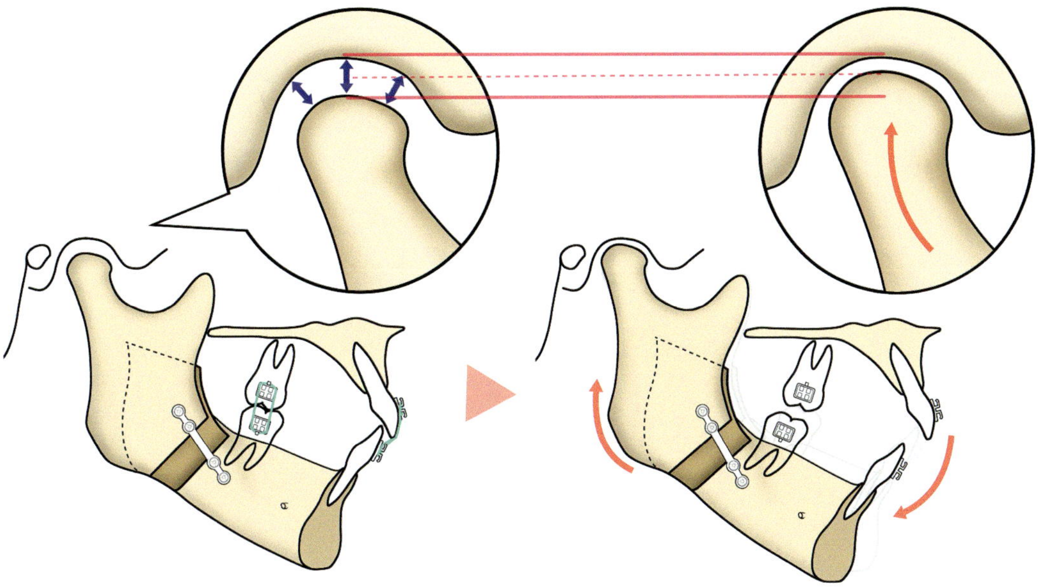

Fig. 9.15 Central Condylar Sag due to inferior traction on the proximal segment during osteosynthesis

1. **Central Condylar Sag**

   The central form can be recognized intraoperatively by the fact that an anterior open bite occurs after RIF when the IMF is opened. The mandible falls back into a class II position (Fig. 9.15). The explanation is assumed to be a slumping back of the condyle into its habitual position. This means that during osteosynthesis the condyles were luxated inferiorly or anteriorly-caudally from their habitual position.
2. **Peripheral Condylar Sag: Type I and II**

   In the peripheral form, two forms are distinguished. First, TMJ compression may occur in the temporomandibular joint in anterior direction by unfavorable retraction during RIF, resulting in an open bite in the posterior region after opening the IMF. This type is sometimes difficult to be diagnosed intraoperatively, because the contact between the condyle and glenoid fossa may be supported by the occlusion. Late relapse from condylar resorption may result in malocclusion. On the long term the mandible falls back into a class II position (Fig. 9.16).

More difficult to visualize is lateral luxation/displacement of the temporomandibular joint head, whereby there is a displacement of the midlines after opening the IMF. This can be very subtle and is more difficult to detect. The condyle is in incorrect relation to the glenoid fossa. Creating the gap between the bone segments in mandibular advancement, a bowing effect may happen by the tension on the condyle and ramus due to forces by rigid fixation. Once the IMF is removed, the tension on the ramus is released causing the condyle to move medially and slide inferiorly on the medial wall of the fossa causing a posterior open bite (Fig. 9.17).

The most serious consequences of condylar sagging are antero-inferior condylar displace-

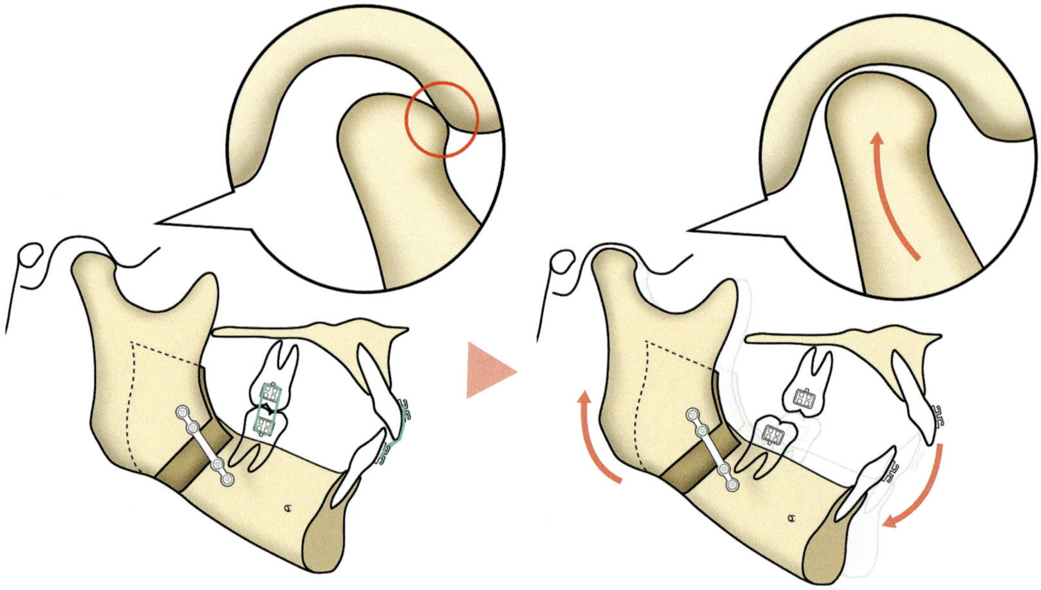

Fig. 9.16 Peripheral Condylar Sag—type I—due to anterior dislocation of the condyle during osteosynthesis Copyright Keisuke Koyama 2020. All rights reserved

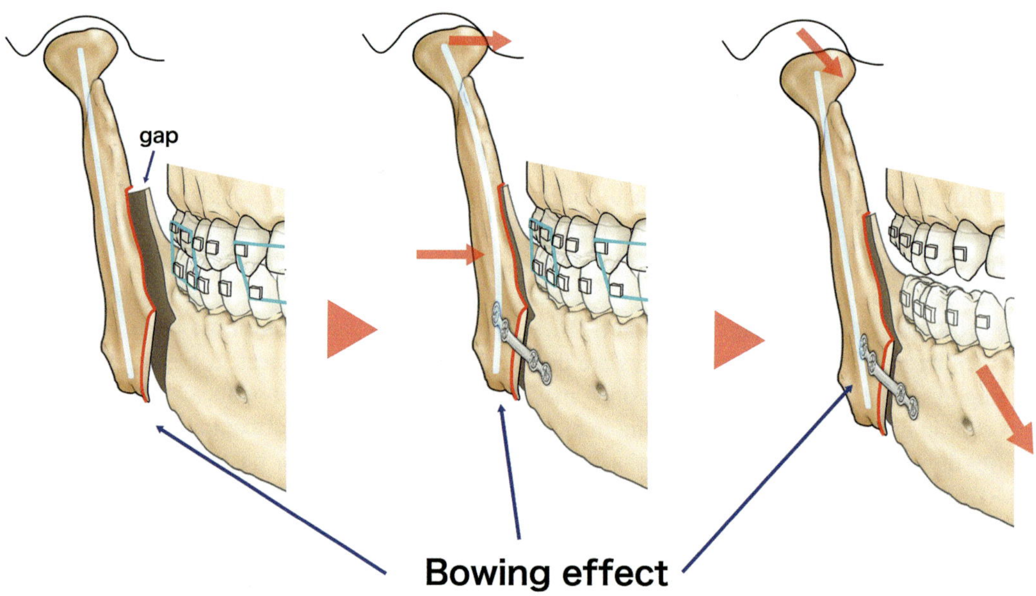

Fig. 9.17 Peripheral condylar sag—type II—due to a bowing effect on the proximal segment (white line). An antero-inferior dislocation of the condyle may result ©Copyright Keisuke Koyama 2020. All rights reserved

ment, condylar resorption, and skeletal instability with an incalculable influence on the postoperative mandibular position [31].

> **Note**
> Malposition of the condyle in the glenoid fossa—condylar sag—can occur as immediate or late change in the position of the condyle after RIF leading to occlusal disturbances.
> Causes:
> Incorrect vector in condylar positioning.
> Intra-articular bleeding, edema, and bending of the proximal segment when applying rigid fixation.

8 Osteosynthesis and Trauma of the Alveolar Nerve

The incidence of neurosensory disturbances of the IAN after rigid osteosynthesis is 1–15% [26, 27].

Experimental studies suggest that rigid internal fixation—primarily compression screw osteosynthesis rather than positioning screw osteosynthesis—can lead to neurosensory disturbances. Positioning screws ensure a constant distance between the split segments and prevent undesirable compression of the IAN.

Incorrect screw placement can compress, constrict, or transect the IAN. In order to avoid this complication, the course of the nerve must be radiologically verified before screw placement, especially in the area of the mandibular base ("base screw").

9 Osteosynthesis and Bone Healing

The aim of rigid fixation is the stability of the mandibular bone segments and a predictable and complication-free bone healing. The fact that rigid fixation enables primary bone healing favors this form of osteosynthesis.

According to *Spiessl* [2], however, it is not the process of bone healing that is decisive for bone consolidation, but rather that a functionally stable fixation of bone segments is guaranteed until bone healing occurs.

> From a clinical perspective, primary intramembranous bony healing is not the true therapeutic goal. It is irrelevant whether bone consolidation is achieved indirectly through secondary differentiation of fibrous or cartilagenous tissues or through direct primary regeneration of osteons. [2]

10 Removal of Osteosynthesis Material

The removal of osteosynthesis plates and screws has been advocated with the argument that osteosynthesis plates act as loadbearing plates without exposing the bone to the full range of physiological stresses and increasing the risk of fractures of the osteosynthesis material. In contrast, the more delicate osteosynthesis plates according to the load-sharing concept of *Champy* et al. [34] reduce the risk of underloading.

The basic argument against removing these implants is that the incidence of infection and other complications is relatively low. In addition, the removal of the implants poses a morbidity risk for the patient. Infections, nerve injuries, and anesthetic complications cannot be excluded. Costs are also caused by this procedure.

The removal of osteosynthesis material should be based on the presence of patient complaints, plate exposure, and loosening or fracture of the implant.

11 Revascularization and Bone Healing

The revascularization of the bone segments and the bone consolidation process takes place in phases [35].

11.1 Immediately Postoperative

The intermedullary circulation between the proximal and distal mandibular segment is interrupted immediately after the mandibular split. The osteotomy margins are avascular.

- Intramedullary circulation between the proximal and distal segments.
- Margins of osteotomy—avascular.

11.2 One Week Postoperative

Hypervascularization of the osteotomy gap and the surrounding soft tissues. No soft tissue reattachment yet, isolated areas of subperiosteal bone formation

- Level of hypervascularization around surgical site.
- No soft tissue reattachment.
- Margins of osteotomy—avascular.

11.3 Two Weeks Postoperative

- Avascular zone at the proximal osteotomy side.
- Necrotic zone at the distal osteotomy side.
- No soft tissue attachment at the distal necrotic zone.

11.4 Three Weeks Postoperative

- Soft tissue reattachment.
- Vascular anastomoses between proximal and distal segment.
- Osteoid formation throughout marrow formation.

11.5 Six Weeks Post-op

The circulation between the osteotomized segments is reconstituted, the soft tissues reattach.

- Circulation reconstituted across the osteotomy site.
- Soft tissue reattachment established.

11.6 12 Weeks Postoperative

Reconstitution of a continuous circulation between the bone segments.

- Circulation between the segments is continuous.

12 Conclusion

Rigid internal osteosynthesis is a prerequisite for early functional treatment in osteotomies of the maxillofacial skeleton. This principle helps to avoid long, functionally disadvantageous intermaxillary fixation. Patient-specific implants help to transfer preoperative planning to the surgical site and help to prevent malpositioning. Depending on the individual initial situation, plate removal should be considered after bony consolidation.

References

1. van Sickels JE, Dolce C, Keeling S, Tiner BD, Clark GM, Rugh JD. Technical factors accounting for stability of a bilateral sagittal split osteotomy advancement: wire osteosynthesis versus rigid fixation. Oral Surg Oral Med Oral Pathol Oral Radiol Endod. 2000;89:19–23.
2. Spiessl B. Chirurgie der Kiefer. In: Naumann HH, editor. Kopf- und Hals-Chirurgie. Indikation, Technik, Fehler und Gefahren. Operations-Manual, vol. 2. Stuttgart: Thieme; 1972.
3. Spiessl B. Osteosynthese bei sagittaler Osteotomie nach Obwegeser-Dal Pont. Fortschr Kieferheilkd Gesichtschir. 1974;18:145–8.
4. Spiessl B. Osteosynthese des Unterkiefers Manual der AO-Prinzipien. Berlin Heidelberg: Springer; 1988.
5. Harris M, Reynolds IR. Fundamentals of orthognathic surgery. Saunders; 1991.
6. Souyris F. Sagittal splitting and bicortical screw fixation of the ascending ramus. J Maxillofac Surg. 1978;6(3):198–203.
7. Spiessl B. Rigid internal fixation after sagittal split osteotomy of the ascending ramus. In: Spiessl B,

editor. New concepts in maxillofacial bone surgery. Berlin, Heidelberg, New York: Springer; 1976.

8. Steinhäuser EW. Bone screws and plates in orthognathic surgery. Int J Oral Surg. 1982;11:209–16.
9. Beukes J, Reyneke JP, Damstra J. Unilateral sagittal split mandibular ramus osteotomy: indications and geometry. Br J Oral Maxillofac Surg. 2016;54(2):219–23.
10. Stacy GC. Recovery of oral opening following sagittal ramus osteotomy for mandibular. J Oral Maxillofac Surg. 1987;45:487–92.
11. Michel C, Reuther J. Orthopädische Chirurgie. In: Hausamen E, Machtens E, Reuther J, editors. Mund-, Kiefer- und Gesichtschirurgie: Operationslehre und – Atlas. Springer; 1995.
12. Spiessl B. The sagittal splitting osteotomy for correction of mandibular prognathism. Clin Plast Surg. 1982;9:491–507.
13. van Sickels JE, Flanary CM. Stability associated with mandibular advancement treated by rigid osseous fixation. Oral Maxillofac Surg. 1985;43:338–41.
14. van Sickels JE, Richardson DA. Stability of orthognathic surgery: a review of rigid fixation. Br J Oral Maxillofac Surg. 1996;34:279–85.
15. Luhr HG. Compression plate osteosynthesis through the Luhr system. In: Krüger E, Schilli S, editors. Oral and maxillofacial traumatology, vol. 1. Chicago: Quintessence; 1982. p. 319.
16. Swift JQ. Mandibular advancement. Atlas Oral Maxillofac Surg Clin North Am. 1993;1:17–27.
17. Lindorf HH. Funktionsstabile Tandem-Verschraubung der sagittalen Ramusosteotomie Operationstechnik, neue Instrumente und Erfahrungen. Dtsch Z Mund Kiefer Gesichts Chir. 1984;8:367–73.
18. Lindorf HH. Sagittal ramus osteotomy with tandem screw fixation. Technique and results. J Maxillofac Surg. 1986;14:311–6.
19. Raveh J, Vuillemin T, Lädrach K, Sutter F. New techniques for reproduction of the condyle relation and reduction of complications after sagittal ramus split osteotomy of the mandible. J Oral Maxillofac Surg. 1988;46:751–7.
20. Kashani H, Rasmusson L. Osteotomies in orthognathic surgery. In: Motamedi MHK, editor. Textbook of advanced Oral and maxillofacial surgery, vol. 3. Intechopen; 2016.
21. Baker DL, Stoelinga PJ, Blijdorp PA, Brouns JJ. Long-term stability after inferior maxillary repositioning by miniplate fixation. Int J Oral Maxillofac Surg. 1992;21(6):320–6.
22. Blomqvist JE, Isaksson S. Skeletal stability after mandibular advancement: a comparison of two rigid internal fixation techniques. J Oral Maxillofac Surg. 1994;52(11):1133–7.
23. Rubens BC, Stoelinga PJ, Blijdorp PA, Schoenaers JH, Politis C. Skeletal stability following sagittal split osteotomy using monocortical miniplate internal fixation. Int J Oral Maxillofac Surg. 1988;17(6):371–6.
24. Borstlap WA, Stoelinga PJW, Hoppenreijs TJM, van't Hof MA. Stabilisation of sagittal split set/back osteotomies with miniplates: a prospective, multicentre study with 2-year follow-up. Int J Oral Maxillofac Surg. 2005;34(5):487–94.
25. Fujioka M, Fujii T, Hirano A. Comparative study of mandibular stability after sagittal split osteotomies: biocortical versus monocortical osteosynthesis. Cleft Palate Craniofac J. 2000;37(6):551–5.
26. Kim JH, Kim SG, Oh JS. Complications related to orthognathic surgery. J Korean Assoc Maxillofac Plast Reconstr Surg. 2010;32:416–21.
27. Kim YK. Complications associated with orthognathic surgery. J Korean Assoc Oral Maxillofac Surg. 2017;43(1):3–15.
28. Jędrzejewski M, Smektała T, Sporniak-Tutak K, Olszewski R. Preoperative, intraoperative, and postoperative complications in orthognathic surgery: a systematic review. Clin Oral Investig. 2015;19:969–77.
29. Tuinzing DB, Swart JGN. Lageveränderungen des Caput mandibulae bei Verwendung von Zugschrauben nach sagittaler Osteotomie des Unterkiefers. Dtsch Z Mund-Kiefer- u Gesichtschir. 1978;3:94.
30. Escobar V, Greenberg AM, Schwimmer A. Mandibular osteotomies and considerations for rigid internal fixation. In: Greenberg AM, Prein J, editors. Craniomaxillofacial reconstructive and corrective bone surgery: principles of internal fixation using AO/ASIF technic. Springer; 2002.
31. Reyneke JP, Ferretti C. Intraoperative diagnosis of condylar sag after bilateral sagittal split ramus osteotomy. Br J Oral Maxillofac Surg. 2002;40(4):285–92.
32. Hall HD, Chase DC, Payor LG. Evaluation and refinement of the intra-oral vertical subcondylar osteotomy. Oral Surg. 1975;33:333–41.
33. Yamauchi K, et al. Condylar luxation following bilateral intraoral vertical ramus osteotomy. Oral Surg Oral Med Oral Pathol Oral Radiol Endod. 2007;104:747–51.
34. Champy M, Lodde JP, Jaeger JH, Wilk A. Bases biomécaniques de l'ostéosynthèse mandibulaire selon la méthode de F.X. Michelet. Revue stomatal chirur maxillofac. 1976;77(1):248–51.
35. Fonsecca RJ, Marciani RD, Turvey TA. Oral and maxillofacial surgery, orthognatic surgery and craniofacial surgery. Saunders; 2009.

Pre- and Peri-operative Care in Orthognathic Surgery - Anesthesiology and CMF-Surgery

10

Pia-Marina Guardiola, Peter Kessler, and Nicolas Hardt

Contents

P.-M. Guardiola (✉)
Departement of Anesthesiology, Intensive Care and Pain Medicine, Hirslanden Klinik St. Anna, Lucerne, Switzerland

P. Kessler (✉)
Department of Cranio-Maxillofacial Surgery, Maastricht University Medical Center, Maastricht, The Netherlands
e-mail: peter.kessler@mumc.nl

N. Hardt (✉)
Kantonsspital Lucerne, Clinic and Policlinic of Cranio-Maxillofacial Surgery, Lucerne, Switzerland

P. Kessler et al. (eds.), *Illustrated Manual of Orthognathic Surgery*,
https://doi.org/10.1007/978-3-031-06978-9_10

Abstract

Modern perioperative care is complex and involves a large number of staff from multiple disciplines. Patient outcomes depend on well-designed processes, consistent clinical practice, and effective communication. The peri- and postoperative care should be a unified process of multiple coordinated steps (Kwon and Laskin, Quintessence Publishing 2001; Kerridge, Best Pract Res Clin Obstet Gynaecol 20(1):23–40, 2006).

The flow of information in the surgical process is based on standardized pre-, peri-, and postoperative checks, notes, and orders in the operating room, the recovery ward, and the normal patient ward.

Preoperative protocol establishes what is thought to be the pathology of the patient and what procedure is planned for the operation an anesthesia.

It indicates that the appropriate preoperative tests have been performed and reviewed. It also confirms the presence of an informed consent document (operative permit). Surgical care provided to a patient requires a written, signed, informed consent document. Often referred to as an "op permit," it is an essential part of the medical record. It must be properly completed prior to any invasive, anesthetic, or other procedure that involves any significant risk to the patient.

Preoperative checks and orders assure that the patient is ready for surgery and all preoperative medical instructions have been performed. All necessary laboratory exams, X-rays, consultations, and permits must be ordered in a timely manner to ensure their availability before surgery. Similarly, preoperative determination of the intubation manner between anesthesia and CMF surgery is essential in particular with regard to possible intubation problems.

Perioperative notes include the anesthesia induction, anesthesia maintenance, and intraoperative ongoing monitoring and documentation of the patient's vital functions, as well as documentation of all perioperative prophylactic measures taken for a successful without adverse events postoperative course.

Keywords

Clinical examination · Anamnesis · Preoperative assessment · Preparations for the surgical procedure · Anesthesiologic protocols · Preoperative check · Medication · Antibiotics · Cortisone · Edema · Preparation for surgery · Intubation · Difficult airway · Documentation · Extubation · Pain management

1 Preoperative Phase

1.1 Anesthesiology: Preoperative Checks

The preoperative check includes at the entrance to the operating room, the surgeons name, the patients ID with birth date, marked operation side, the existence of all necessary laboratory examinations, medical examinations including allergies, the execution of the preoperative medical orders with regard to the medicamentous prescriptions and a pre-existing continuous medication and confirms the existence of the patient's approval of the operation and anesthesia [1, 2].

1.2 Pre-op Medical Examination for Orthognathic Procedures

The preoperative examination serves to the differentiation between patients without and with systemic diseases (diagnosis-related examination) as well as to the classification of the surgical risk (intervention-specific examination).

1.3 Orthognathic Procedures (Mandibular +/− Maxillary Osteotomies)

Are to be attributed to surgical risk class B like, e.g., large laparoscopic surgery, large spinal surgery, joint replacement, carotid surgery, endovascular and vascular prosthesis. Surgical interventions of risk class B/C in healthy patients <60 years require an intervention-specific examination.

The basic examination includes the following:

1. Laboratory analysis.
   Hematology: Small blood count-Indices—RBC/WBC/Hb.

> **Note**
> Anemia management standards:
> Hemoglobin under <12 g/l ⇨ no elective surgery.

Coagulation-Indices: INR.
Electrolytes + Creatinine: Na—K.

2. Height and weight.
3. Further preoperative parameters include:

- ECG findings.
- Preoperatively prescribed drugs.
- Presence of organ-specific X-ray documents and X-ray findings.
- Informed Consent: Anesthesia and the operative procedure.

4. NPO Status: Liquid and Food Care.
   In elective procedures, a dietary NPO of 6 h is necessary before the procedure. For clear liquids, a grace period of 2–4 h applies. Permanent medications are taken on the day of surgery with a sip of water.

2 CMF Surgery: Preoperative Checks

Checking the completeness of the preoperative radiologic documentation, the preoperative documentation of the planning documents and the surgical technical aids for maxillofacial osteotomy.

- Maxillofacial X-rays:
  - Cephalometric X-rays.
  - Panorama X-ray.
  - Lateral cephalometric X-ray.
  - Cone-beam computed tomography (CBCT).
  - Multi-slice computed tomography (MSCT).
- Cephalometric Analysis.
- 3D Imaging and 3D Planning
- Maxillofacial—technical aids:
  - Intermaxillary splints, wafers, etc.

3 Anesthesiology

3.1 Preoperative Medications: Have to Be Continued as a General Rule

Especially:

- Antiarrhythmics.
- Anticonvulsants.
- Steroids.
- Thyroid hormones.
- Parkinson therapy.
- Contraceptives.

Others Have to Be Paused:

- Discontinuation of platelet aggregation inhibitors (7–10 days before surgery) is possible if allowed by the general practitioner or cardiologist.
- Antidiabetics have to be adapted.
- Antidepressants.
- Oral anticoagulants—after feedback with general practitioner.
- Ginko-compounds—as they effect coagulation.
- Antihypertensive medications such as calcium antagonists, ACE inhibitors and Angiotensin II antagonists.
- Diuretics.

3.2 Procedure in Patients with Platelet Aggregation Inhibitors

Aspirin—ASA Acetylic Salicylic Acid
For primary prophylaxis: should be discontinued 10 days before surgery.

Aspirin—ASA Acetylic Salicylic Acid
For secondary prophylaxis has to be continued.

Plavix and Analogs
Usually set off 7–10 days before surgery, after feedback with GP or cardiologist.

4 Anesthesia and CMF Surgery: Preoperative Assessment

- Intubation form.
- Intubation difficulties.
- Estimation of ITN difficulties.
- Patients positioning.

4.1 Intubation Form: Decision with CMF Surgeon

4.1.1 Types of Endotracheal Tubes (ETT): Intubation

- Oro-tracheal Intubation/Standard tube/Preformed Tube.
- Naso-tracheal intubation.
- Tracheostomy Tubes.

4.1.2 Intubation: Technique

- Standard procedure: Laryngoscopy.
- Optic enhanced Laryngoscopy (Type-C-MAC).
- Fiber-optic Intubation/awake or sleeping.

4.1.3 Naso-tracheal Intubation: In CMF Operations

Naso-tracheal intubation is indicated in following CMF operations:

- Interventions on the lower jaw, upper jaw and upper floor and tongue.
- Surgically necessary intermaxillary wiring/fixation—IMF.
- For oral intubation barriers.

> **Note**
>
> Naso-tracheal Intubation is the standard for maxillofacial osteotomies:
>
> Reasons are:
>
> Intraoperative occlusion setting associated with intraoperative intermaxillary fixation.

4.2 Intubation Problems

Any intubation problems in maxillofacial procedures require mutual preoperative information between anesthesia and CMF surgery and the mutual professional coordination of the procedure.

4.2.1 Difficult Airway: Definition

Intubation is considered difficult if it is "difficult or impossible" to perform direct laryngoscopy and to introduce the endotracheal tube into the larynx and trachea [3–5].

All hospitals must have algorithms for difficult airways, which have to be followed to ensure patients safety.

Generally associated with a difficult airway in CMF surgery are:

- Anatomical oropharyngeal bottlenecks and obstacles or functional changes.
- Oropharyngeal malformations.
- Obstacles due to pre-intervention: scarring and stricture by scarring.
- Post-tumor states.
- Injuries: Scarcity stricts/synechia.
- Endonasal hyperplasia/septum deviations/endonasal malformations.
- Cervical neck mobility impairment.

> **Note**
>
> Iatrogenic injuries with bleeding and swelling associated with intubation attempts.

- Functional movement restrictions of the oral opening due to
  - Jaw joint diseases/arthrosis/ankylose/juvenile arthritis/myofascial pain syndrome/jaw joint diseases with mouth-opening disabilities such as joint discopathy like discus luxation and joint osteoarthritis.
- Skeletal variants of facial skull growth (skeletal dysgnathias).
  - Isolated mandibular hypoplasia/hyperplasia/retrognathia/prognathia.
  - Combined mandibular–maxillary retrognathias/prognathias.
- Macroglossia.

- Extreme obesity.
- Carious front teeth: Compromised sight with the laryngoscope.

Specific problems associated with a difficult airway in orthognathic maxillofacial osteotomies are

Skeletal Dysgnathias

Since patients with skeletal dysgnathias may have altered size relations of the jaw compartments and/or movement restrictions of the oral opening, possible intubation difficulties must be expected.

> **Note**
>
> Indications of difficult laryngoscopy and intubation in CMF Operations are:
>
> - Obesity.
> - Mandibular retrognathia/prognathia/maxillary hyperplasia.
> - Oral opening restriction <30 mm.
> - Impaired neck mobility.
> - Low thyro-mental or sterno-mental distance.

4.2.2 Estimation of ITN Difficulty

Mallampati Test [6, 7]

The test allows conclusions to be drawn about the size of the tongue in relation to the oropharynx and thus to potential obstacles in laryngoscopy. The examination should be carried out on the watchful, upright sitting patient, who opens his mouth as far as possible and stretches out his tongue as much as possible (Fig. 10.1).

Upper Lip Bite Test [8].

Mandibular Protrusion Test [9]

Determining whether the patient can bite the upper lip with the lower incisors? If the patient cannot do so, intubation is most likely to be associated with difficulties (Fig. 10.2).

> **In the Case of Predictable Difficult Intubation**
>
> 1. Optic laryngoscopic device with C-Mac and D-Blade and a pre-bent tube with an introducer.
> 2. Consider fiber-optic intubation at awake patient.

Class 1

Shows mandibular advancement beyond the upper teeth. Lower incisors can be protruded anterior the upper incisors.

Class 2

Shows that the mandible cannot be advanced beyond the upper teeth. The lower incisors can be brought edge to edge with the upper incisors.

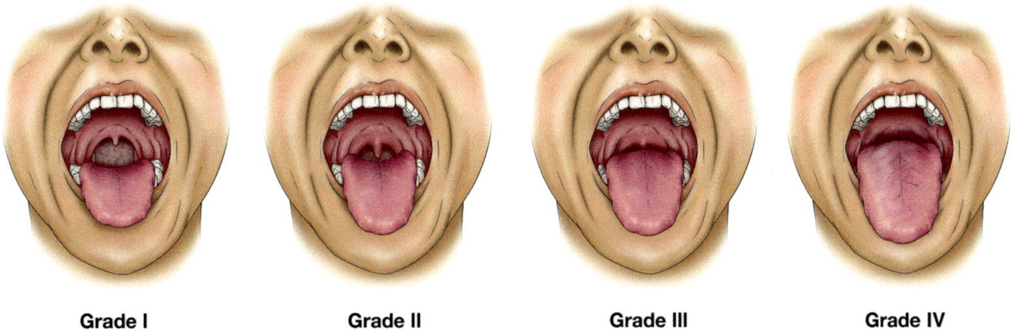

Fig. 10.1 Modified Mallampati classification. Graduation of the visibility of oropharyngeal structures: palate arches and tonsils depending on size and form of the tongue. Grade I: soft palate, uvula, mouth, and front and rear tonsil bed visible. Grade II: soft palate and uvula visible. Grade III: soft palate and base of the uvula visible. Grade IV: soft palate not visible. ©Copyright Keisuke Koyama 2021. All rights reserved

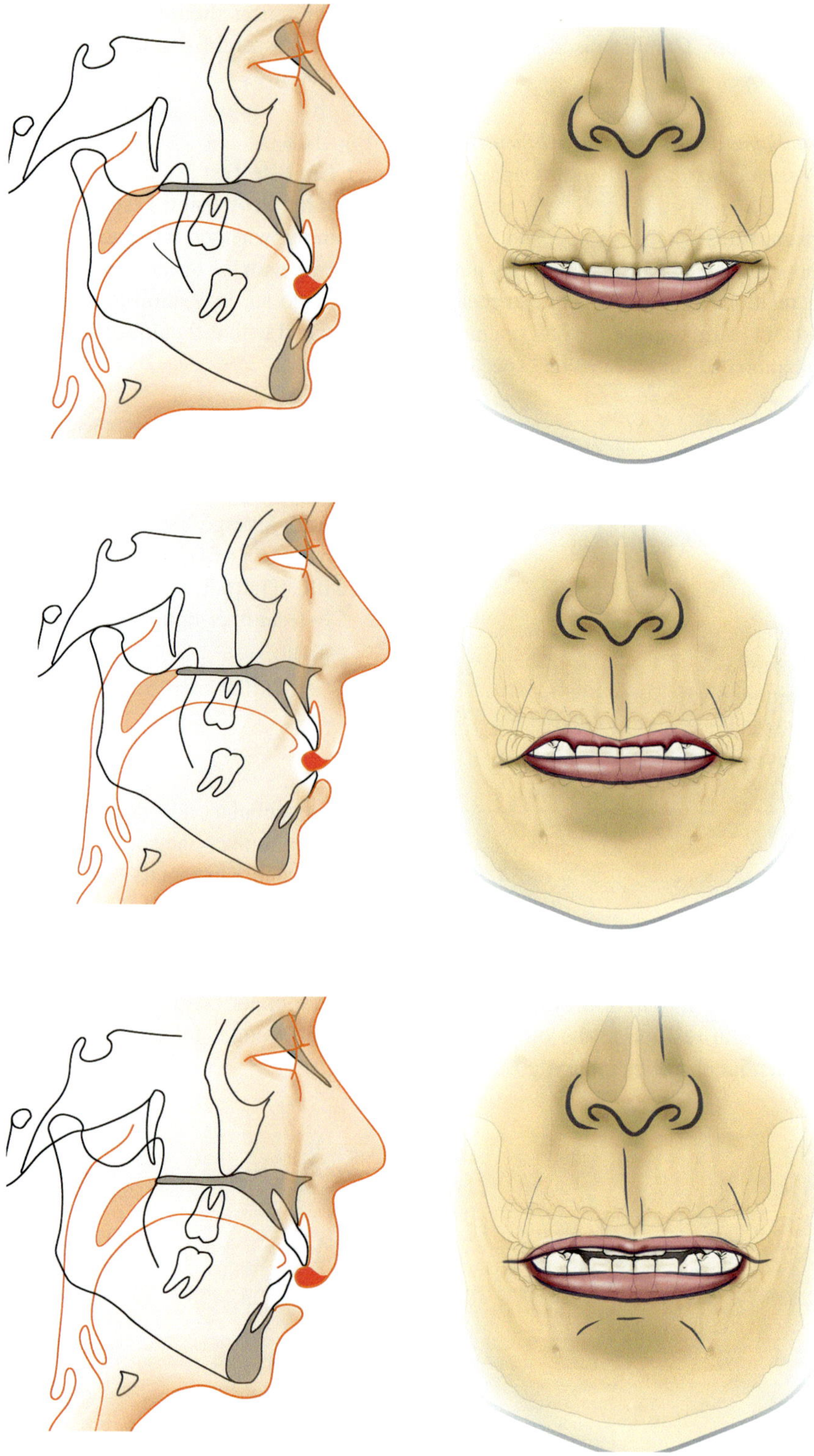

Fig. 10.2 Upper lip bite test: Class 1—Lower incisors can bite upper lip above the vermillion line Class 2—Lower incisors can bite below the vermillion border Class 3—Cannot bite upper lip

Class 3

Shows that the lower incisors cannot reach the upper teeth. The lower incisors cannot be brought edge to edge with the upper incisors.

Advancement of the mandible may be considered a favorable sign for intubation without complications in association with moving of the tongue (Fig. 10.3).

4.2.3 Anamnestic ITN Difficulties

Of great importance are also targeted questions and pre-existing data on intubation difficulties in previous anesthesia or pre-surgery on the mouth, nose, larynx, or trachea.

Patients with known intubation problems in previous anesthesias are often in possession of an anesthesia card with an exact identification of the problem encountered [10].

4.3 Patients: Positioning: Determination with CMF Surgeon

The so-called "sniffing position" or Jackson position is considered optimal position for anesthesia initiation and intubation.

The patient lies flat on the back, his head is lightly underlaid with an intubation cushion or upholstery ring. Due to additional reclination, the airways are open to the maximum.

The oral cavity, pharynx, and larynx form an almost straight axis and thus release the view of the larynx (Fig. 10.4).

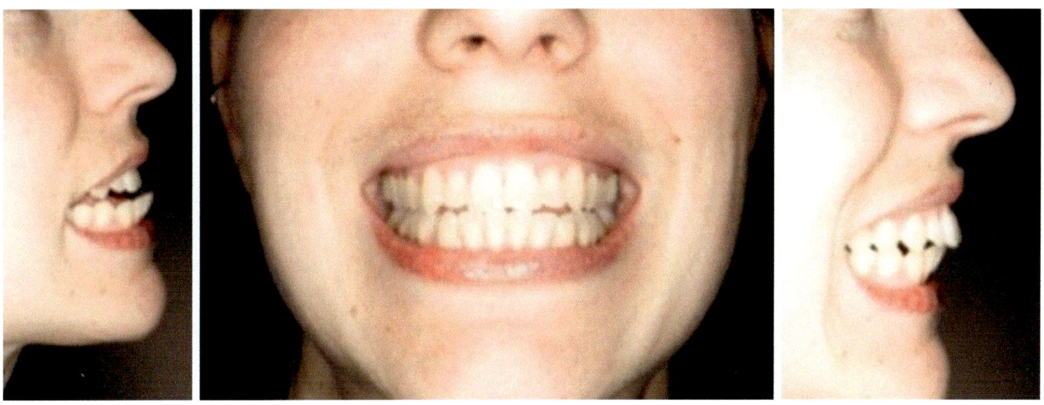

Fig. 10.3 Mandibular Protrusion Test

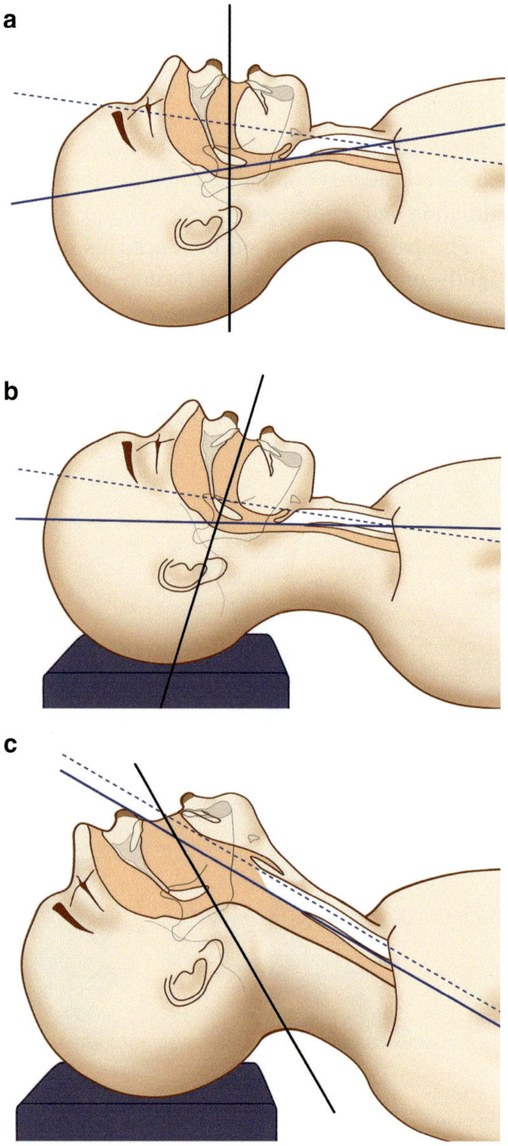

Fig. 10.4 Course of the intubation axis (**a**) Head in body axis without vertical displacement or flexion-extension (**b**) Head in elevated position without flexion-extension (**c**) Head in elevated position with maximum extension opens a straight intubation pathway ©Copyright Keisuke Koyama 2021. All rights reserved

5 Perioperative Phase: Anesthesia procedure in CMF Surgery

The actual anesthesia consists of 5 phases:

- Preparation: iv line, basic monitoring and if necessary enhanced monitoring.
- Anesthesia Induction.
- Maintenance.
- Recovery, Emergence.
- Documentation.

5.1 Preparation

- Check allergies and drugs.
- Check anesthetic equipment.
  - Connection of monitoring.
  - Peripheral-venous access.
  - Infusion start.
- Monitoring.
- Basic Monitoring

Continuous measurement of vital parameters:

- ECG.
- Puls oximetry.
- Non-invasive blood pressure measurement.
- Capnometry.
- Inspiratory O_2 concentration.
- In- and expiratory measurement of inhalation anesthetics, if used.
- Respiratory parameters and pressures.
- Temperature.
- Neuromuscular monitoring.
- BIS monitoring.
- Advanced Monitoring at ITN
  - Invasive blood pressure measurement-artery.
  - Cerebral blood flow and O_2 consumption.
  - Monitoring urinary output with urinary catheter.

5.2 Anesthesia Induction

- Preoxygenation O_2 by mask.
- Opioid administration.
- Induction with administration of hypnotic.
- Administration of muscle relaxants.
- Intubation (oral/nasal).
- Connecting respirator and respiratory monitor.
- Auscultation of both lungs.
- Fixation of the tube.
- Tube cuff pressure control.
- If needed administer vasoactive drugs.

5.2.1 Critical Moments: Tubs Displacement/Disconnection

Accidental causes:

- Head-bearing change with release of the external tube fixation.
- Intraoral manipulations with dislocation of the oro-tracheal tube.

Throat after Intubation

The throat can be tamponed to prevent blood from flowing into the stomach or into the lungs.

5.3 Maintenance: ITN Anesthesia

- Continuation of ITN—preferably with target controlled total intravenous anesthesia.
- Administration of opioids as required.
- Repeat doses of relaxants if required.
- Normo-ventilation with a PEEP of approx. 5 cm H_2O.
- Measure blood loss.
- Maintain body temperature.
- Longer interventions.
  - Control of patients positioning.
  - Continuous cuff pressure measurement.
  - Measure urinary output.

5.4 Recovery: Emergence

5.4.1 Requirements for Anesthetic Discharge

- Steady contact: anesthesia and surgeon—for estimating the duration of the surgery.
- With the onset of the wound closure—reduction-removal of the anesthetics.
- At the end of the operation increase inspiratory oxygen concentration.
- Test the muscle relaxant lasting effect and eventual need for reversal or antagonists.

5.4.2 Extubation Criteria

- Sufficient spontaneous ventilation.
- Normal respiratory frequency.
- TOF 100%—Muscle relaxation recovery.
- Existing protective reflexes.
- Normal temperature.
- Stable circulation.
- No bleeding.

5.4.3 Measures before Extubation

- Removal of all swabs and possible suction.
- Nasal careful suction/continuity test.
- In wound secretion, blood and saliva, immediate suction, bleeding control.
- If blood enters the stomach, it should be extracted perioperatively via a gastric tube to prevent postoperative vomiting.

5.4.4 Extubation

- The extubation takes place—after operations in the area of the respiratory tract—only when awake patient with sufficient protective reflexes and unhindered passage of the breathing air.

5.5 Documentation

All vital parameters, blood losses and measures taken by the anesthesia staff and special events and complications, are carefully recorded in the anesthesia protocol.

5.5.1 Anesthesia Protocol

- Induction and intubation including occurring ITN problems as well as the laryngological visual relations.
- Perioperative drugs and anesthetics.
- Vital signs are displayed at least every 5 min.
- Ventilation parameters every 20 min or in case of changes.
- Fluids administered and estimated blood loss.

The documentation of special surgical measures, in particular of

- Drains.
- Specimens.
- Surgical Complications.

6 Perioperative Phase: Prophylactic Measures in CMF Surgery

6.1 Perioperative Prophylaxis with Antibiotics

The aim of perioperative antibiotic prophylaxis is the prevention of postoperative wound infection for patients undergoing maxillafacial osteotomies.

Execution: Task of the anesthetist.

As a rule of thumb for perioperative antibiotic prophylaxis in cranio-maxillary procedures:

- Antibiotic protection only for >2 h of surgery.
- Antibiotic administration <24 h—time: 30–60 min before starting surgery.
- For preparations with a standard dosing of 2×/d, single-shot prophylaxis is sufficient even for longer procedures.
- Repetition of antibiotic administration after >3 h surgical time.
- Prolongation of antibiotic therapy only in case of pre-existing infection.

A possible perioperative antibiotic regimen can be as follows:

Antibiotics: Cefazolin and Metronidazole at the initiation continuing postoperatively with Amoxicillin-Clavulanic Acid

> Cefazolin 1.5 g i.v. single shot.
> + Metronidazole 500 mg i.v.—intravenous Single shot.

6.1.1 Alternative Proposals

For a possible postoperative antibiotic regime:

Antibiotics: *Aminopenicillin* + Beta-lactam antibiotics.

> Ampicillin 2 g i.v. single shot.
> + Sulbactam 1 g i.v. single shot.

6.1.2 Alternative Proposals in Cases of Allergy

In case of allergy to beta lactams: clindamycin.
In case of allergy to beta lactams: clindamycin + aminoglycoside.
In case of allergy to beta lactams: glycopeptides.

In the case of present risk factors, almost all inpatients have an indication of perioperative antibiotic prophylaxis during an operation.

6.2 Perioperative Pain Prophylaxis

6.2.1 Basic Pain Therapy

- Ibuprofen (NSAR).
- Metamizol.

6.2.2 Enhanced Pain Therapy

Peaks in intensity in the early postoperative period:

- iv opioids in the recovery room

6.2.3 Severe Pain Therapy

Expected postoperative pain exacerbation can well be handled with:

"Patient-controlled analgesia"
- with opioids, such as Fentanyl or Hydromorphin,
- Ketamin infusion.

6.3 Perioperative Prophylaxis against Swelling

In contrast to the early postoperative pain, the postoperative facial swelling reaches the characteristic maximum 48–72 h after surgery. These symptoms can affect intensively the patient's quality in the postoperative phase of well-being.

As a rule, the postoperative facial swelling usually present for 2–3 weeks, which then subsides down to some residual edema at 3–4 weeks post-surgery.

Perioperative swelling prophylaxis for the operating area:

0.1 mg/kg iv Dexamethasone before surgery and every 6–8 h after

or,

125 mg iv Prednisolone (Prednisone) every 8 h.

6.4 Postoperative Nausea and Vomiting: PONV Prophylaxis

6.4.1 Influencing Factors

Opioids.

Female gender.

Nonsmoker status.

History of nausea and vomiting after anesthesia.

History of motion sickness.

Perioperatively low blood pressure.

Pain.

Psychological stress.

Full urinary bladder.

6.4.2 Prophylaxis: Reducing Emetogenic Influence

With anamnestically known PONV [11].

Prophylactic administration of 0.1 mg/kg dexamethasone.

5-HT3-antagonist (Type: Ondansetron)

Avoid low blood pressure.

Avoid pain and stress.

Preferably administer non-opioid analgesics.

7 Conclusion

Anesthesiologist and surgeon form a team and coordinate optimally to maximize patient safety. The procedure corresponds to a fixed sequence, which should be more or less spread out depending on the anamnesis. On the day of the operation, the briefing and the time-out procedure fulfill the necessary communication in the team for the maximum safety of the patient.

References

1. Guidelines for the Provision of Anaesthetic Services (GPAS). Guidance on the provision of anaesthetic services for postoperative care. Chapter 4. London: The Royal College of Anaesthetists RCoA; 2019.
2. Standards for basic anesthetic monitoring. ASA. Committee on Standards and Practice Parameters (CSPP), 2020.
3. American Society of Anesthesiologists–ASA. Practice guidelines für postanaesthetic care. Anesthesiology. 2002;96(742)
4. Apfelbaum J, et al. Practice guidelines for Management of the Difficult Airway Updated Report by the American Society of Anesthesiologists Task Force on Management of the Difficult Airway. Anesthesiology. 2013;118:1–20.
5. Larsen R. Anästhesie. München: Elsevier; Urban und Fischer; 2013.
6. Mallampati SR, Gatt SP, Gugino LD, et al. A clinical sign to predict difficult tracheal intubation: a prospective study. Can Anaesth Soc J. 1985;32:429–33.
7. Samsoon GL, Young JR. Difficult tracheal intubation: a retrospective study. Anaesthesia. 1987;42(5):487–90.

8. Detsky ME, Jivraj N, Adhikari NK, Friedrich JO, Pinto R, Simel DL, Wijeysundera DN, Scales DC. Will this patient be difficult to intubate?: the rational clinical examination systematic review. JAMA. 2019;321(5):493–503.
9. Takenaka I. Mandibular protrusion test for prediction of difficult mask ventilation. Anesthesiology. 2001;94(5):935.
10. Dörges V, Bein B. Klinisches Management des Schwierigen Atemweges. Anasth Intesiv Notf. 2006 Sep;41(9):564–75.
11. Apfel CC, Läärä E, Koivuranta M, Greim CA, Roewer N. A simplified risk score for predicting postoperative nausea and vomiting: conclusions from cross-validations between two centers. Anesthesiology. 1999;91(3):693–700.

Postoperative Care in Orthognathic Surgery

11

Peter Kessler, Veronique C. M. L. Timmer, and Nicolas Hardt

Contents

P. Kessler (✉) · V. C. M. L. Timmer
Department of Cranio-Maxillofacial Surgery, Maastricht University Medical Center, Maastricht, The Netherlands
e-mail: peter.kessler@mumc.nl; v.timmer@mumc.nl

N. Hardt (✉)
Kantonsspital Lucerne, Clinic and Policlinic of Cranio-Maxillofacial Surgery, Lucerne, Switzerland

Abstract

Postoperative care of patients undergoing orthognathic surgery requires special attention, as surgical procedures are located in the airway entry zone and may compromise it. Special attention must be paid to postoperative bleeding, swelling, and airway obstruction.

P. Kessler et al. (eds.), *Illustrated Manual of Orthognathic Surgery*,
https://doi.org/10.1007/978-3-031-06978-9_11

Postoperative pain management is absolutely essential to make the patient feel safe. This is even more important if the patient has received intermaxillary fixation after surgery.

Keywords

Postoperative patient management · Pain · Medication · Recovery · Monitoring · Wound care · Diet · Mobilization

1 Postoperative Management

Inpatient care is highly dependent on the type of procedure, age, and condition of the patient. General principles of medical management are outlined below.

Postoperative management is divided into immediate postoperative observation and monitoring in the recovery ward and postoperative care in the normal ward.

After extubation in the OR and ensuring safe spontaneous breathing, the patient is transferred to the recovery ward for further observation. On the part of the OR team (anesthesia/OMF surgeon), information and instructions can be provided during the sign-out procedure in the OR, digitally and in the form of OR notes and orders.

Postoperative care instructions consider the impact of surgery and anesthesia on the patient's condition. Postoperative orders ensure that the findings and effects of the surgery are appropriately addressed to ensure patient safety.

1.1 Postoperative Instructions

Essential information during sign-out procedure:

- Relevant general medical diagnoses and findings.
- Procedure(s) performed.
- Intermaxillary situation, occlusion, fixation.
- Estimated/measured blood loss.
- Postoperative pain medication.
- Continuation of antibiotic therapy, specify dosage, and medication.
- Patient positioning.
- Food intake and quality.
- Special measures in the wound area, e.g., cooling.
- Information to relatives.

Optional—usually noted in the anesthesia protocol:

- Anesthetics used.
- Infusion amounts.
- Fluid balance.
- Laboratory results.

1.2 For the Later Postoperative Phase

- Food buildup.
- Removal of the urinary catheter.
- Gastric tube removal.
- Laboratory checks.
- Control of food intake.
- Postoperative X-ray control.

- Medication management.
- Expected discharge date.
- First outpatient follow-up.

1.3 Postoperative Management in the Recovery Room

Postoperative management in recovery includes immediate cardio-pulmonary monitoring, oxygen saturation measurement, and respiratory control/assurance.

If necessary, laboratory parameters may be checked. Specifically, observation and monitoring includes the following parameters:

> **NotePostoperative recovery monitoring includes three cardinal measures:**
>
> - Stabilization of the postoperative patient.
> - Timely detection and treatment of complications.
> - Initiation of postoperative treatment.

1.3.1 Standard Basic Monitoring

- Continuation of infusion therapy, temperature measurement.
- Fluid balance, urine output.
- O_2 insufflation—application of 2–4 l O_2/min on average.
- Documentation of vital signs.
  - Balancing of drainage losses, if applied.
  - Laboratory results, if indicated.

1.3.2 Clinical Examination

- Response to response.
- Respiration—Breathing.
- Respiratory rate.
- Arterial O_2 saturation by pulse oximetry.
  - If necessary: blood gas analysis.
  - Auscultatory lung findings.

1.3.3 Cardiovascular Function

- Heart rate and pulse.
- Blood pressure.
- ECG assessment.

1.3.4 Neuromuscular Function

- Muscle strength assessment.
- Relaxation surplus: Nerve Stimulator.
- Vigilance and orientation ability.
- State of consciousness

1.3.5 Pain Level

- Pain level: location and intensity of pain—visual analog scale.
- Effect of pain therapy.

1.4 Controlling the Surgical Area in Orthognathic Surgery

- Edema of the face.
- Tongue swelling.
- Swallowing ability.
- Pressure dressing intact.
- Intraoral weeping.
- IMF stability, occlusion, wafer.

1.5 Final Clinical Assessment

After final clinical assessment and satisfactory course without complications, the patient is transferred to normal ward with further instructions. The patient usually remains in the recovery room for 3 h.

1.5.1 Example I: CMF-Surgery [1]

Postoperative monitoring in the recovery room

Surgical Procedure: BSSO and Le Fort I osteotomy.

Level of consciousness: responsive but sleepy.

Vital signs: RR 105/65, P 100, R 16.

In and outs:

IV: 1100 mL.

Foley: 2200 mL.

NG: 200 mL.

Labs: Hct: 29%.

PE: RRRs murmurs, gallops.

Lungs: Bibasilar rales.

Abdomen: BS × 4.

Head and neck:

Moderate facial edema, pressure bandage intact,

Minimal intraoral oozing, MMF stable.

Assessment:

Satisfactory postop results and progress.

Postoperative care on the normal ward.

- Patient positioning and mobilization.
- Antibiotic regime.
- Pain management.
- Antiedematous therapy.
- PONV therapy—opening of IMF, wire cutter.
- Resumption of an existing permanent medication.

Antiedematous physical therapy.

Nutrition.

Wound treatment.

Wound control.

Drainage removal.

Laboratory controls.

X-ray controls.

1.5.2 Example II: Orthognathic Surgery *(Adapted from* [1]*)*

Postoperative arrangement after transfer to the ward using the example of monomaxillary surgery on the mandible: BSSO

Positioning of the patient

Upper body/head elevated 30°.

Medication.

Continuation of antibiotic therapy for at least 24 hours.

Pain medication based on NSAIDs.

Repeat dexamethasone dose of 8 mg 10 and 20 hours after surgery.

Thermo-/Physical therapy.

Cooling of the wound area: cold packs or cooling mask.

Nutrition.

Start feeding with water, tea and water-based ice cream.

Build up nutrition—from the 2nd/third day with soft food rich in protein and vitamins.

Special notes on postoperative therapy.

Physical postoperative antiedematous treatment to reduce swelling.

Regular intermittent application of ice or chilled gel compresses to the surgical area—face-cheek-perioral—for the first 3 days after surgery, automatic cooling systems have proven their worth.

Sleeping for 1–2 weeks after surgery with the upper body/head elevated at a 30° angle.

Application of special light compression bandages as directed by the surgeon.

Postoperative pain management: See Chap. 10.

Regular evaluation of pain intensity (VAS)

Choice of medication: primarily according to pain intensity.

Choice of NSAIDs: According to type of surgery and any contraindications. Possible drug combination on recommendation of the pain team.

> **Note**
>
> Chronic pain patients:
>
> Include pre-existing pain medication in postoperative pain therapy on the ward.

For detailed planning of individual postoperative pain treatment, please consult Chap. 10.

2 Postoperative Therapy of Postoperative Nausea and Vomiting (PONV)

The risk of PONV is generally 20–30%. The risk of PONV should be taken very seriously, especially after operations in which spontaneous or reflex opening of the mouth is restricted or impossible due to intermaxillary fixation. Anesthetic and surgical procedures must be adapted to this. For anesthetic procedures, intravenous methods have proven beneficial, as has the targeted administration of antiemetics.

During induction of anesthesia and postoperatively, dexamethasone is used not only as an antiphlogistic but also as an antiemetic, e.g., in combination with serotonin (5-HT3) receptor antagonists, such as ondansetron.

Nausea and vomiting should be treated immediately, as there is a high risk of recurrence.

2.1 On the Recovery

10–20 mg Propofol i.v. fractionated by anesthesiologists—attention respiratory depression.

2.2 On the Ward

Ondansetron i.v. or Dimenhydrinat. (histamine receptor antagonist). For dose information, please remember maximum doses, age reference, and weight relation.

For further information please consult Chap. 10.

2.3 Postoperative Drug Thrombosis Prophylaxis

Thromboprophylaxis is part of perioperative patient management for any procedure under general anesthesia and is subject to strict recommendations in every hospital.

Low-molecular-weight heparins (LMWH) or unfractionated heparins (UFH) have proven themselves.

2.3.1 Indication

The risk of thrombosis should be assessed preoperatively. History of family history of thrombosis should be included in peri- and postoperative drug management. Gender, age, and weight and physical fitness play a major role. In addition to medicinal measures, physical aids are obligatory for thrombosis prophylaxis.

3 Restart of a Pre-Existing Continuous Medication

3.1 Cardiovascular Medication

Stable circulatory conditions: Restart/continue immediately postoperatively.

Unstable circulatory conditions: dose reduction or temporary pause and restart after cardiology consult.

3.2 Antidiabetics in Diabetes Patients

Restart in general after the onset of oral food intake.

Exceptions:

Metformin: restart 48 h postoperatively.

Insulin: Measure basal insulin and blood glucose, after first food intake initiation with insulin and correction according to schedule, thereafter according to preoperative schedule.

3.3 Corticosteroid Medication

For continuous therapy above the Cushing's threshold dose: Dose adjustment postoperatively depending on extent of surgery.

Below Cushing's threshold dose: Continue immediately postoperatively at the usual dose.

3.4 Postoperative Hydration and Oral Nutritional Supplementation

Fluid intake: Aim for neutral fluid balance to motivate patients to drink early in the process.

With trouble-free drinking, continue i.v. volume therapy only when medically indicated.

3.5 Dietary Structure

Aim for early oral nutrition.

Nutrition by gastric tube only, if oral nutrition currently is unforeseeable.

From day 2–3: soft protein- and vitamin-rich diet.

4 Wound Care in Orthognathic Surgery

4.1 Postoperative Considerations

- Minimizing bacterial colonization of intraoral wounds during the early healing phase.
- Avoidance of trauma to the intraoral wounds and immobilization of the wound margins.
- Intraoral wounds present challenges due to the need to protect healing tissues when ingesting solids of different textures and various types of fluids at different temperatures. In addition, there is the presence of many types of microorganisms that can cause opportunistic infections.
- The primary goal of intraoral wound care is to create optimal conditions for the natural healing processes of the wound to occur.
- Patients should avoid disturbing the wound, especially during the first 3–7 days.
- Cleanliness of the mouth is essential for good healing, as a clean wound heals better and faster.

4.2 Intraoral Wound Treatment

4.2.1 Oral Hygiene

- The mouth should be thoroughly cleaned after each meal and rinsed with warm salt water (half a teaspoon of salt in an 8 ounce glass of warm water).
- Disinfectant mouth rinse 4–6 times daily until healing is complete and normal oral hygiene is possible again.
- Patients should be encouraged to brush their teeth three times a day. Use a small, soft pediatric toothbrush.
- Consumption of dairy products should be avoided for the first 10 days.
- Alcohol and tobacco: Consumption of alcohol and tobacco should also be avoided for the first 2 weeks after surgery, as they promote infection of the wound and delay healing.
- Antibiotics and intraoral wounds: The need for antibiotics for intraoral wounds should be a clinical decision based on the type of procedure and risk for infection, as well as the patient's immune status and health.
- Removal of drains from day 3 onward.
- Suture removal of intraoral sutures on postoperative day 8.

5 Conclusion

Pre-, peri-, and postoperative care of the patient are integral parts of the success of orthognathic surgery. Not only medical professionals but also patients evaluate the treatment according to these criteria.

Reference

1. Kwon PH, Laskin DM. Clinician's manual of oral and maxillofacial surgery. Quintessence Publishing; 2001.

Part III

Bilateral Ramus Split Osteotomies (BSSO) - Surgical Principles

Principles of the BSSO – Clinical Aspects

12

Peter Kessler, Nicolas Hardt, and Suen An Nynke Lie

Contents

Abstract

The bilateral splitting osteotomy—BSSO—according to Obwegeser–Dal Pont has become the standard therapy worldwide for cutting the mandible in all forms of mandibular positional correction (Obwegeser Dtsch Zahn Mund Kieferheilk 23:1, 1955; DalPont Minerva chir 1, 1958). The success of this technique depends on anatomical conditions, but also on the technically correct execution. An exact analysis of the local conditions intraoperatively, but also the choice of instruments plays a role.

The main goal of the step-shaped sagittal splitting of the lower jaw with intraoral access was on the one hand to reduce the complication rate of previous techniques using extraoral approaches, on the other hand to eliminate the problem of insufficient contact surfaces of the osteotomized bone segments and a reduction in the risk of inferior alveolar nerve damage.

Keywords

Principles of BSSO · Bilateral sagittal splitting osteotomy · Transoral approach · Access to the spaces · General rules in sagittal splitting · Obwegeser · Dal pont · Hunsuck · Epker

P. Kessler (✉) · S. A. N. Lie
Department of Cranio-Maxillofacial Surgery, Maastricht University Medical Center, Maastricht, The Netherlands
e-mail: peter.kessler@mumc.nl; suen.lie@mumc.nl

N. Hardt (✉)
Kantonsspital Lucerne, Clinic and Policlinic of Cranio-Maxillofacial Surgery, Lucerne, Switzerland

P. Kessler et al. (eds.), *Illustrated Manual of Orthognathic Surgery*,
https://doi.org/10.1007/978-3-031-06978-9_12

1 Transoral Approach to the BSSO—*Line of Thoughts*

In principle, the surgical technique can be divided into logical surgical steps (Figs. 12.1, 12.2, 12.3, 12.4):

- Intraoral access at the front edge of the ascending mandible in the retromolar region by mucosa incision.

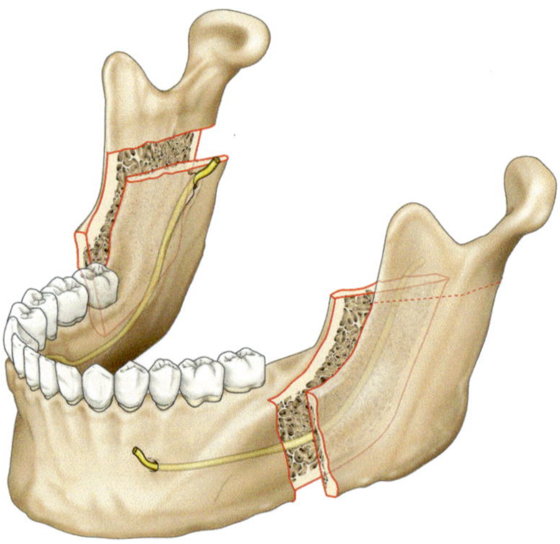

Fig. 12.1 Principle of the bi-sagittal retro molar osteotomy according to Obwegeser–Dal Pont—BSSO [3, 4]

- Creation of a sub periosteal access medially between ramus and pterygoid muscle (lingual approach/lingual tunnel).
- Identification of the mandibular foramen and the inferior alveolar nerve.
- Creation of a horizontal osteotomy above the mandibular foramen with subsequent cutting of the inner/lingual cortex of the ramus [1, 2] (Fig. 12.2).
- Creating a lateral-vertical (buccal) osteotomy with cutting of the cortex until cancellous bone is reached [3]. Pay attention to a sufficient osteotomy of the lower jaw margin (Fig. 12.3).
- Connecting osteotomy line between the lingual and buccal osteotomies and splitting of the ramus into a medial (distal) and lateral (proximal) segment (Fig. 12.4).
- After complete osteotomy and sufficient mobilization of the split segments, the tooth-bearing mandibular segment is adjusted to the maxilla according to the preoperative planning in the intended mandibulo-maxillary position and intermaxillary fixation is applied. Wafers/splints can be used, if needed.
- Depending on the initial diagnosis, the joint-bearing mandible part is now manually guided into the articular fossa and held in position until osteosynthesis is completed.
- Finally, the functionally stable osteosynthesis of the segments is performed.

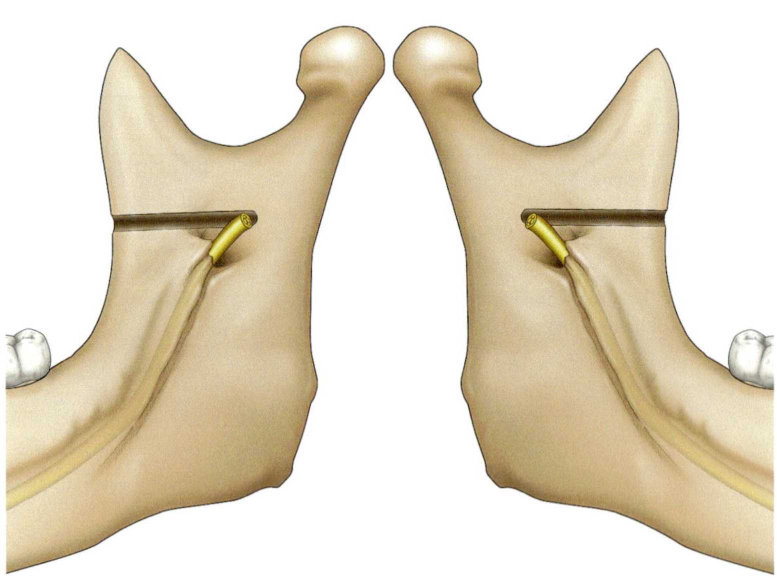

Fig. 12.2 Creating a horizontal (lingual) osteotomy line above the mandibular foramen with osteotomy of the lingual cortex until cancellous bone is visible. Hunsuck-Epker modification [2].

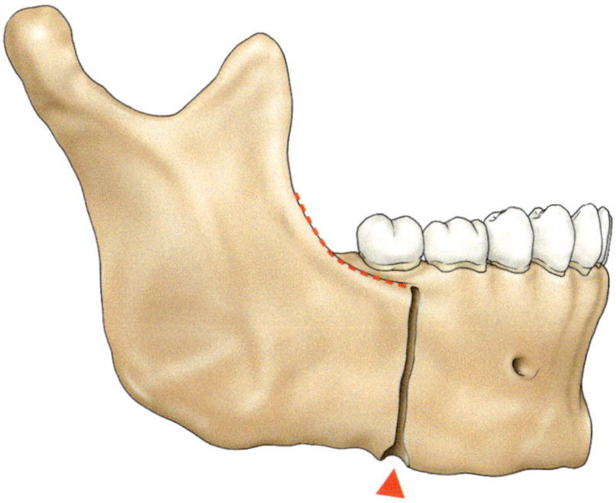

Fig. 12.3 Lateral-vertical (buccal) osteotomy with cutting through the cortex to the cancellous bone including the mandibular margin acc. Dal Pont [3]

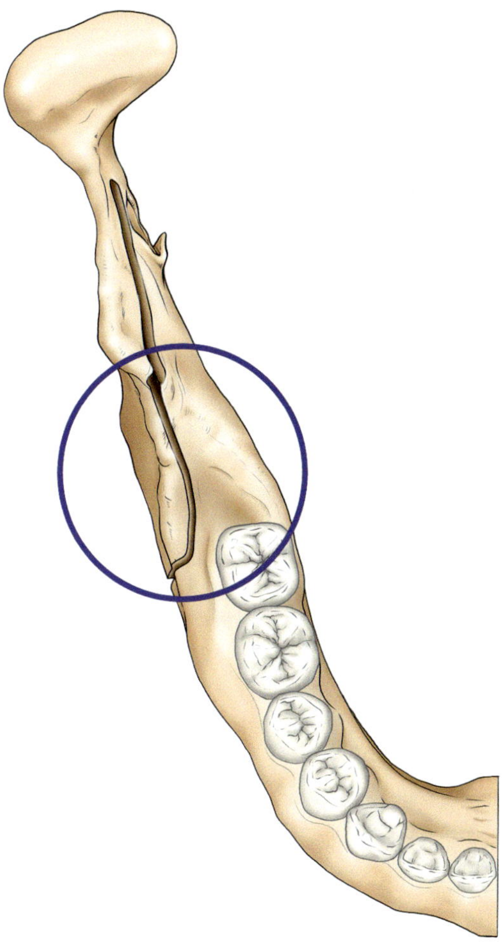

Fig. 12.4 Application of the sagittal connecting osteotomy and splitting the mandibular ramus

2 Conclusion

If the surgical steps for preparing the sagittal split are carefully followed, splitting the mandible in the mandibular angle region should not be a problem. Note that the split on the lingual side can take an arbitrary course.

References

1. Epker BN. Modification in the sagittal osteotomy of the mandible. J Oral Surg. 1977;35:157–9.
2. Hunsuck EE. A modified intraoral sagittal splitting technic for correction of mandibular prognathism. J Oral Surg. 1968;26(4):250–3.
3. DalPont GL. Osteotomia retromolare per la correzione della progenia. Minerva Chir. 1958;1
4. Obwegeser H. Zur Operationstechnik bei der Progenie und anderen Unterkieferanomalien. Dtsch Zahn Mund Kieferheilk. 1955;23:1.

Relation of Cortical Versus Cancellous Bone – The Crucial Ratio

13

Peter Kessler, Nicolas Hardt, and Suen An Nynke Lie

Contents

Abstract

The sagittal ramus osteotomy has become the standard procedure due to the large contact area of the split bone segments and the associated optimal conditions for bone healing with sufficient bone overlap. However, due to the intrabony course of the inferior alveolar nerve (IAN) throughout the whole length of the osteotomy this surgical technique is closely associated with a potential injury of the IAN. Thus, temporary postoperative lesions occur up to 87% and permanent lesions between 3% and 39%. In order to reduce the risk of injury, the most precise knowledge of the anatomical course of the IAN within the osseous-mandibular structures is absolutely essential. The neurovascular bundle of the IAN enters lingually through the mandibular foramen into the mandibular canal. Depending on the split on the lingual side, the IAN will be more or less exposed to a risk of trauma.

Keywords

Anatomy of the mandible · Cortical bone · Cancellous bone · Sagittal split · Mandibular canal · Third molar · Anatomical variations · Bad split

P. Kessler (✉) · S. A. N. Lie
Department of Cranio-Maxillofacial Surgery, Maastricht University Medical Center, Maastricht, The Netherlands
e-mail: peter.kessler@mumc.nl; suen.lie@mumc.nl

N. Hardt (✉)
Kantonsspital Lucerne, Clinic and Policlinic of Cranio-Maxillofacial Surgery, Lucerne, Switzerland

P. Kessler et al. (eds.), *Illustrated Manual of Orthognathic Surgery*,
https://doi.org/10.1007/978-3-031-06978-9_13

1 The Mandibular Canal: A Crucial Structure of Lower Resistance

The mandibular canal (MC), including the canal neurovascular structures, plays a key role in the surgical implementation of osteotomies of the mandible, especially the bilateral sagittal splitting of the mandible—BSSO (Fig. 13.1).

The mean maximum diameter of the MC is 2.52 mm. It contains neurovascular structures such as the inferior alveolar nerve with a diameter of 1.84 mm, the inferior alveolar artery with a diameter of 0.42 mm, and the inferior alveolar vein with a diameter of 0.58 mm [1].

- Location and topography of the mandibular canal

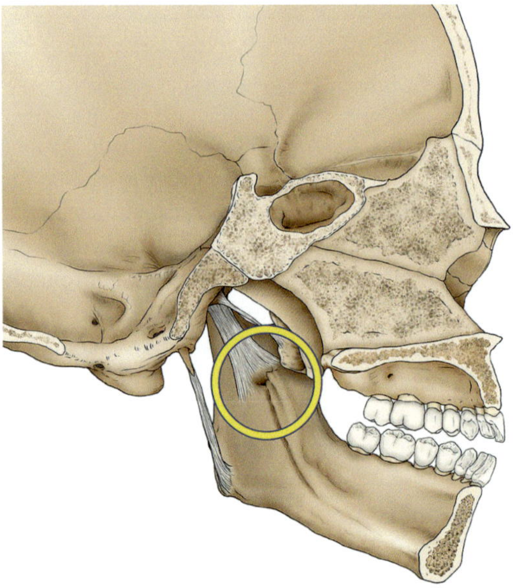

Fig. 13.1 The third branch—the inferior alveolar nerve—of the trigeminal nerve (N.V) entering the mandible at the mandibular foramen

The MC is a canal that allows the inferior alveolar neurovascular bundle to traverse the mandible to supply the dentition, mandibular bone, and soft tissue around the gingiva and lower lip.

The MC is usually well separated from the surrounding cancellous bone by its denser bone wall.

Within the mandible from the proximal to the distal end, the MC first runs medially along the inner side of the lingual cortical bone (facies interna) and then turns successively at the level of the third molar in a more caudal-lateral direction and runs in the anterior 2/3 thirds of the mandible close to the lateral (buccal) cortical bone (facies externa) to the exit of the IAN on the buccal side at the mental foramen (Fig. 13.2) [2].

- In the posterior two-thirds, the mandibular canal is closer to the inner surface of the mandible, and in the anterior third, it is closer to its outer surface [2].
- Anatomical preparations of the sagittal split of the mandible show that both an impacted third molar (M3) and the IAN—which runs directly under the M3—remain in the medial (distal) segment during sagittal splitting (Fig. 13.3) [3].
- Course Variants of the MC and Branching Patterns of the IAN

The MC is not a single canal, but an anatomical structure with multiple branches and variations. Thus, a second canal or an additional retromolar canal may also be located in the corpus mandibulae (Fig. 13.4) [5].

Basically, three intra-mandibular anatomical variants of the MC canal course can be distinguished and classified [1].

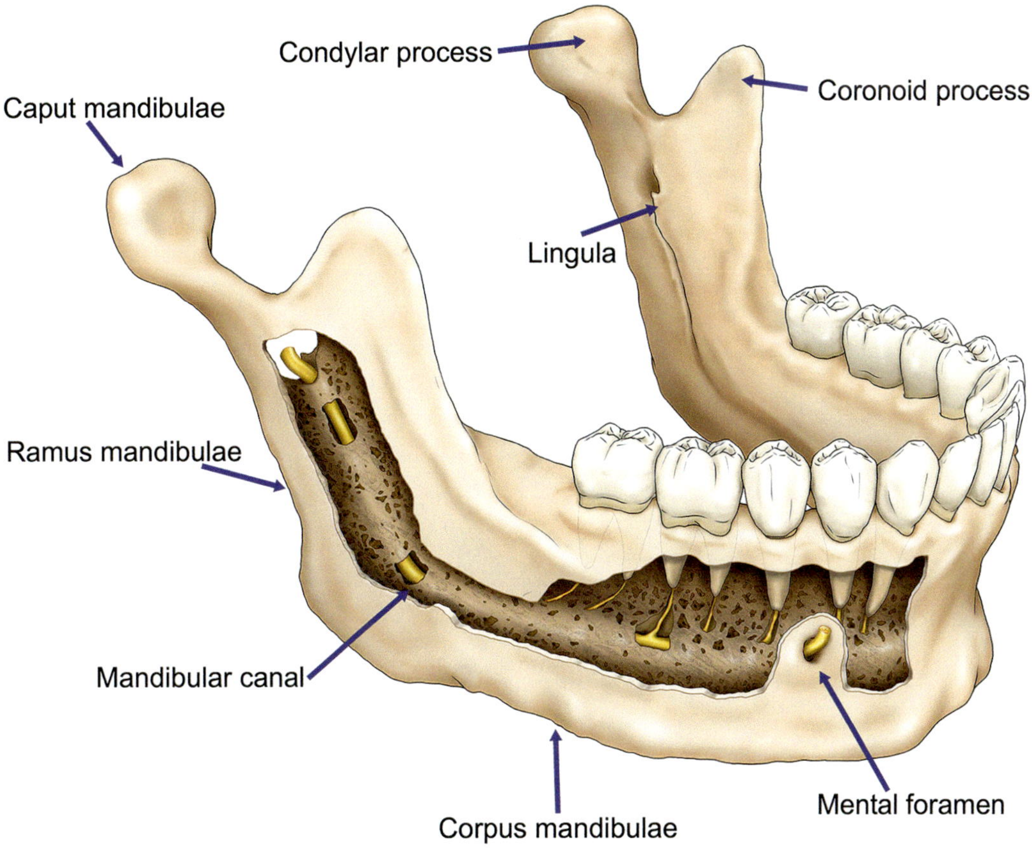

Fig. 13.2 Course of the IAN within the mandibular canal

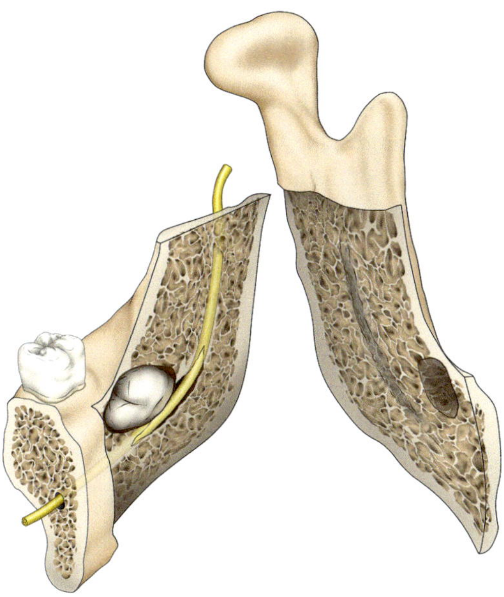

Fig. 13.3 The impacted M3 and the underlying IAN remain after sagittal split in the tooth-bearing distal segment

2 Anatomical Variants of the MC: Canal Course

Type 1

The MC with the IAN is a single, large structure located in a bony canal and passing very close to the root tips.

Type 2

The MC with the IAN passes closer to the mandibular base and the main nerve has small branches emerging from the canal which are connected with the root tips.

Type 3

The MC with the IAN has a main branch of the nerve innervating the posterior region of the mandible, while a lower branch traverses the mandible to the anterior region (Fig. 13.4).

- Mandibular Canal and Sagittal Splitting—BSSO

a

b

c

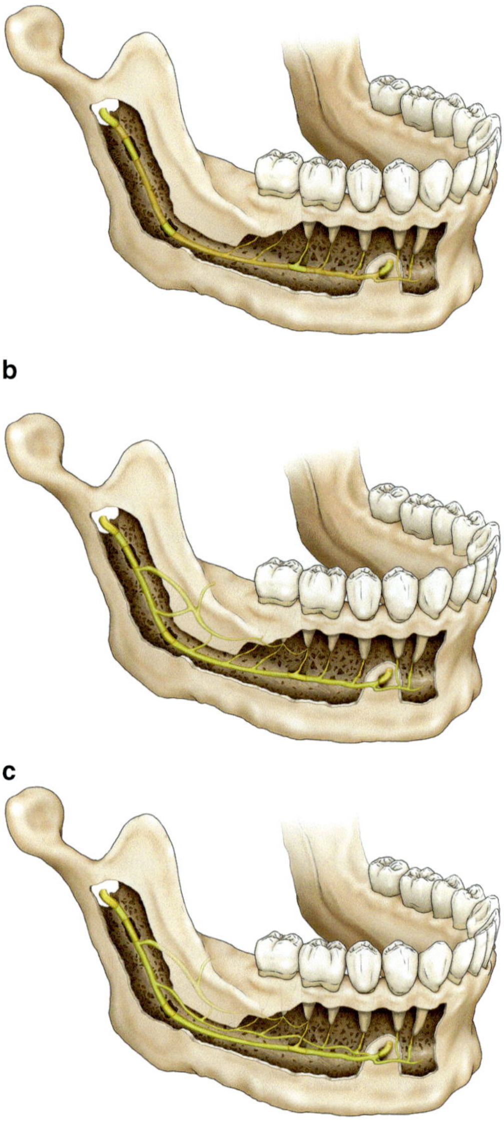

Fig. 13.4 Anatomical variations of the intra-mandibular course of the mandibular canal (MC) and the branching of the IAN showing types a, b, and c of the mandibular canal [4]. (**a**) IAN runs in a single MC (**b**) IAN of a single MC with an accessory canal innervating the retromolar area (**c**) IAN runs in a double MC.

The canal derives its clinical significance from the potential for injury to the neurovascular bundle with the IAN in the sagittal splitting of the mandible throughout the osteotomy site [6–8].

Potential cause of MC injury in BSSO is:

- Low cancellous bone thickness lateral to the nerve canal to the buccal mandibular cortical plate [7, 8].

Temporary postoperative lesions occur in up to 87% and permanent lesions in 3% to 39%.

Note

Median bone thickness lateral to the nerve canal to the buccal mandibular cortical plate (CBCT).

- <4 mm immediately posterior to the mental foramen
- Increased to <6 mm over the next 30 mm.
- Then decreased to <3 mm at the level of the mandibular foramen.

3 Conclusion

Therefore, preoperative determination of the exact location of the MC is indicated in orthognathic surgery of the mandible by using cone-beam tomography (CBCT). For detailed information see Part II.

References

1. Kamburoğlu K, Ozen T, Balcioglu HA, Kurt B, Kutoglu T, Ozan H, Kilic C. The position of the mandibular canal and histologic feature of the inferior alveolar nerve. Clin Anat. 2010;23:34–42.
2. Hollinshead WH. Anatomy for Surgeons for the head and neck. Harper and Rowe; 1982.
3. Wolfe SA, Berkowitz S. Plastic surgery of the facial skeleton. Lippincott, Williams and Wilkins; 1989.
4. Carter RB, Keen MS. The intramandibular course of the inferior alveolar nerve. Journal of Anatomy. 1971;108(3):433–40.
5. Haas LF, Dutra K, Porporatti AL, Mezzomo LA, De Luca CG, Flores-Mir C, et al. Anatomical variations of mandibular canal detected by panoramic radiography and CT: a systematic review and meta-analysis. Dentomaxillofac Radiol. 2016;45(2):20150310.
6. Rich J, Golden BA, Phillips C. Systematic review of preoperative mandibular canal position as it relates to postoperative neurosensory disturbance following the sagittal split ramus osteotomy. Int J Oral Maxillofac Surg. 2014;43(9):1076–81.
7. Valdec S, Borm JM, Casparis S, Damerau G, Locher M, Stadlinger B. Vestibular bone thickness of the mandible in relation to the mandibular canal-a retrospective CBCT-based study. Int J Implant Dent. 2019;5(1):37.
8. Hur SM, Kim H, Kim H. Topography and spatial fascicular arrangement of the human inferior alveolar nerve. Clin Implant Dent Relat Res. 2013;15(1):88–95.

Anatomical Reference Points – Indispensable Aids

14

Peter Kessler, Nicolas Hardt, and Suen An Nynke Lie

Contents

Abstract

The basis of a precise and uncomplicated sagittal split is a controlled and systematic approach. Cornerstones of the orientation are topographical-anatomical points/landmarks, which should be surgically identified in *every case and at all times* in order to be able to constantly have orientation for the surgical process.

This prevents disorientation and possible complications caused by loss of control, which the novice will throw off course. Step by step and according to the rules the surgical process must strictly be followed. It is divided into five sections.

Keywords

Anatomy of the mandible · Topography · Anatomical reference points in BSSO · Identification of the mandibular foramen · BSSO relevant clinical and topographic anatomy

See Fig. 14.1.

P. Kessler (✉) · S. A. N. Lie
Department of Cranio-Maxillofacial Surgery, Maastricht University Medical Center, Maastricht, The Netherlands
e-mail: peter.kessler@mumc.nl; suen.lie@mumc.nl

N. Hardt (✉)
Kantonsspital Lucerne, Clinic and Policlinic of Cranio-Maxillofacial Surgery, Lucerne, Switzerland

P. Kessler et al. (eds.), *Illustrated Manual of Orthognathic Surgery*,
https://doi.org/10.1007/978-3-031-06978-9_14

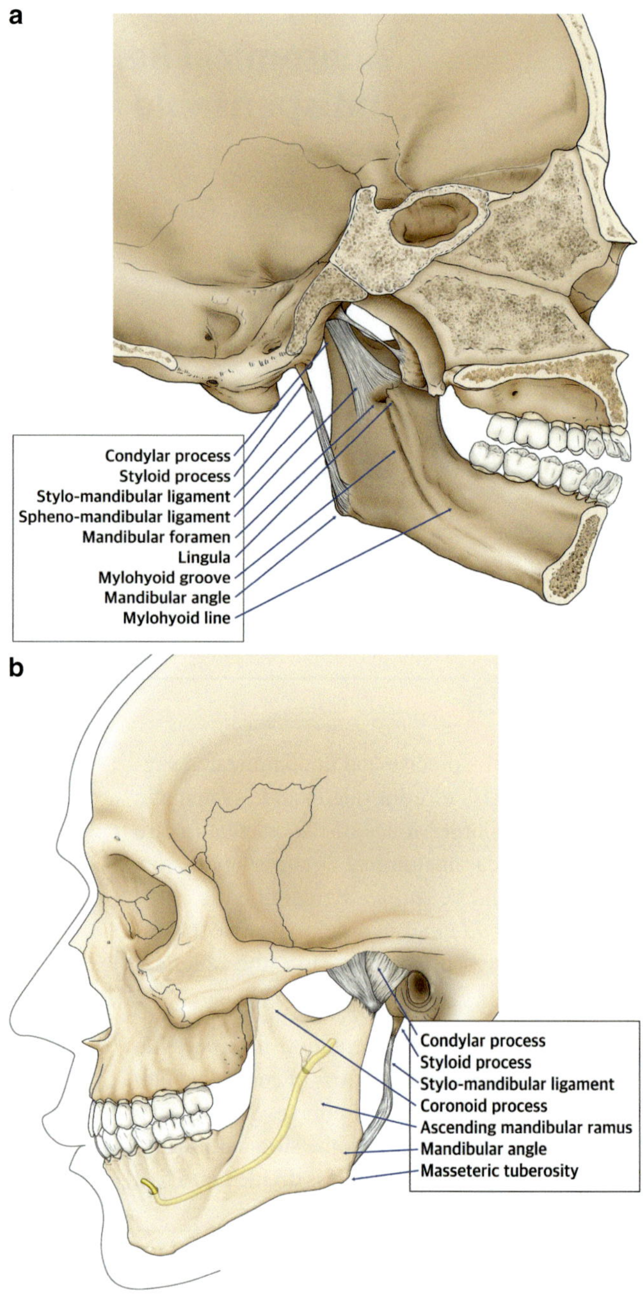

Fig. 14.1 Anatomically–topographically important landmarks in the area of the preparation of the mandibular sagittal split osteotomy [1] (**a**) lingual aspect (**b**) lateral-buccal aspect ©Copyright Keisuke Koyama 2020. All rights reserved

1 Conclusion

The complex anatomy consisting of different soft and hard tissues in the mandibular angle region must be understood in order to identify the landmarks required to gain the necessary orientation intraoperatively to successfully split the mandible.

Reference

1. Ferner H, Staubesand J. Sobotta/Becher Atlas der Anatomie des Menschen. Urban & Schwarzenberg; 1972.

General Rules in Sagittal Splitting – Five Steps

15

Peter Kessler, Nicolas Hardt, and Suen An Nynke Lie

Contents

Abstract

The operation for sagittal splitting of the mandible is composed of a logical sequence of surgical steps that must be consistently followed during each splitting procedure in order to operate successfully, with clarity and safely.

Five surgical steps can be distinguished, from incision to osteosynthesis. Even the incision can be decisive for obtaining a sufficient overview of the surgical area, which is located on both sides of the ascending mandibular branch. The spaces between the masticatory muscles and the mandible must be created technically in such a way that the overview is not impeded or even made impossible by bleeding or remaining soft tissue attachments. The identification of the vascular and nerve bundle at the mandibular foramen must be ensured. Only then is the mandible split with usually three osteotomy lines lingually, buccally and the connection cut successful.

P. Kessler (✉) · S. A. N. Lie
Department of Cranio-Maxillofacial Surgery, Maastricht University Medical Center, Maastricht, The Netherlands
e-mail: peter.kessler@mumc.nl; suen.lie@mumc.nl

N. Hardt (✉)
Kantonsspital Lucerne, Clinic and Policlinic of Cranio-Maxillofacial Surgery, Lucerne, Switzerland

P. Kessler et al. (eds.), *Illustrated Manual of Orthognathic Surgery*,
https://doi.org/10.1007/978-3-031-06978-9_15

Keywords

Principles of the BSSO · Mucoperiosteal incision · Bilateral sagittal splitting osteotomy (BSSO) · Transoral approach · Access to the spaces · Anatomical reference points in BSSO · Identification of the mandibular foramen · Systematic approach · BSSO relevant clinical and topographic anatomy · Surgical steps · Creation of bone cuts · Mandibular canal · Avoidance of iatrogenic fractures · Avoidance of caudal mandibular step formation · Instruments

1 Surgical Approach

The mucosa-periosteal incision starts at the ventral aspect of the coronoid process (*crista temporalis of the muscular process*) and runs in the retromolar region laterally in the sulcus between the belly of the masseteric muscle somewhat laterally of the external oblique line (*linea obliqua externa*) in anterior direction up to the level of the first/second molar.

A pronounced lateral-vestibular incision of the mucosa in the retromolar and buccal vestibule prevents injuries to the lingual nerve and provides sufficient cuff tissue for subsequent mucosal closure (Fig. 15.1). The buccal artery and vein cross the mucoperiosteal incision line and must be coagulated (Spiessl 1974).

Lead structure: External oblique line.

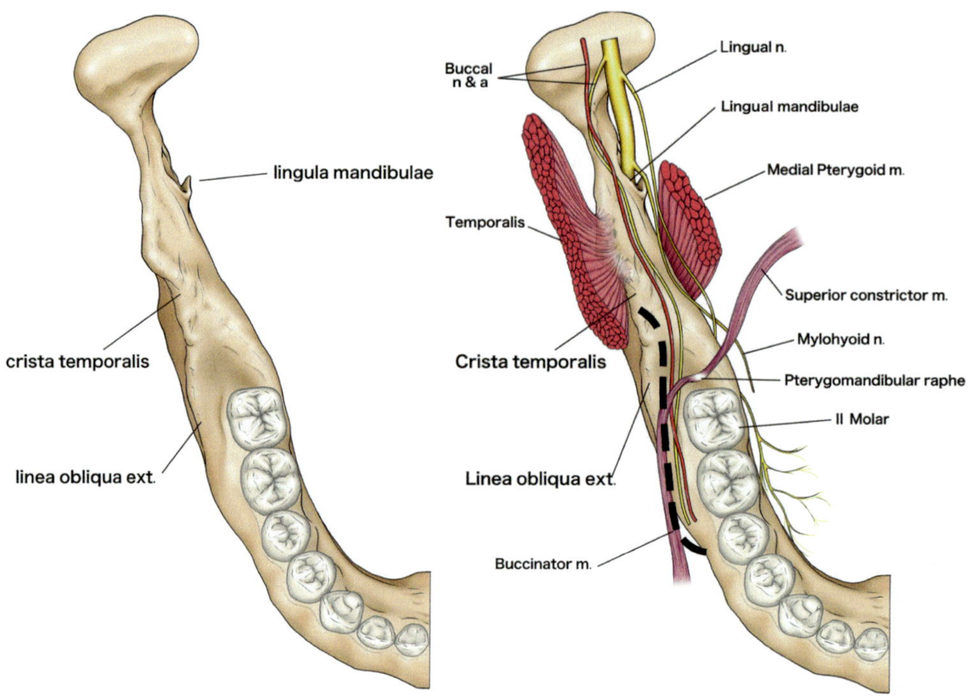

Fig. 15.1 View of the mandibular jaw from above with the relevant anatomical structures in order to create the incision correctly. Incision line is marked in black

2 Access to the Lateral Side of the Ascending Ramus: Submasseteric Space

Anterior Aspect of the Ascending Ramus
Gentle dissection of the soft tissues beginning in the retromolar region upwards to the tendon insertion of the temporal muscle. The base of the coronoid process must be thoroughly dissected from the tendinous attachment of the temporal muscle.

Submasseteric Space
Gentle approach to the space between the ascending ramus medially and the masseteric muscle laterally. Pay attention not to harm the periosteal/perimuscular tissues.

Landmarks

- Semilunar/mandibular notch (*incisura semilunaris*) cranially.
- Base of the condylar process (*processus condylaris*) dorsally.
- Mandibular angle to the attachment of the masseteric muscle at the masseteric tuberosity latero-inferiorly (*angulus mandibulae, tuberositas masseterica*).

> Lead structures: Semilunar notch—base muscular process—base condylar process.

3 Access to the Medial Side of the Ascending Ramus: Pterygo-Mandibular Space

Anterior Aspect of the Ascending Ramus
Gentle dissection of the soft tissue attachments on the lingual side of the ascending ramus beginning downward from the coronoid process strict subperiosteally to the retromolar region, where the body of the mandible gets wider due to the alveolar process.

Pterygo-Mandibular Space
Subfascial space between the lingual side of the ascending ramus laterally and the medial pterygoid muscle (*musculus pterygoideus medialis*) medially. Pay attention not to harm the periosteal/perimuscular tissues, especially along the edge of the internal oblique line (*linea obliqua interna, sulcus mylohyoideus*) in the retromolar region.

Landmarks

- Internal oblique line (*linea obliqua interna*).
- Semilunar/mandibular notch (*incisura semilunaris*).
- Lingula and the neurovascular bundle of the IAN at the mandibular foramen.
- Posterior edge of the ascending ramus.

> Lead structures: Semilunar notch—internal oblique line—lingula.

4 Creation of the Osteotomy Lines

4.1 Upper Horizontal Osteotomy (Lingual Osteotomy)

Anterior Aspect of the Ascending Ramus
On the lingual side about 1 cm inferior to the mandibular/semilunar notch and about 4–6 mm above the mandibular foramen parallel to the occlusal plane of the mandible.

Anterior-Posterior Length of the Osteotomy
The internal oblique line will be cut horizontally up to the mandibular sulcus which lies posteriorly to the mandibular foramen (acc. *Hunsuck).*

Point of Orientation: About 1 cm Inferior to the Semilunar Notch
Note:

The outer surface of the ramus is kept in view to ensure the depth of the lingual osteotomy.

One should take into account that the inner cortical layer is concave and curved.

4.2 Lower Vertical Osteotomy (Buccal Osteotomy)

Pre-Masseteric Space
Vertical osteotomy of the lateral cortex from the pre-masseteric submandibular notch at the height of the second molar (M2) reaching the anterior end of the external oblique line.

Caudo-Cranial Length of the Osteotomy
Depending on the shape of the mandibular body, it can be from convex to concave. The length of the osteotomy and also the depth of the osteotomy must correspond to these shapes and can be shorter for convex shapes than for concave ones.

Lead structures: second molar tooth on buccal side.

4.3 Sagittal Connecting Osteotomy

Retromolar Region
Osteotomy starts at the anterior edge of the lingual osteotomy and runs downward to the cranial end of the buccal osteotomy parallel to the buccal cortex, but well inside along the cortico-cancellous border (about 5 mm medially).

Leading Structures
Reference Point: Bone Cut Medial to the Oblique Line

Cutting Length
From the intersection of the lingual-horizontal cut to the intersection of the vertical-buccal cut. Length is depending on the location of the aforenamed osteotomies. Depth of the osteotomy should not exceed 10 mm.

Point of orientation: Buccal cortex—osteotomy medially along the external oblique line.

5 Reference Points for Osteosynthesis

5.1 Bi-Cortical Screws

Two/three screws at the superior border parallel to the upper edge of the proximal segment. At least one screw has to pass through the oblique line (“Obliqua-screw”).

Alternatively two screws can be applied at the superior border and a third screw at the base of the jaw, about 6–8 mm above the lower edge of the mandible (“Base screw”). In this form of osteosynthesis the three screws should be equidistant.

Screw size 2 mm, length depending on the mandibular width.

5.2 Mono-Cortical Screws and Miniplates

Standard is a 4-hole plate with a bar in different design shapes, two screws posterior to the buccal split of 5 mm length, two screws anteriorly to the split of 7 mm length. Plate position on or parallel to the oblique line.

Screw size 2 mm, and plate profile accordingly.

Plate length depending on indication for surgery and mandibular advancement/setback.

Focus on plates, screws, and instrumentation (screw driver).

6 Conclusion

The consecutive sequence of the five steps outlined above greatly facilitates the procedure of sagittal splitting of the mandible and makes this procedure, which can never be 100% controlled, safe.

Further Reading

Bell HW, Proffit WR, White RP. Surgical correction of dentofacial deformities, vol. 1-3. Saunders; 1980.

Fonsecca RJ, Marciani RD, Turvey TA. Oral and maxillofacial surgery, orthognathic surgery and craniofacial surgery. Saunders; 2009.

Michel C, Reuther J. Orthopädische Chirurgie. In: Hausamen E, Machtens E, Reuther J, editors. Mund-, Kiefer- und Gesichtschirurgie. Operationslehre und Atlas; Springer, 1995.

Spiessl B. Osteosynthese bei sagittaler Osteotomie nach Obwegeser/Dal Pont. In: Schuchardt K (Hrsg) Fortschritte der Kiefer- und Gesichts-Chirurgie, Bd XVIII. Thieme, Stuttgart New York, 1974;S 145–8.

Steinhäuser EW. Bone screws and plates in orthognathic surgery. Int J Oral Surg. 1982;11:209–16.

BSSO Relevant Clinical and Topographic Anatomy (Studies and Variations)

16

Peter Kessler, Nicolas Hardt, and Suen An Nynke Lie

Contents

P. Kessler (✉) · S. A. N. Lie
Department of Cranio-Maxillofacial Surgery, Maastricht University Medical Center, Maastricht, The Netherlands
e-mail: peter.kessler@mumc.nl; suen.lie@mumc.nl

N. Hardt (✉)
Kantonsspital Lucerne, Clinic and Policlinic of Cranio-Maxillofacial Surgery, Lucerne, Switzerland

Abstract

Detailed knowledge of topographic conditions is required for all surgical procedures. Measurements and landmarks help to make the preoperative planning first mentally one's own and then to implement it intraoperatively. In routine, these measurements will not be necessary every time, but they can be

P. Kessler et al. (eds.), *Illustrated Manual of Orthognathic Surgery*,
https://doi.org/10.1007/978-3-031-06978-9_16

a useful aid for orientation and for gaining confidence in the sagittal splitting of the mandible.Measurement points and anatomical orientation aids serve to transfer the virtual reality of computerized planning to the surgical site.

Keywords

BSSO relevant clinical and topographic anatomy · Principles of the BSSO · Bilateral sagittal splitting osteotomy · Transoral approach · Access to the spaces · Measurement · Anatomical landmarks · Anatomical reference points in BSSO · Identification of the mandibular foramen · Anatomical orientation · Surgical steps · Obwegeser · Dal Pont · Hunsuck · Epker · Creation of bone cuts · Short lingual osteotomy (SLO) · Mandibular canal · Surgical variants

1 Topography of the Mandibular Foramen (Fig. 16.1)

Anatomically important structures for orientation during the BSSO are

- The mandibular foramen—**MF**
- The lingula—**La** and
- The mandibular sulcus—**SuC**

2 Topographic and Metric Relations on the Lingual Side of the Ascending Mandibular Ramus

2.1 Position of the Anti-Lingula Opposite to the Lingula/Mandibular Foramen

Possible strategy, if the mandibular foramen is difficult to find or after loss of orientation (e.g. bleeding): After dissection of the submasseteric space definition the anti-lingula on the lateral side of the ascending ramus can be helpful as the first point of orientation for the topographic position of the mandibular foramen (Fig. 16.2).

The relative position of the lingula in the lingual side in relation to the position of the anti-lingula is posterior-inferiorly.

The mandibular sulcus and the channel entrance of the IAN are clearly *below* the level of the anti-lingula.

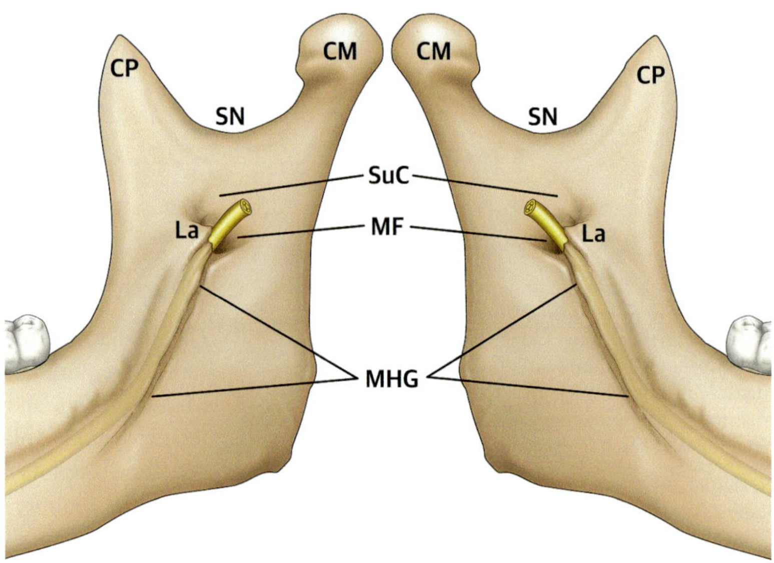

Fig. 16.1 Topographic anatomy of the mandibular foramen and lingual aspect of the ascending mandibular ramus. CM condyle of the mandible, CP coronoid process, SN semilunar notch, SuC sulcus colli, MF mandibular foramen, MHG mylohyoid groove, La lingula. ©Copyright Keisuke Koyama 2020. All rights reserved

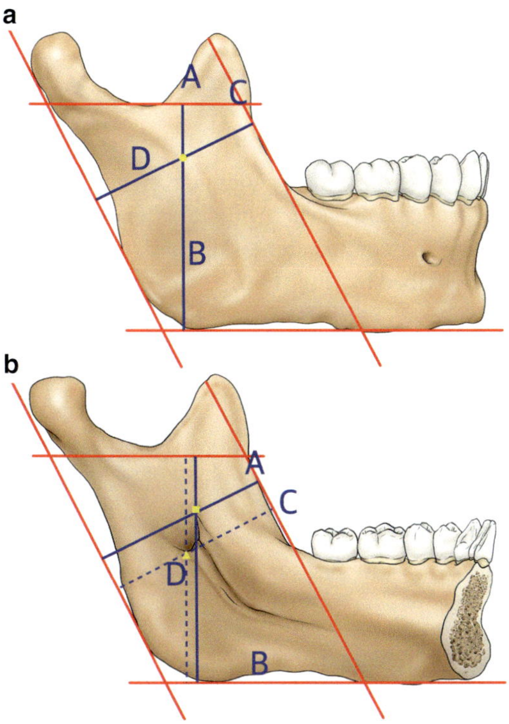

Fig. 16.2 Anatomical relationship of anti-lingula on the latera/buccal side (a) to the mandibular foramen on the lingual side (b) of the ascending ramus [1].©Copyright Keisuke Koyama 2020. All rights reserved. **Circle** = Position of the anti-lingula—crossing point line A/B—C/D. **Square** = Position superior border of the mandibular foramen (lingula)—crossing point line A/B—C/D. **Triangle** = Position inferior border of the mandibular foramen

2.2 Vertical and Horizontal Measurements Between the Mandibular Foramen and the Borders

The average distance between the mandibular foramen/the lingula and anterior border of the ascending ramus measures 16.8–23.2 mm. The distance to the posterior border of the ascending ramus is 10.0–17.8 mm. The vertical distance to the semilunar notch measures 14.1–25.2 mm, whereas the vertical distance between the lower border of the mandible to the lingula is 18.6–42.5 mm (Fig. 16.3) [1].

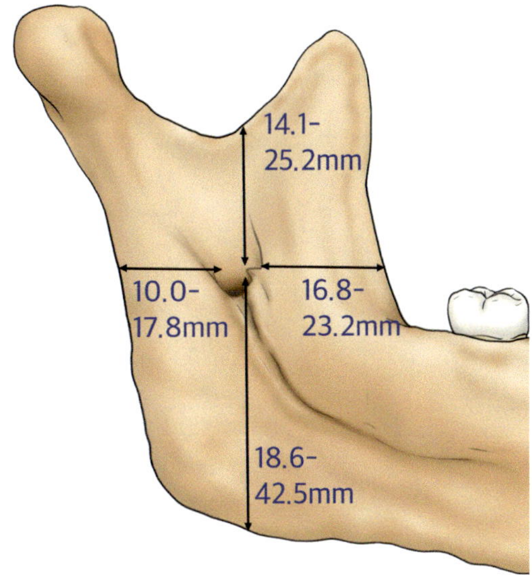

Fig. 16.3 Measures as indicating the distances between the mandibular foramen/lingula and the surrounding borders of the mandible. ©Copyright Keisuke Koyama 2020. All rights reserved

3 Topographic Determination of the Lingual Osteotomy

The Point X is a safe and easy to find anatomical reference point to determine the vertical level of the lingual bone cut in the BSSO. Point X indicates the deepest site in the concave structure of the anterior aspect of the ascending ramus (Fig. 16.4). The wider the mandibular ramus, the closer to the mandibular foramen the horizontal BSSO cut should be attempted.

The horizontal plane defined by point X–X1–X2 runs directly across the entrance point of the neurovascular bundle of the IAN (Fig. 16.5). Any lingual osteotomy should be made at least 4 mm above this line.

Note

Ideally the horizontal osteotomy on the lingual side should not be more than 4 mm above the line Point X–X1–X2

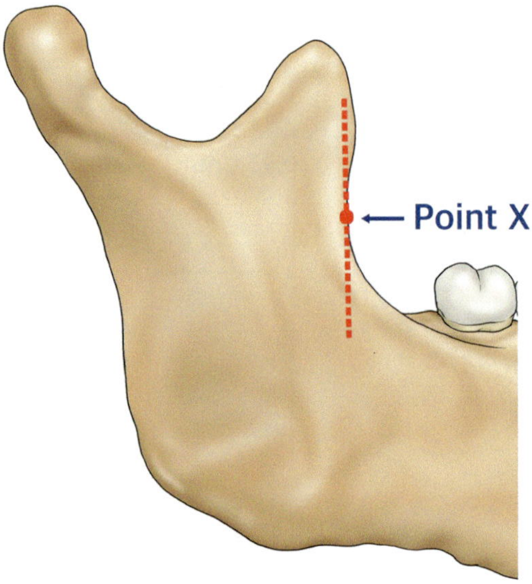

Fig. 16.4 Localization of point X at the deepest point of the concave anterior edge of the ascending mandibular ramus.

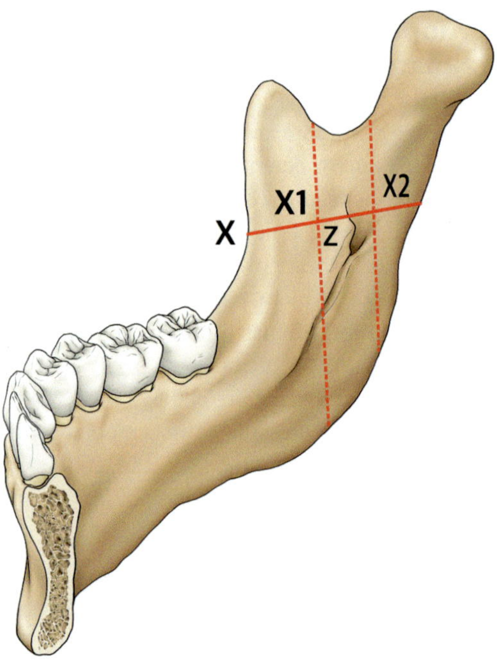

Fig. 16.5 The line point X–X1–X2 runs directly above the entrance of the mandibular canal. Point Z marks the lingula.

4 Lingual Osteotomy Line and Cortex Fusion above the Mandibular Foramen

The ideal lingual osteotomy line is about 4 mm above the mandibular foramen in the anterior, cortico-cancellous part of the ascending ramus which is a continuation of the inner oblique line as described by (Fig. 16.6).

> **Note**
>
> The higher the osteotomy line is placed above the lingula, the more difficult the splitting

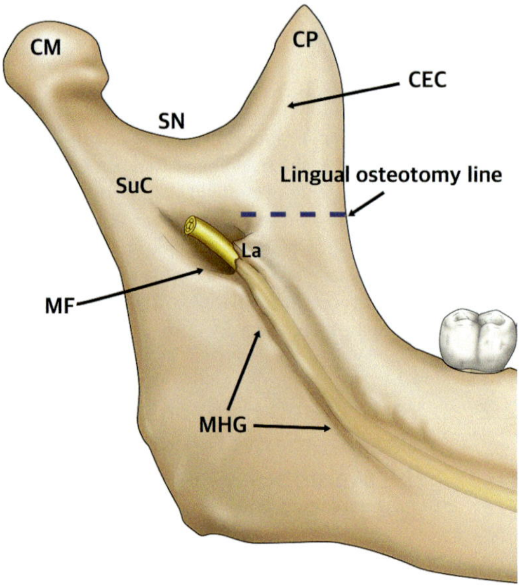

Fig. 16.6 Ideal position of the lingual osteotomy line ca. 4 mm above the lingula: La. CM condyle of the mandible, CP coronoid process, SN semilunar notch, SuC sulcus colli, CEC crista endocoronoidea, MF mandibular foramen, MHG mylohyoid groove.

5 The Neurovascular Bundle

The neurovascular bundle can be injured at the entry into the mandibular canal and within the canal at any time by preparation of the lingual tunnel, performing of the lingual osteotomy, splitting of the mandible, as well as after splitting by rough manipulation and later during rigid osteosynthesis (Fig. 16.7).

5.1 Care of the Neurovascular Bundle

The neurovascular entrance point should be visualized intraoperatively and the neurovascular bundle should be in the tooth bearing (distal) mandibular segment after splitting [1, 3].

6 BSSO and Vascular Structures in the Vicinity of the Lingual Aspect of the Ascending Ramus

The maxillary artery is embedded in the deep lobe of the parotid gland dorso-medially of the neck of the condylar process. During its course several smaller arteries are branching off, including the inferior alveolar artery. The latter faces downward, leaving the parotid gland to enter the mandibular canal at the mandibular foramen and to provide endosteal supply. Before the inferior alveolar artery enters the mandibular foramen, the vessel gives off two branches, the lingual and the mylohyoid arteries.

The lingual branch follows the lingual nerve to supply the mucous membrane of the floor of the mouth. The mylohyoid branch runs in the

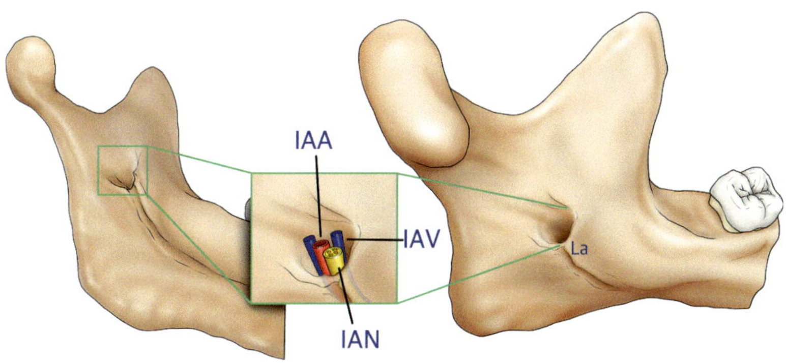

Fig. 16.7 Neurovascular structures of the mandibular foramen. IAN inferior alveolar nerve—situated right behind the lingula, IAA inferior alveolar artery, IAV inferior alveolar veins.

mylohyoid groove then ramifies on the undersurface of the mylohyoideus to vascularize the periosteum of the lower inner mandibular cortex.

These branches of the inferior alveolar artery are supplemented in the floor of the mouth by the deep lingual artery, a direct branch of the external carotid artery. The blood supply to the inner cortex is tiered, above and below the mylohyoid muscle.

The blood flow through the mandibular periosteum could easily maintain a sufficient blood supply to the teeth of the mobile segment even when the labial periosteum was degloved (Fig. 16.8) [2].

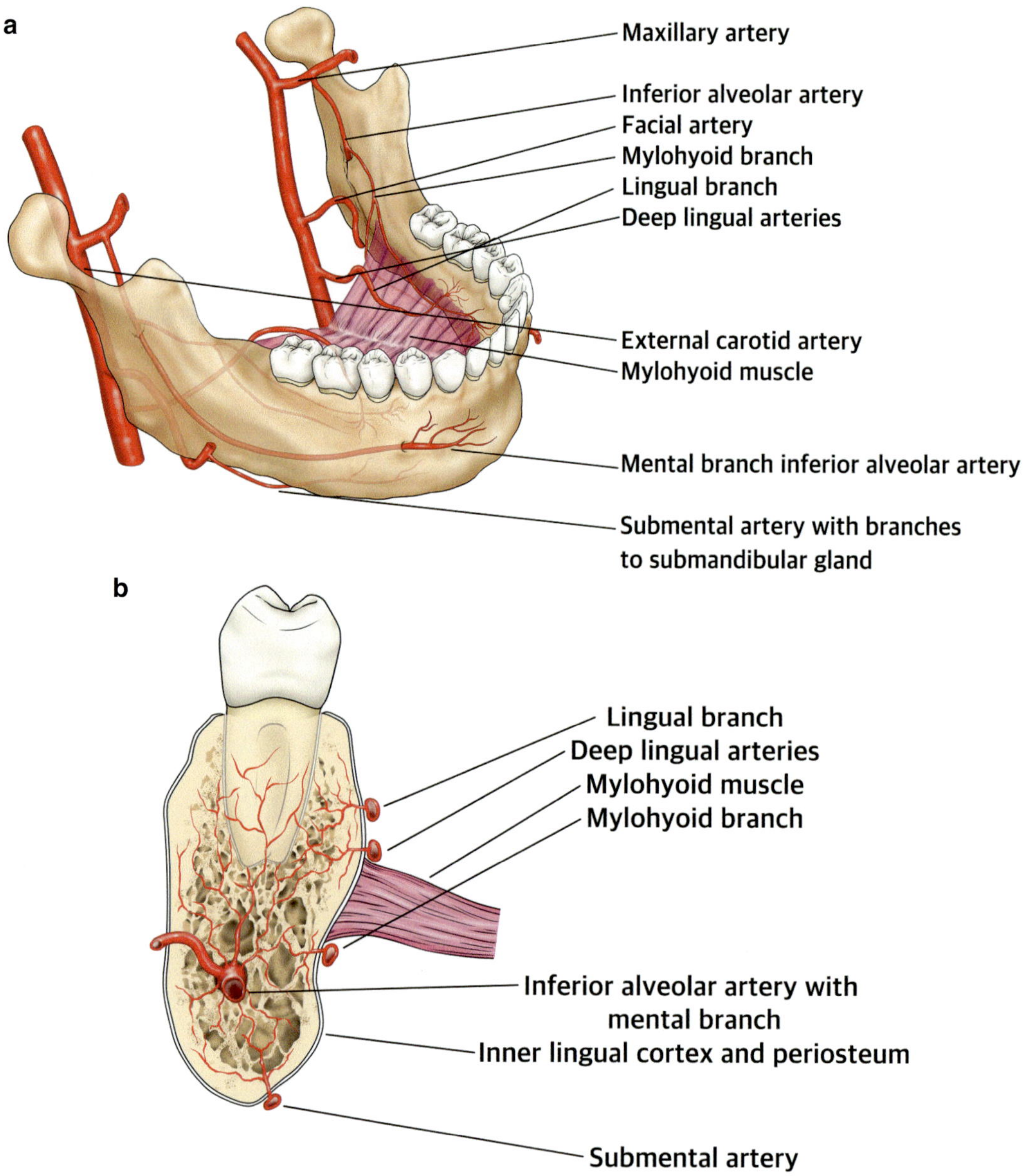

Fig. 16.8 The inner cortex and lingual periosteum of the mandible and floor of the mouth are supplied by a three-tiered distribution of vessels, best seen on an oblique lingual view of the mandible (**a**) and in cross section in the area of parasymphysis (**b**).

7 Variants of the Upper Horizontal Osteotomy (Lingual Osteotomy)

It corresponds to the anatomical—topographical findings that the flail—to dumbbell-shaped ramus cross-section in anterior-posterior extension has a very variable transverse bone thickness, accompanied by an equally variable width of the cancellous bone layer (Fig. 16.9).

This anatomical fact led to Hunsuck's recommendation to limit the lingual osteotomy to the anterior cortico-cancellous area of the ascending ramus. The often bi-cortical sulcus colli (SuC) is not suitable for controlled splitting of the mandible.

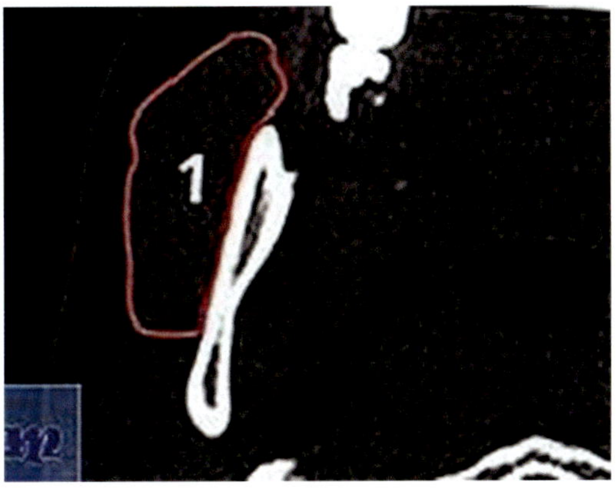

Fig. 16.9 Horizontal CT-scan of the right ascending mandibular ramus above the lingula. 1 = masseteric muscle

Transversal radiological distance measurements of the ramus at the level of the mandibular foramen show the greatest bone width in the anterior ramus region. The transverse bone distance values in the anterior ramus range from 3.0 mm (14%) to <7.0 mm (27.5%) [8]

The average anterior ramus thickness is 4.9 mm with a standard deviation of +/− 1 mm.

In the area of the posterior ramus margin, the average transverse width is approximately 50% of the anterior measurement with a correspondingly reduced cancellous bone layer.

In the median ramus section—at the level of the mandibular foramen—the bone width is only about 1/3 of the average anterior bone width accompanied by a very narrow layer of cancellous bone. See Figs. 16.9 and 16.10.

> **Note**
> Transversal radiological bone distance measurements in the region of the ascending ramus are not representative for a true assessment of the existing cancellous/cortical bone ratio

Fig. 16.10 Different types of lingual osteotomy. Shortening of the lingual bone cut will lead to less bone overlap. (**a**) Bone cut to the posterior end of the ramus. Note the bi-cortical sulcus colli region. (**b**) Bone cut on the anterior cortico-cancellous area of the ascending ramus as suggested by *Hunsuck*. ©Copyright Keisuke Koyama 2020. All rights reserved

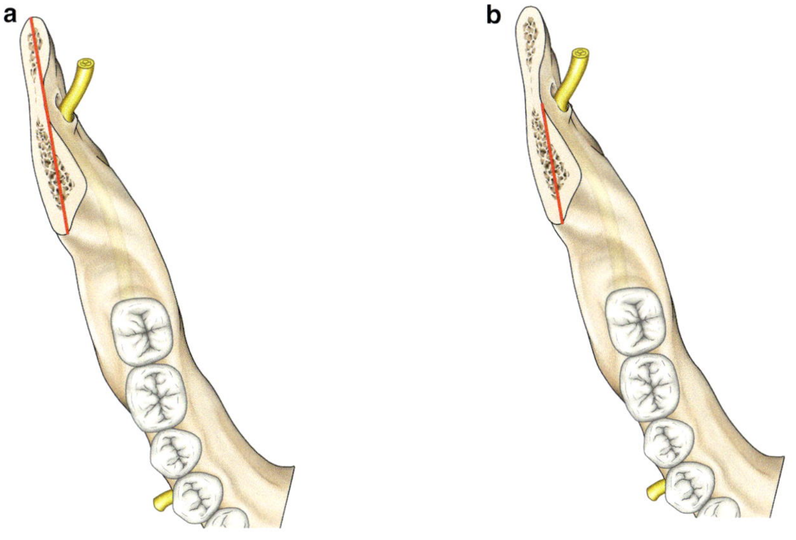

Note
The width of the individual cancellous bone layer in the middle and posterior ramus section—the presumptive splitting region—is significantly less than in the anterior part of the ascending ramus

8 Variants of the Vertical Osteotomy (Buccal Osteotomy)

There are different variants of lateral vertical bone cut in the inferior rim area when performing a BSSO. These variations concern both the vertical length of the osteotomy and the anterior-posterior or sagittal positioning of the osteotomy.

We distinguish between short and long sagittal splits, whereby the starting point at the osteotomy of the lingual side is not changed. However, the length of the connecting osteotomy between the lingual and buccal osteotomy line changes.

Variations in length of the vertical osteotomy [5]:

(a) a more buccal bone cut.
(b) central bone cut.
(c) lingual bone cut.

Follow-up examinations by CT showed that the bone cuts during a BSSO are often not placed exactly as planned. The vertical buccal cut reached the caudal cortex in all cases, but only reached the lingual cortex (inferior border osteotomy) in 38% of the splits [7].

For splitting the inferior mandibular border, types b) and c) have proven to be the most suitable, as the inferior split of the mandibular margin is technically the best option for a reliable osteotomy of the buccal and lingual segments (Fig. 16.11) [4, 5].

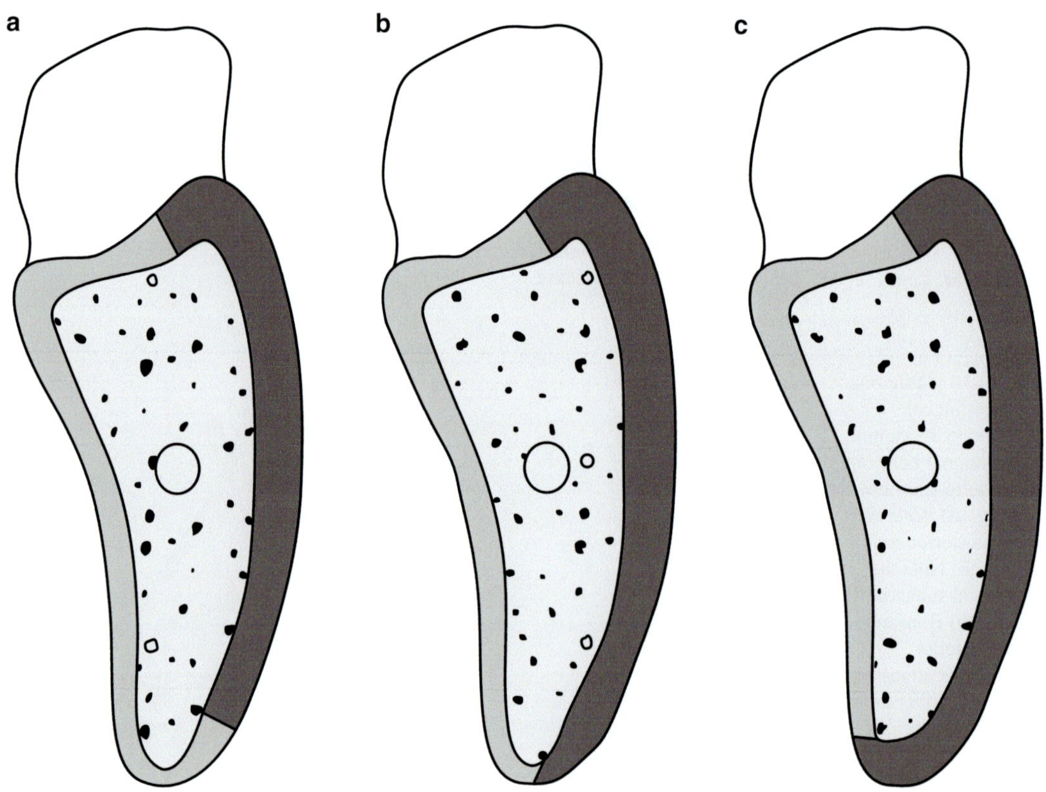

Fig. 16.11 Different types of vertical buccal bone cuts [5] (**a**) without inferior border osteotomy, (**b**) with touching the inferior border, (**c**) including inferior border osteotomy

Moving the vertical buccal osteotomy to a region with a greater buccolingual volume and more cancellous bone may facilitate the splitting process. On the other hand, shortening the sagittal splitting path to a region with less buccolingual thickness and less cancellous bone will increase the risk of uncontrolled mandibular fracture.

9 Variant of the Sagittal Osteotomy

The corticotomy and removal of the narrow edge of the external oblique line up to the visible border between cancellous bone and lateral buccal cortex considerably facilitates the marking and determination of depth of the buccal sagittal osteotomy lines (Fig. 16.12) [6, 9, 10]

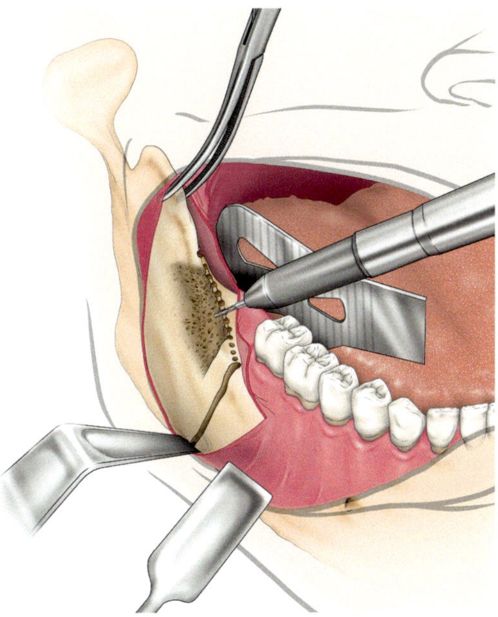

Fig. 16.12 Corticotomy of the edge of the external oblique line up to the visible border between cancellous bone and lateral cortex.

10 Conclusion

Taking into account the local anatomical conditions and observing a consistent surgical technique, the sagittal split of the mandible is achieved in a predictable manner. Anatomical variations can be understood and specific situations can be addressed intraoperatively to avoid a bad split of the mandible or unnecessary damage to important structures.

References

1. Aziz SR, Dorfman BJ, Ziccardi VB, Janal M. Accuracy of using the antilingula as a sole determinant of vertical ramus osteotomy position. J Oral Maxillofac Surg. 2007;65(5):859–62.
2. Beukes J, Reyneke JP, Damstra J. Unilateral sagittal split mandibular ramus osteotomy: indications and geometry. Br J Oral Maxillofac Surg. 2016;54(2):219–23.
3. Bell WH, Levy BM. Revascularization and bone healing after anterior mandibular osteotomy. J Oral Surg. 1970;28:196–203.
4. Pilling E, Schneider M, Mai R, Eckelt U. Präoperative Lagebestimmung des Canalis mandibulae vor sagittaler Ramusosteotomie des Unterkiefers. Mund Kiefer Gesichtschir. 2004;8(1):18–23.
5. Dreiseidler T, Bergmann J, Zirk M, Rothamel D, Zöller JE, Kreppel M. Three-dimensional fracture pattern analysis of the Obwegeser and dal Pont bilateral sagittal split osteotomy. Int J Oral Maxillofac Surg. 2016;45(11):1452–8.
6. Houppermans PNWJ, Verweij JP, Mensink G, Gooris PJJ, van Merkesteyn JPR. Influence of inferior border cut on lingual fracture pattern during bilateral sagittal split osteotomy with splitter and separators: A prospective observational study. J Craniomaxillofac Surg. 2016;44(10):1592–8.
7. Böckmann R, Schön P, Neuking K, Meyns J, Kessler P, Eggeler G. In vitro comparison of the sagittal split osteotomy with and without inferior border osteotomy. J Oral Maxillofac Surg. 2015;73(2):316–23.
8. Farhad BN, Daljit SG. Orthognathic surgery: principles, planning and practice. Wiley & Blackwell; 2011.
9. Spiessl B. Osteosynthese des Unterkiefers. Rekonstruktive Chirurgie, Teil III. New York, Tokyo: Springer,Berlin,Heidelberg; 1988.
10. Steinhäuser EW. Educational course on surgical methods in orthognathic surgery, vol. 8. Luzern, Switzerland; 1973. p. 4.

Strategic Surgical Approach and Technical Details

17

Peter Kessler and Nicolas Hardt

Contents

P. Kessler (✉)
Maastricht University Medical Center, Department of Cranio-Maxillofacial Surgery, Maastricht, The Netherlands
e-mail: peter.kessler@mumc.nl

N. Hardt (✉)
Kantonsspital Lucerne, Clinic and Policlinic of Cranio-Maxillofacial Surgery, Lucerne, Switzerland

P. Kessler et al. (eds.), *Illustrated Manual of Orthognathic Surgery*,
https://doi.org/10.1007/978-3-031-06978-9_17

Abstract

The splitting technique, which has been modified and perfected over decades, has largely eliminated previous complications such as vascular bleeding, irregular osteotomy procedures, and unexpected fractures, as well as postoperative malpositioning of the mandibular condyles resulting in postoperative relapse.

There is still a residual surgical risk of temporary and sometimes unavoidable permanent an- or hypoesthesia of the lip and chin. This is due to the immediate proximity of the alveolar neurovascular bundle to the osteotomy site, which may result in a lesion of the nerve even with the utmost caution.

Keywords

Anatomy of the mandible · Topography · Anatomical reference points in BSSO · Incision · Identification of the mandibular foramen · BSSO relevant clinical and topographic anatomy · Surgical approach · Lingula · Lingual tunnel · Osteotomy lines · Horizontal lingual osteotomy · Vertical buccal osteotomy · Sagittal osteotomy · Mandibular split · Sagittal split · Mandibular margin · Osteotomes · Spreader · Lindemann burr · Piezo surgery

1 Anatomical Basis of Mandibular Bone Splitting

1.1 Splitting Technique of the Ramus in the Borderline between Lateral Cortical and Cancellous Bone

The design of the bone cuts and the splitting behavior of the ramus to be expected is based on the knowledge of the ratio and relation of cancellous bone mass between the mandibular nerve canal and the lateral cortex in the pre-angular, angular, and supra-angular regions of the mandible. The decisive anatomical relationships can be excellently depicted on three-dimensional X-ray images.

Accordingly, the topography of the mandibular canal must be taken into account in the sagittal splitting of the mandibular angle and ramus, i.e., the splitting occurs strictly in the boundary zone between the lateral cortical bone layer, the cancellous bone mass, and the mandibular canal.

Bone cross-sections mostly provided by cone-beam CT data provide the guidelines for performing an atraumatic osteotomy within the lateral aspect of the mandibular angle.

In view of the risk of nerve injury, the lateral margin is divided into a pre-angular (1), angular (2), and supra-angular (3) section (Fig. 17.1) [1, 10, 11].

There is minimal to no cancellous bone between the wall of the nerve canal and lateral cortex in the angular and supra-angular regions (**c** and **d**) [1, 11].

In the angular and post-angular sections, there is generally only a small layer of cancellous bone between the canal and the lateral cortex. In the pre-angular zone, the supply of cancellous bone is usually greater, but the course of the mandibular canal approaches the buccal cortical lamella, so the risk of injury to the inferior alveolar nerve (IAN) is also present here (a, b) [1].

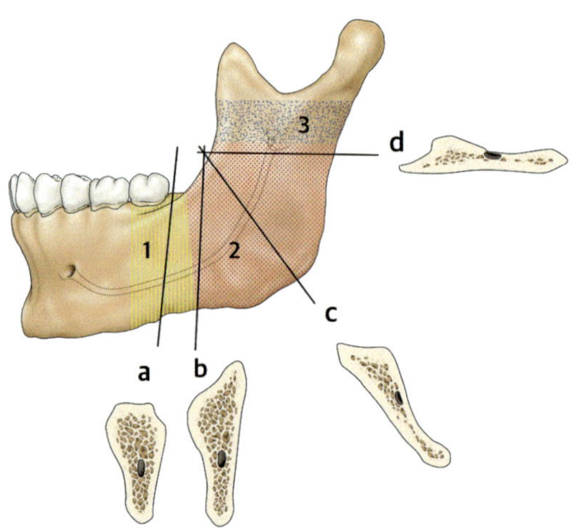

Fig. 17.1 Relationship of the mandibular canal to the lateral cortex in the pre-angular (1), angular (2), and supra-angular (3) regions relevant for performing the mandibular split (**a**, **b**, **c**, and **d**). ©Copyright Keisuke Koyama 2020. All rights reserved

2 Sagittal Split Osteotomy of Mandible (BSSO)—Surgical Technique Surgical Access

2.1 Intraoral Mucoperiosteal Incision

A mouth spreader/bite block on the contra-lateral side ensures the maximum mouth opening.

The oral mucosa is infiltrated buccally and lingually in the region of the mandibular angle with a local anesthetic containing a vasoconstrictive additive, e.g., epinephrine solution in a concentration of 1:100,000 for better intraoperative hemostasis and pain control.

The cheek is stretched with two wound hooks of matching length, e.g., Langenbeck hooks, in cranio-lateral and bucco-caudal direction. Then a continuous mucoperiosteal incision is made down to the bone—beginning from the base of the coronoid process, then continued lateral of the external oblique line of the ramus downwards to the mandibular vestibule and ending in the region between the first and second molar (Fig. 17.2).

It is advisable to leave 7–8 mm wide strip of the non-keratinized alveolar epithelium in the molar and retromolar region—to facilitate subsequent suturing.

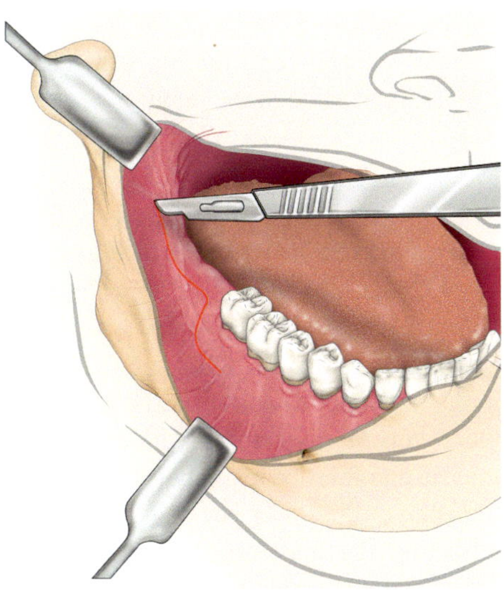

Fig. 17.2 Preparing the surgical site in the lower jaw after insertion of the mouth spreader/mouth prop on the left. The extension of the mucoperiosteal incision extends from the anterior edge of the coronoid process (*temporal crista of the coronoid process*) to the vestibular crista buccinatoria in the region of the first/second molar.

In order not to lose bone contact when exposing the edge of the ascending ramus, the incision can also be performed in two sections [12].

After careful incision the mucosa and periosteum are dissected laterally starting at the external oblique line and extending the dissection to the lower mandibular border, and to the insertion of the tendon of the masseteric muscle.

For a better overview, the incision can be extended cranially to the end of the coronoid process (modification acc. to [10]).

This is followed by subtle hemostasis and, optionally, selective diathermy of the buccal artery, which crosses the ramus at the level of the jaw angle.

> **Note**
> The incision should not be too lateral in the proximal area to avoid injury to the buccinator muscle and possible herniation of the buccal fat pad.
> (*Corpus adiposum buccae*).

> **Note**
> The pronounced lateral-vestibular placement of the mucosal incision in the posterior vestibule prevents injury to the lingual nerve and provides sufficient cuff tissue for subsequent wound closure.

2.2 Exposure of the Ramus and the Buccal Region of the Second and Third Molars

Dissection of the periosteum begins along the anterior border of the ramus and follows the external oblique line upwards to the base of the coronoid process and caudally to the mandibular vestibule, exposing the oblique line including the retromolar region and the lateral crista buccinatoria (Fig. 17.3).

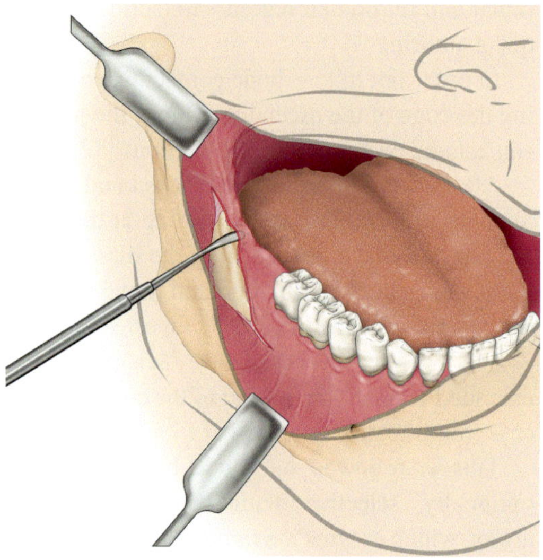

Fig. 17.3 Subperiosteal exposition of the lateral-buccal aspect of the mandibular ramus.

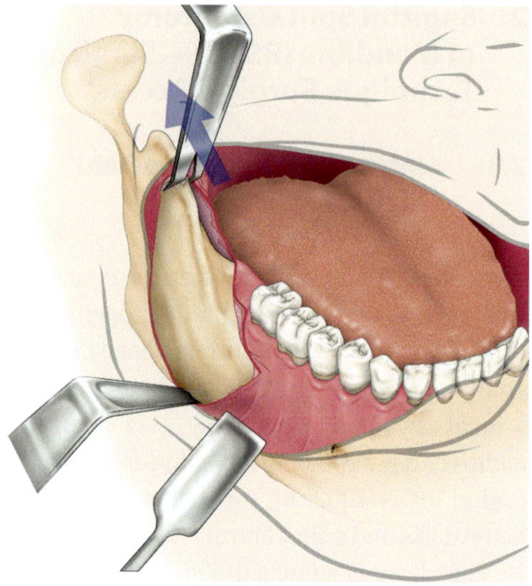

Fig. 17.4 Exposure of the coronoid process with a V-shaped rectangular retractor—dovetail retractor, which is positioned and pushed up in the anterior and inferior part of the coronoid process.

2.3 Anterior and Inferior Exposure of the Coronoid Process

After exposure of the anterior edge of the ramus, two Langenbeck hooks are inserted into the upper edge of the incision to retract the mucosa and visualize the insertion of the tendon of the temporal muscle to the coronoid process.

Note
A relatively small relief incision in the area of the tendon insertion of the temporal muscle improves access to the coronoid process.

A blunt dissector is then used to detach the tendinous attachments from the coronoid process in cranial direction. A dovetail hook (ramus hook) is then placed on the exposed inferior edge of the bone (*crista temporalis of the coronoid process*) and the hook is pushed upwards manually to remove the muscle and tendon attachments of the temporal muscle until the coronoid notch is exposed (Fig. 17.4).

A curved Kocher clamp/Zatinsky clamp/aortic clamp is then attached to the coronoid process to act as a self-sustaining retractor of the abovementioned soft tissues.

Note
The extensive elevation of the coronoid tendon attachments improves the access to the lingual side of the ramus.

2.4 Exposure of the Lateral Side of the Ramus (Sub-Masseteric Space)

Starting anteriorly in the region of the second molar a subperiosteal space is created using a blunt curved dissector in direction masseteric muscle and inferior mandibular border, exposing the edge of the lower jaw and the jaw angle and retracting the masseteric muscle laterally. The muscle attachment at the mandibular angle itself is not detached to avoid unnecessary devascularization of the proximal ramus.

The posterior margin of the ramus can be exposed optionally, if a classical osteotomy according to Obwegeser is intended to protect the

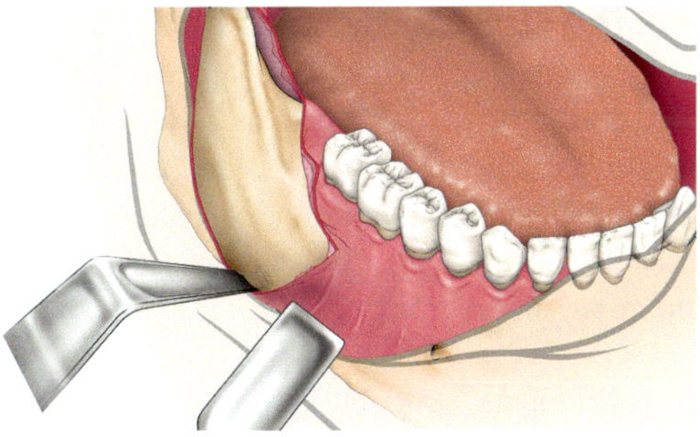

Fig. 17.5 Exposure of the inferior mandibular rim, curved channel retractor inserted.

delicate retromandibular structures with a curved channel retractor (Fig. 17.5) .

2.5 Exposure/Dissection of the Lingual Side of the Ramus (Pterygomandibular Space)

To expose the lingual side of the ramus, a clamp is first fixed to the coronoid process to secure the soft tissue position as explained above.

The dissection is performed below the level of the sigmoid arch (*incisura semilunaris*), which is palpated with the blunt dissector.

After crossing the internal oblique line by careful dissection, the dissector is guided close to the bone—strictly in a subperiosteal plane—in dorsal direction and parallel to the occlusal plane of the mandible to create a space between the medial surface of the ascending ramus and the neurovascular bundle on the lingual side of the so-called lingual tunnel. Notice that the ascending ramus is concave here (Fig. 17.6).

The pterygomandibular periosteal reflection on the lingual side is then widened to a subperiosteal tunnel and the medial bone surface is exposed directly to the lingula and the mandibular foramen identifying the neurovascular bundle.

Then the question is whether to use the lingual osteotomy according to Obwegeser or Hunsuck, the short lingual osteotomy—SLO.

In case of the Obwegeser variant the lingual dissection has to be continued to the posterior edge of the ascending ramus.

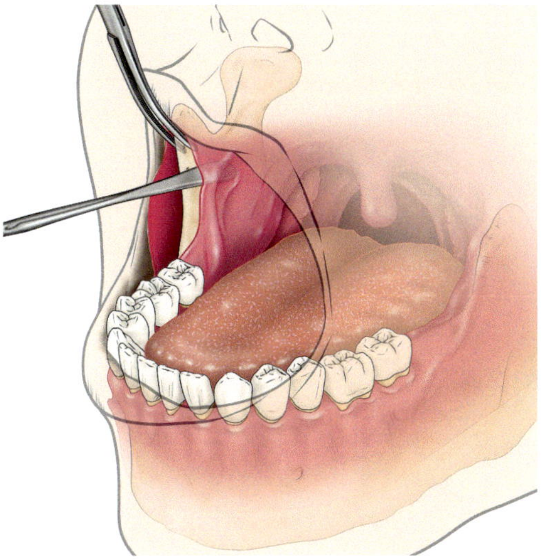

Fig. 17.6 A blunt curved periosteal dissector is used to create a strictly subperiosteal tunnel on the lingual side of the mandibular ramus to expose the medial surface of the ramus. Tissue retraction with a clamp positioned at the coronoid process.

The Hunsuck variant ends at a point immediately posterior to the neurovascular bundle. A narrow channel retractor is then placed in the subperiosteal tunnel to protect the medial vascular nerve bundle (Fig. 17.7) [4, 8, 9]

Note

Care should be taken to avoid damage to the IAN, artery, and vein enclosed in a periosteal fibrous bundle when dissecting the lingual tunnel.

Nevertheless, unpleasant venous bleeding may occur during preparation in the lingula area, but will stop after insertion of a channel retractor.

In clinical practice, the channel retractor is positioned approximately parallel to the mandibular occlusal plane at approximately a 45 ° angulation to the vertical.

Excessive soft tissue retraction on the lingual side is unnecessary and can cause stretching of the IAN as well as distortion or distension of the vessels over the sharp edge of the mandibular foramen (Fig. 17.8).

Note

In practice, a clear access is achieved after inserting the narrow channel retractor and by pivoting the channel retractor 45° to the vertical plane.

The channel retractor then lies parallel to the mandibular occlusal plane.

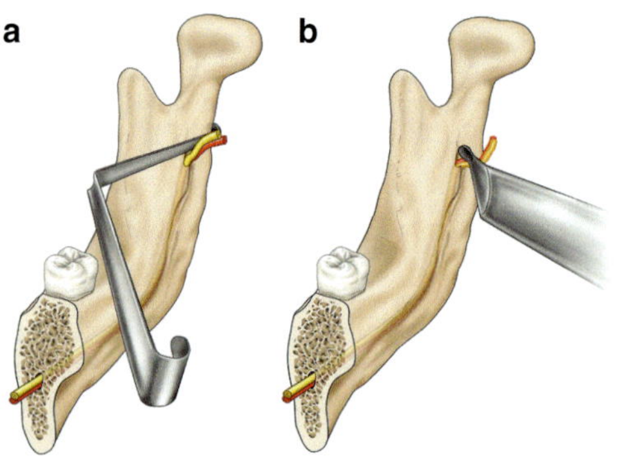

Fig. 17.7 The correct position of the channel retractor with adequate soft tissue retraction is a prerequisite for sufficient visualization and accessibility for the lingual osteotomy and avoids injuries to the neurovascular bundles. (**a**) Obwegeser, (**b**) Hunsuck.

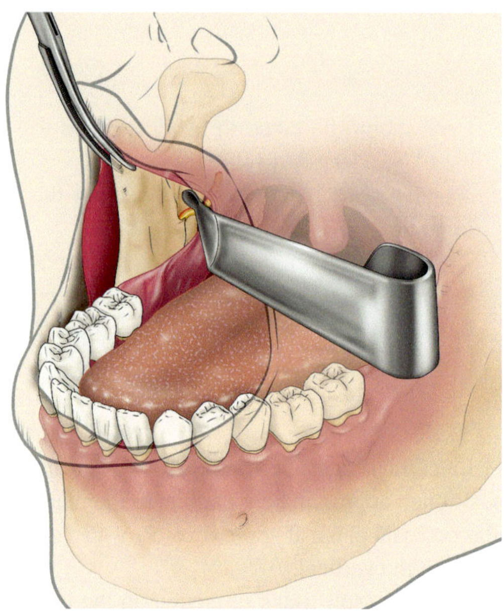

Fig. 17.8 Inserted channel retractor for visualization of the lingual ramus side and the neurovascular bundle. Care should be taken that the neurovascular bundle is not damaged by the channel retractor due to excessive retraction.

3 The Osteotomy Lines

The design of the bone cuts and the subsequent splitting of the mandibular ramus are based on the knowledge of the ratio of cancellous bone to cortical bone in the pre-angular, angular, and supra-angular regions.

- Instruments suitable for a mandibular osteotomy:
  Drills in the following order: Lindemann burr long—milling cutter/round burr—Lindemann burr short.
- Oscillating saw for the sagittal bone cut.
- Piezoelectric bone surgery.

In principle, the sagittal osteotomy requires three osteotomy lines to mark the borderline between cortical and cancellous bone (Fig. 17.9):

(a) Horizontal bone cut—lingual cortex of the ascending ramus.
(b) Vertical bone cut—lateral buccal cortex—mandibular body.
(c) Sagittal bone cut—oblique line—region of the ascending ramus.

3.1 Horizontal Bone Cut—Horizontal Osteotomy

Before making the horizontal bone incision, it is recommended that, e.g., a Seldin retractor be inserted into the lingual subperiosteal tunnel superior to the lingula and then rotated by 45° to the vertical (Fig. 17.10). This will stretch the periosteum in a tent-shaped manner in the area of the foramen (see identification technique of the mandibular foramen—Chap. 14).

For safe localization of the mandibular foramen at the tip of the lingual tunnel, it is recommended to estimate the plane and length of the planned osteotomy line with a blunt nerve probe, which is placed in the foramen under direct visualization (Fig. 17.11) [7]

After clear dissection of the surgical field, the first osteotomy is usually the horizontal bone cut on the lingual side.

If burrs are used: The horizontal osteotomy through the lingual cortex to a depth equal to half

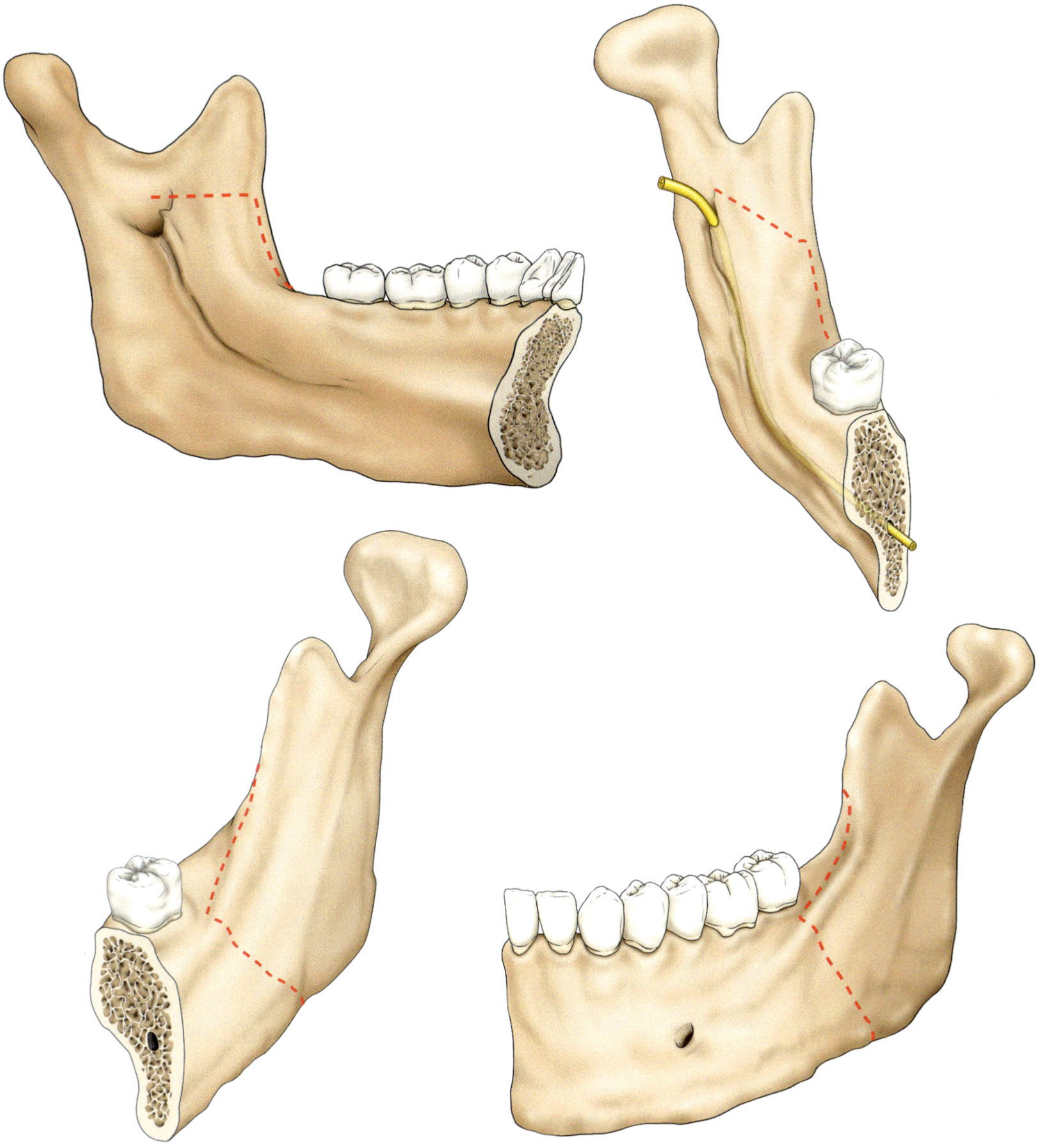

Fig. 17.9 Bone cuts for sagittal splitting of the mandible.

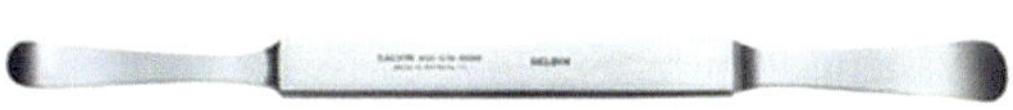

Fig. 17.10 Seldin retractor

the medio-lateral thickness of the ramus can be performed with the long Lindemann burr. The linguo-medial cortex cut is made approximately 1 cm below the mandibular notch, parallel to the occlusal surface of the lower row of teeth. Starting point of the osteotomy: In or slightly above the lingula (Fig. 17.11).

According to Obwegeser the entire width/length of the inner cortex of the ascending ramus has to be cut as well as the inner cancellous bone layer including the posterior edge of the ramus.

The Hunsuck technique commonly used today for the short lingual osteotomy (SLO) is in the same plane but ends somewhat cranially and distally of the mandibular foramen (Fig. 17.12).

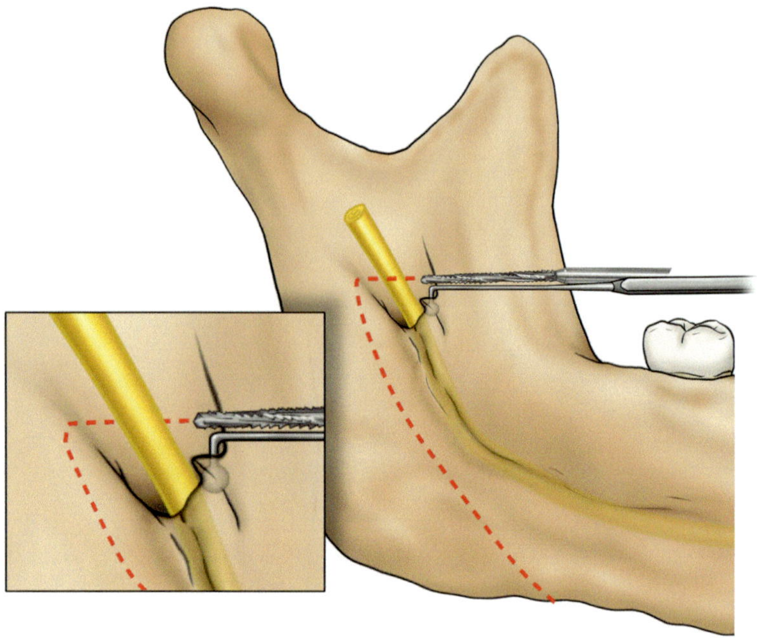

Fig. 17.11 Lateral view of the nerve probe placement in the mandibular foramen and the position of the burr. ©Copyright Keisuke Koyama 2020. All rights reserved

Note

The identification of the mandibular foramen is crucial for the creation of the horizontal osteotomy on the lingual side.

For the determination of the distance between the foramen and the osteotomy line, see detailed technique in Chap. 8.

The horizontal osteotomy should be as low as possible, close to the lingula. In this region, there is usually sufficient cancellous bone between the cortical lamellae to facilitate separation/splitting (Fig. 17.13).

Note

The closer the bone cut is located towards the mandibular notch, the lower the chance that the sagittal split of the proximal ramus is successful.

(see detailed technique in Chap. 8).

Note

If a protruding internal oblique line obstructs the clear arrangement of the bone cuts, a pear- or round-shaped burr is used to make a groove in the internal oblique line to enable a correct horizontal bone section.

3.2 Vertical Bone Cut—Vertical Osteotomy

The vertical cut on the buccal side of the mandible lies in the region of the second molar or slightly more anterior or posterior to the base of the masseteric muscle basically perpendicular to the occlusal surface and primarily affects the lateral cortex [3]

The depth of the bone cut should just reach the cancellous bone layer.

A buccal channel retractor is placed vertically opposite the center of the second molar with its tip below the lower margin of the mandible to protect the soft tissues of the cheek and the facial artery and vein crossing over the mandibular rim in this region.

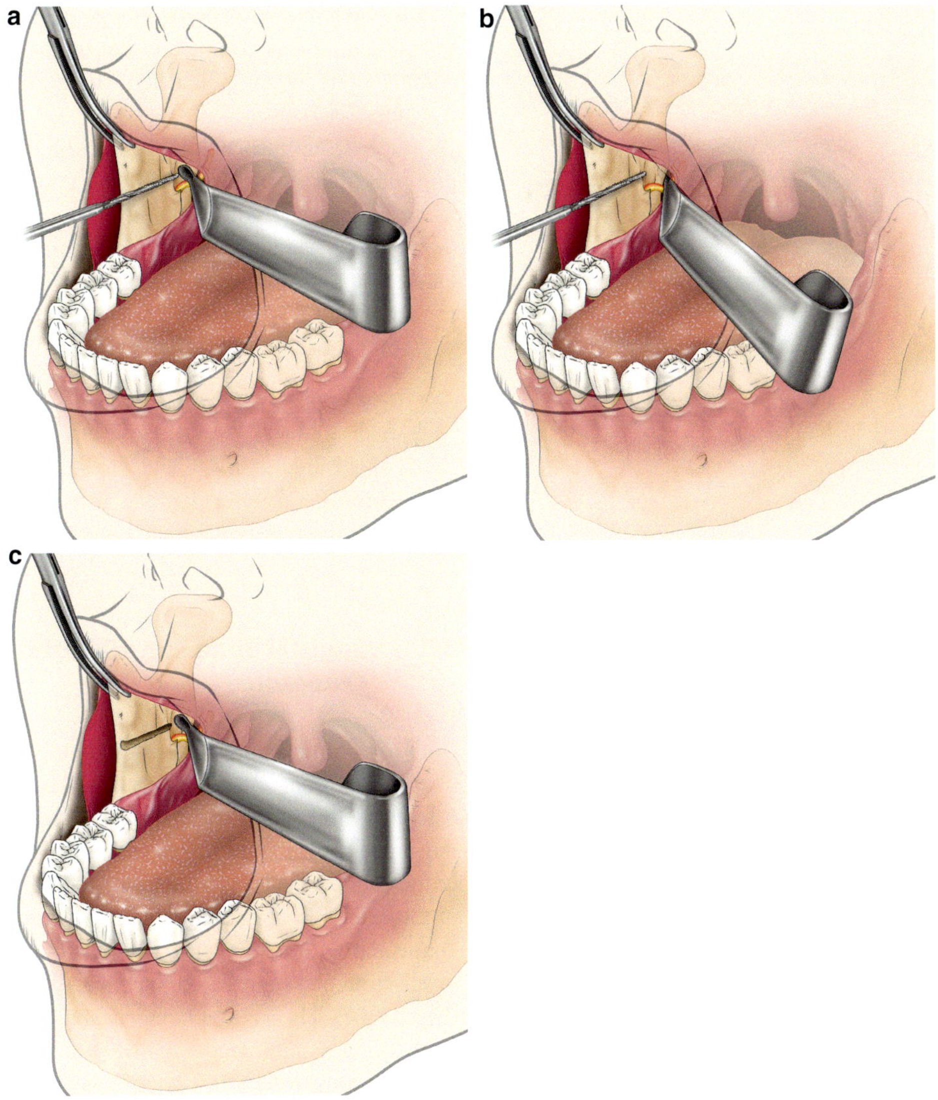

Fig. 17.12 Horizontal bone cut directly above the mandibular foramen (lingula) and the inferiorly placed neurovascular bundle. Note the two possible positions of the channel retractor: (**a**) posteriorly to the lingula (Hunsuck) or (**b**) behind the ascending ramus (Obwegeser) (**c**) Short lingual osteotomy—SLO.

A fissure drill or the long Lindemann burr is then used to cut vertically and downward through the thick outer cortical bone to a depth of about 2 mm until the vascularized cancellous bone becomes visible in the bone cut (Figs. 17.14, 17.15A, B).

Care should be taken to ensure that the osteotomy is not made too deep into the cancellous bone, since the mandibular canal and IAN are located near the lateral cortex.

Note
Due to the proximity of the inferior alveolar nerve (IAN) to the buccal mandibular cortex in the area of the first molar, the anterior vertical osteotomy should be stopped as soon as a cancellous bone hemorrhage occurs in the osteotomy channel indicating that the buccal cortex has been completely severed.

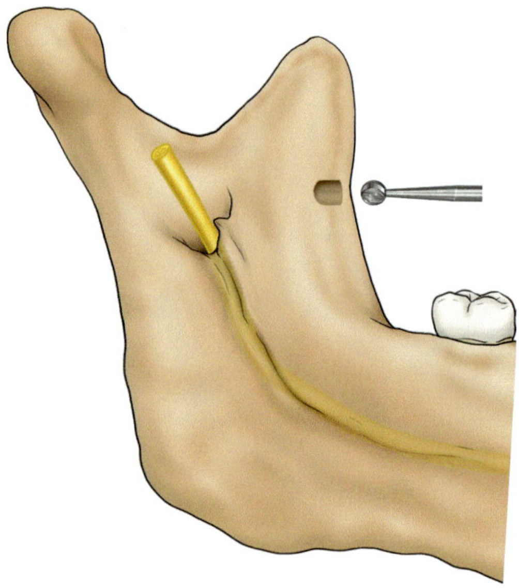

Fig. 17.13 Removal of a protruding internal oblique line with a burr in the preplanned horizontal osteotomy plane.

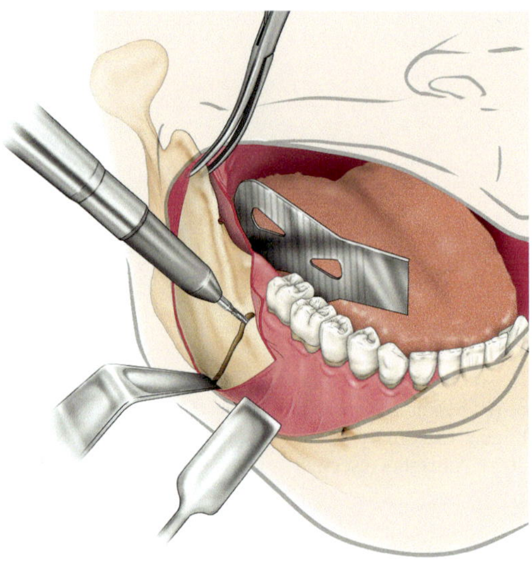

Fig. 17.14 After insertion of a curved channel retractor, the vertical osteotomy including the cortical mandibular margin (inset) is performed with the short or long Lindemann burr.

As indicated in Fig. 17.14, the vertical cut is not made directly through the cortical bone, but at an angle of 45° to the surface.

Likewise, the thick cortical edge of the lower mandibular rim is completely cut until the cancellous bone layer is reached—to a depth of 2–3 mm.

The osteotomy of the basal mandibular margin ends shortly before the lingual cortex. This measure is important and must be performed with care. When adjusting the drill, care must be taken not to overstretch the soft tissue of the cheek (Figs. 17.14 and 17.15a, b) [2, 15]

Note
To check the completeness of the vertical osteotomy, a fine, narrow osteotome should be used to gently follow the bone incision.

3.3 Sagittal Bone Cut—Sagittal Osteotomy

Both osteotomies, the lingual horizontal and vertical buccal bone cuts, are connected by a third osteotomy line. A round burr can be used to mark the connecting line through a series of drill holes in the sagittal plane parallel to the medial aspect of the external oblique line. These holes are then connected with a short drill to create a continuous, straight sagittal connecting bone cut (Fig. 17.16). The sagittal bone cut should be parallel to the sagittal plane of the ramus and the depth of this osteotomy should not reach the mandibular canal [13, 14]

Note
The corticotomy of the narrow edge of the oblique external line up to the visible border between cortical and cancellous bone considerably facilitates the marking and placement of the sagittal bone cut.

The direction and path for the subsequent sagittal splitting are thus determined. The two buccally and lingually inserted channel retractors provide firm support.

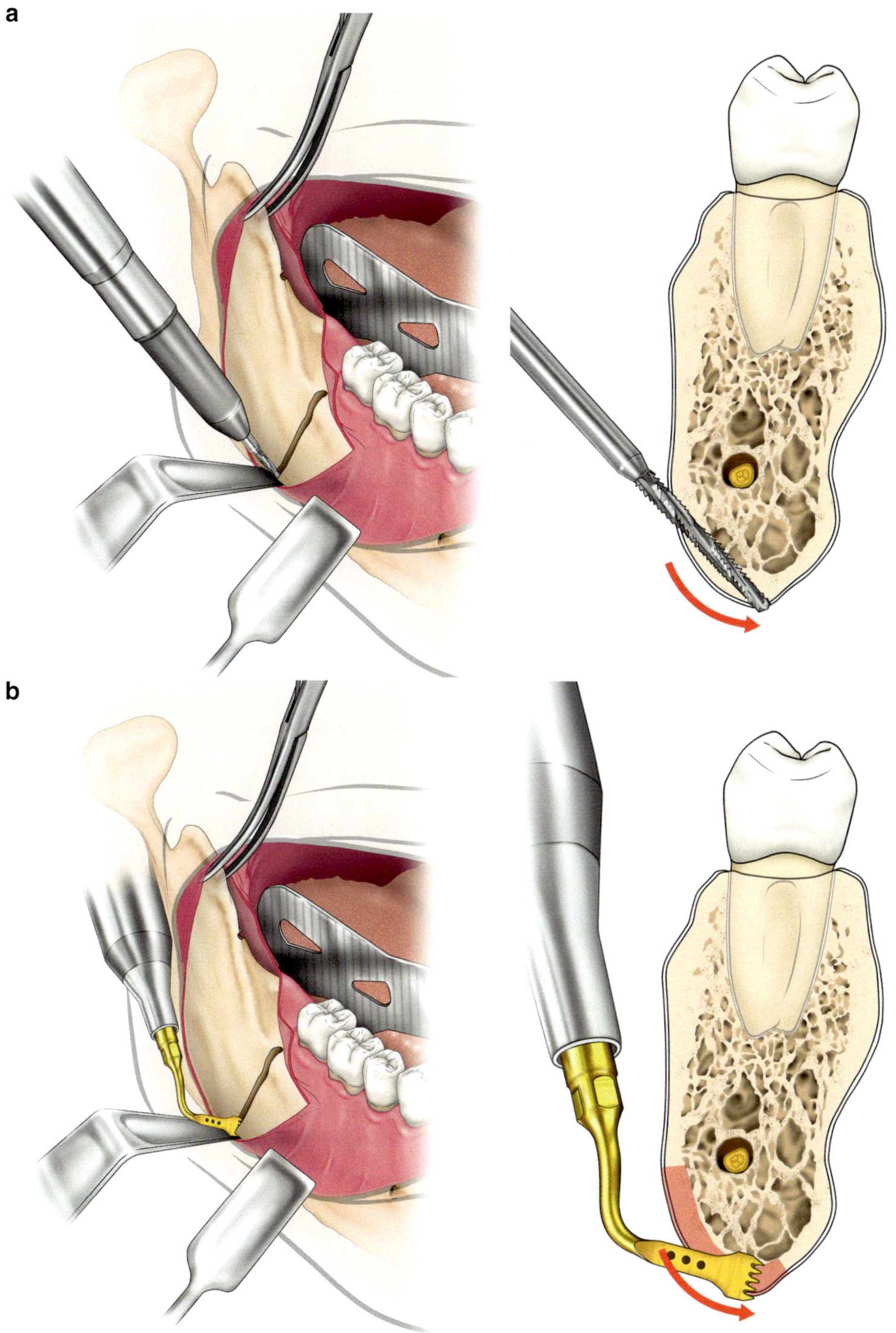

Fig. 17.15 After insertion of a curved channel retractor, the vertical osteotomy is performed with the short or long Lindemann burr. The mandibular margin is cut with the short Lindemann burr (**a**) Alternatively Piezo surgery can be applied (**b**)

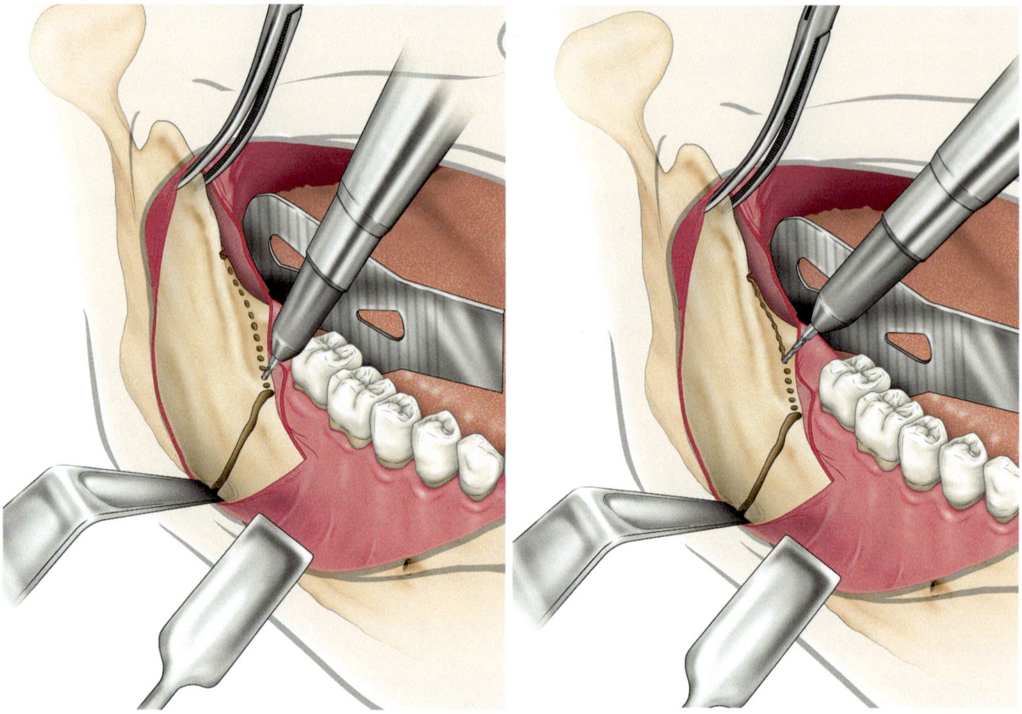

Fig. 17.16 Corticotomy of the edge of the oblique external line up to the visible border between cortical and cancellous bone close to the lateral cortex [12, 14].

4 Sagittal Splitting

- Splitting technique of the ramus in the borderline between lateral cortex and cancellous bone.
- Correct sequence of splitting with thin and wide osteotomes/chisels.
- Modification Hunsuck instead of splitting the posterior ramus margin—the short lingual osteotomy (SLO).

Before the actual splitting begins, the proximal and distal transitions between the bone cuts are separated with fine osteotomes. A narrow osteotome with a finely tapered blade first completes the transition from the sagittal to the vertical osteotomy with light hammer blows in an inferior direction towards the mandibular margin as well as the transition from the sagittal to the horizontal osteotomy in the proximal region [13].

Note

Correct transitions between the three osteotomy lines:

The transition of the horizontal (lingual) cut and the transition of the vertical buccal cut in the sagittal osteotomy line should be selectively deeply cut with a short burr and worked out to facilitate subsequent sagittal splitting along the horizontal and vertical sections with fine osteotomes.

4.1 Pre-Angular Section

The actual sagittal split osteotomy then begins in the pre-angular section, where the cancellous layer and the lateral cortex have approximately the same width, and is performed with especially thin Lambotte osteotomes of different widths: The standard osteotomes have a width of 8, 10, and 12 mm.

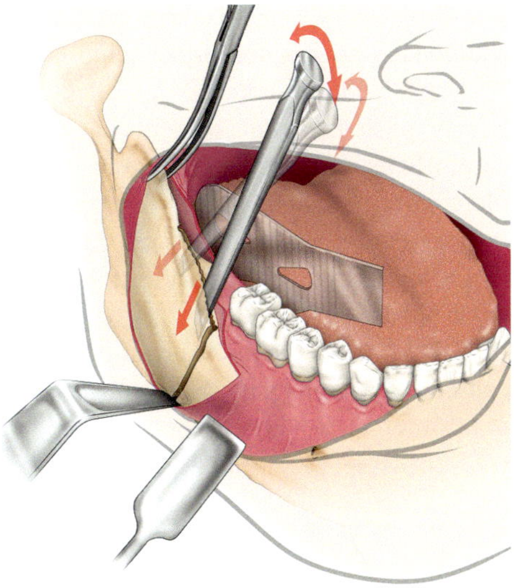

Fig. 17.17 A chisel can be used to deepen the drill cuts.

The fine osteotomes—no. 8 or 10—are used to deepen the cortical drill cuts—starting at the intersection of the sagittal connecting osteotomy and the vertical buccal osteotomy in the region of the first and second molars, respectively. The medial and lateral segments are then separated continuously from pre- to post-angular (Figs. 17.17 and 17.18).

Two Lambotte flat osteotomes alternate to deepen the sagittal osteotomy gap. One osteotome is alternately loosened and re-inserted into the gap parallel to the remaining osteotome—behind the previously placed osteotome—for further splitting and the medial and lateral segments are separated progressively from anterior to posterior - better visibility.

The remaining osteotome continuously determines the direction of splitting by holding it under tension while rotating it carefully so that the osteotomy gap is widened step by step and the splitting process is visually controlled, so that the now free second osteotome can be safely reattached. Initially, the osteotomes should not be guided too medially and too deep to exclude the possibility of transection of the alveolar neurovascular bundle.

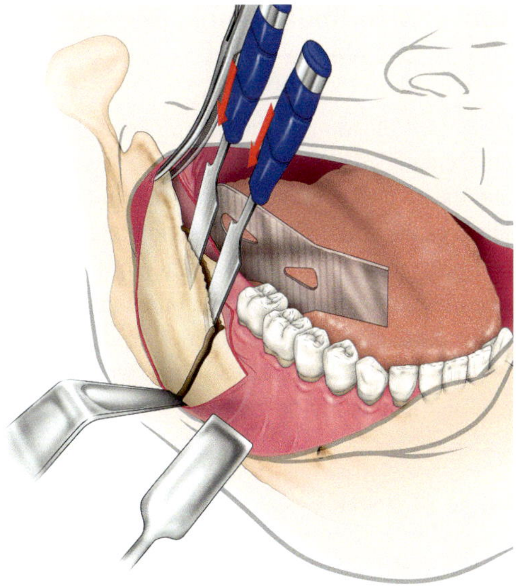

Fig. 17.18 The osteotomes (1 and 2) are impacted alternately for partial splitting of the lateral and medial cortex segments.

4.2 Angular and Supra-Angular Section

Very thinly ground osteotomes or chisels—straight or slightly curved—are used in the angular and supra-angular sections, since there is little or no cancellous bone between the wall of the nerve canal and the lateral cortex.

Here, post-angular splitting is started directly at the lingual horizontal bone cut. A 5 mm osteotome is placed at an angle. Basic direction: connecting line between the mandibular midline and the external oblique line.

The osteotome penetrates to the interface of the cortical bone under light, short hammer blows. After reaching this layer, the osteotome is swiveled into the sagittal (parallel to the outer surface of the ascending ramus).

Gently into the depth, the bone is split either to the posterior of the mandibular foramen [4, 8] or including the posterior margin of the jaw [5, 9].

4.3 Mandibular Angle Beneath the Nerve Canal

After identification of the nerve canal osteotomes are then guided angularly between the lateral cortex and the spongy intramedullary bone in the sagittal plane of the mandible to the mandibular margin—compacta to facilitate the separation of the mandibular margin. The neurovascular bundle must be safe in the distal mandibular segment (Fig. 17.19).

After extensive splitting—up to well below the alveolar canal—wide osteotomes, e.g., 12 mm osteotomes with round wooden handles e.g., are additionally inserted for further splitting.

These wide osteotomes are then used to slowly push the two segments apart and, by carefully twisting the osteotomes, achieve complete inferior and posterior separation of the last trajectory connections of the segments, while visualizing and protecting the neurovascular bundle.

This procedure helps to avoid the "bad split" caused by incompletely osteotomized segments at the inferior mandibular border.

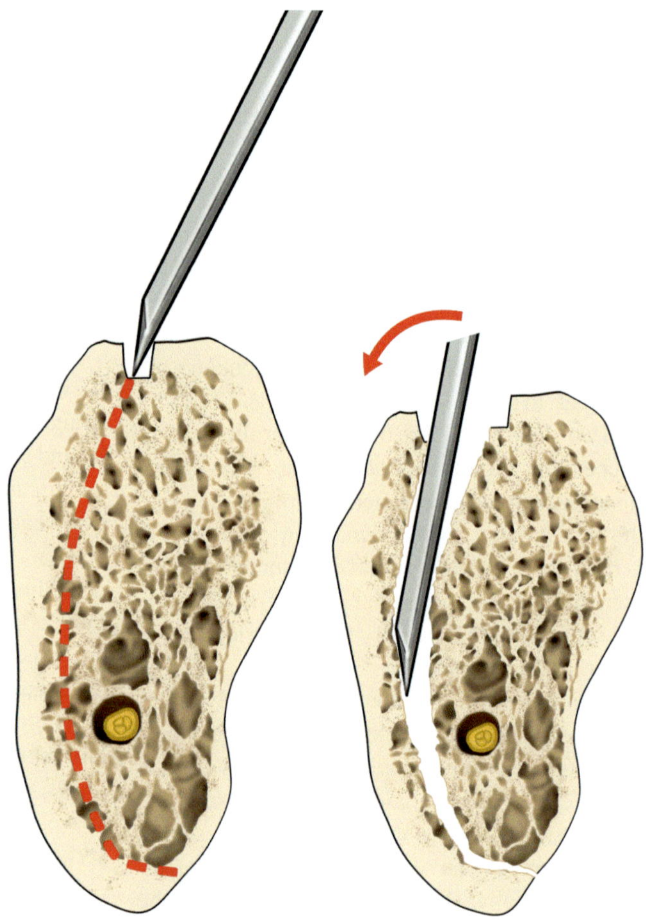

Fig. 17.19 The cross-sectional view demonstrates the course of a complete continuous lateral cortex split to avoid splintering (Hunsuck effect) and nerve injuries [12]

4.4 Advanced Splitting

If the splitting of the buccal and lingual cortex segment is largely advanced, a wider osteotome—no. 10—that widens the osteotomy gap and smaller osteotomes are used alternately as indicated above.

The wider osteotome is left and immediately behind it, smaller osteotomes continue the splitting at the mandibular angle/margin. The osteotome should be directed towards the inner surface of the cortex of the proximal fragment because of the cutting blade of the instrument.

4.5 Splitting of the Mandibular Margin

A fine tapered curved sharp osteotome is then used to split the inferior mandibular rim—starting from the lower part of the vertical osteotomy.

The osteotome is inserted between the partially split bone segments in the area of the lower vertical osteotomy. When separating the mandible margin, the osteotome is pressed lightly against the distal segment to direct the splitting pressure against the inner surface of the proximal segment (Fig. 17.20) [1, 15].

The osteotome is used in the area of the lower vertical bone cut in partially split bone segments. During the separation of the mandibular margin, the osteotome is pressed slightly against the distal segment to direct the splitting pressure against the inner surface of the proximal segment (Figs. 17.20 and 17.21) [1, 6, 13, 15].

Two osteotome technique: The rotation of the wide osteotomes is slow but continuous—preferably anticlockwise on the right side and clockwise on the left side until the ramus fragments begin to split (Fig. 17.20).

One osteotome technique: If only a single wide osteotome is used to spread the segments, the osteotome must be inserted and rotated progressively from the anterior buccal cut beginning to the linguo-medial end of the bone cut (Fig. 17.22).

Alternative splitting techniques often refer to the instrumentation used. The Smith separator and spreader are popular instruments to use when the classic osteotomes do not fit well in the hand (Figs. 17.22 and17.23). A combination of spreader and osteotome is also possible.

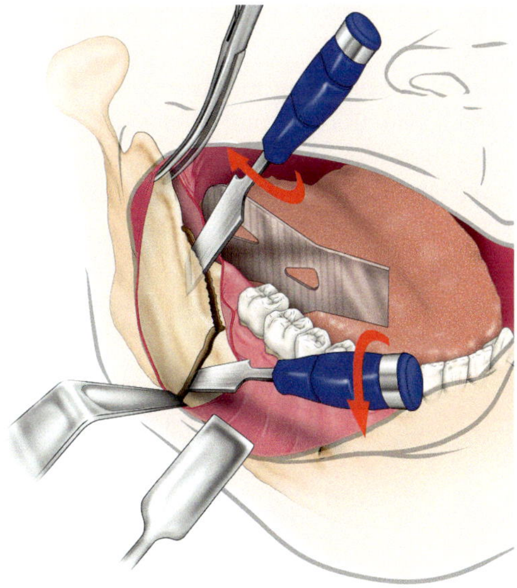

Fig.17.20 Splitting of the inferior mandibular margin.

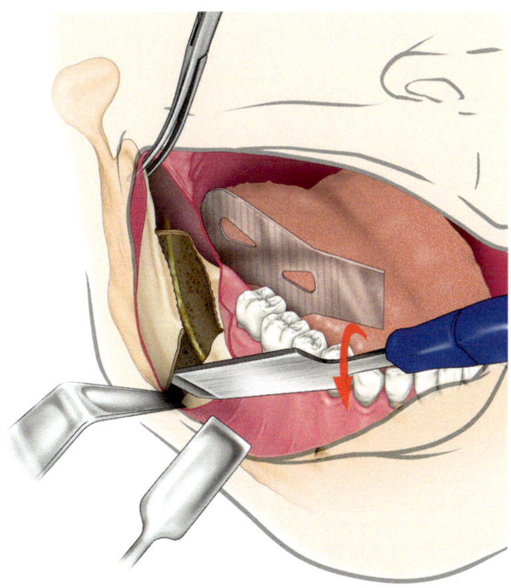

Fig. 17.21 Wide osteotomes inserted into the osteotomy gap, which are rotated alternately for definitive division of the two segments.

Note

- If bleeding due to vascular injury has occurred as a result of the splitting, a folded hemostatic fleece is placed on the bleeding site and the two bone segments are temporarily repositioned and compressed with a clamp.
- Electrocautery should be avoided.

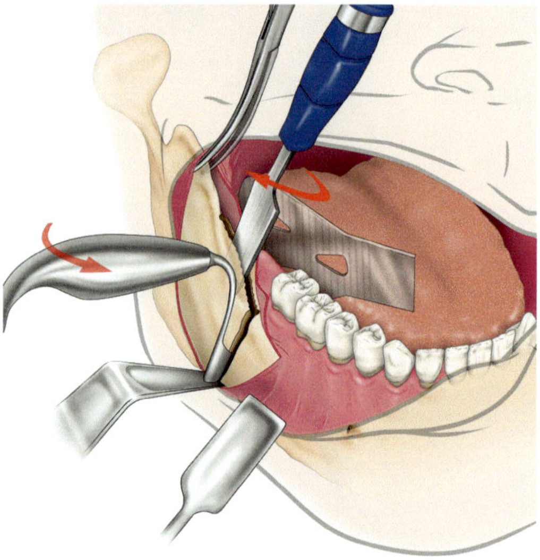

Fig. 17.22 Careful splitting using one osteotome and the Smith separator.

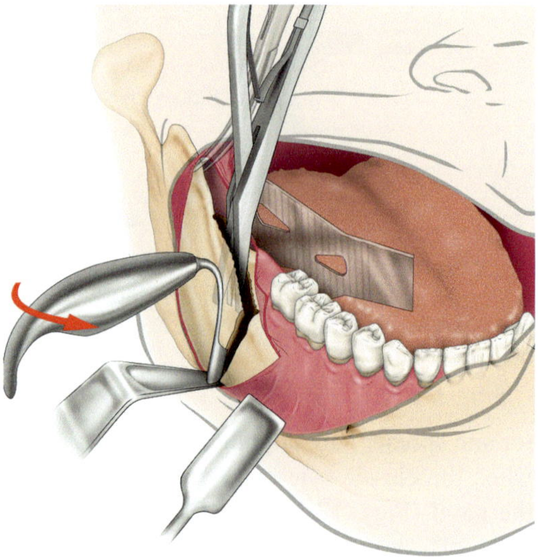

Fig. 17.23 Careful splitting using the spreader and the Smith separator.

4.6 Difficulties in Mandibular Splitting

If the separation of the proximal and distal segments is difficult:

- Use a 5 mm chisel/small osteotome to cut through the presumably resistant lower and angular cortical edge of the osteotomy in the dorsal osteotomy region.
- With a thin chisel/osteotome in the area of the buccal vertical osteotomy, the splitting of the mandibular margin is repeated between the buccal cortical plate and medullary bone in order to separate remaining osseous connections mostly in the area of the mandibular base.

Note

- If there is resistance to the separation of the segments with the wide osteotomes, it should be checked again whether the separation of the cortical structures on all sides has been completely successful.
- In case of recognizable splitting problems, it is better to stop the surgical procedure first and identify the problem.
- The problem should be diagnosed and solved in order to avoid an "unfortunate splitting."
- If the jawbone is very cortical, force must be used occasionally, then this should preferably be done in the axial direction of the instrument (osteotome) without rotating it.

4.7 After the Split

After splitting the mandible, a wide osteotome is inserted and rotated in the anterior region of the sagittal osteotomy and the osteotome is rotated to check the position of the neurovascular bundle, the completeness of the osteotomy, and resistant, adherent tendon and muscle attachments.

Ideally, the IAN after splitting is either completely in the medial distal segment or may be

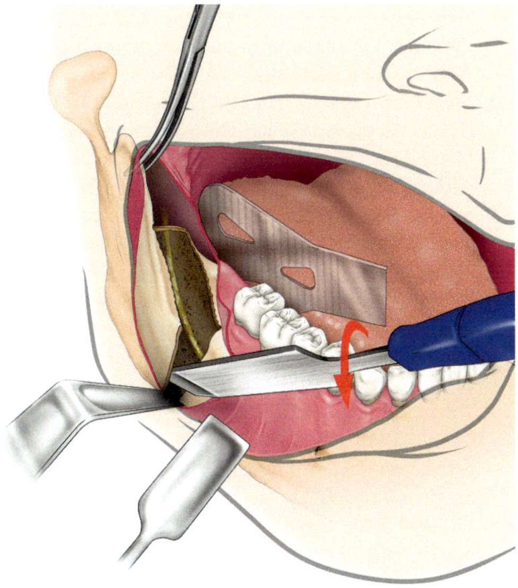

Fig. 17.24 The osteotome is inserted into the osteotomy gap and the gap is expanded by rotating it.

more or less visible in the operation field or adherent to the lateral proximal segment (Fig. 17.24).

If the nerve is partially located in the proximal segment, the nerve is carefully released from the cancellous bone with the blunt dissector, e.g., dissector acc. to Freer, to allow medial repositioning of the nerve.

If the alveolar neurovascular bundle is trapped in the mandibular canal of the proximal segment and the planned segment movement is minimal, it may be unnecessary to expose the nerve in the proximal segment and release it from the surrounding trabecula.

However, in the case of major segmental displacements, repositioning of the nerve is inevitable due to the nerve strain that might occur. Again blunt dissectors must be used.

If the neurovascular bundle is exposed within an incomplete split, the split is first completed with fine osteotomes or chisels in the infra-nerval segment of the mandible and then the nerve is repositioned. Utmost care is obligatory.

Occasionally, inferior detachment of soft tissue attachments of the pterygo-masseteric loop is required to allow the proximal and distal bone fragments to move independently and passively (Fig. 17.24).

Note

- The neurovascular bundle is to be visualized. It should be in the distal segment on the medial side.
- If the mandible is to be advanced, the medial pterygoid muscle is detached from the inferior mandibular border to reduce the risk of relapse.
- If the mandible is to be set back, judicious stripping of the pterygomasseteric sling may be an important consideration to prevent posterior displacement of the condylar segment.
- The cortex of the mandibular margin should be completely severed.
- For control purposes, the osteotomy gap should be clearly expanded and a fine osteotome should be used to gently test the complete cut of the cortical mandibular margin.
- With an index finger placed on the anterior edge of the proximal segment, the distal tooth-bearing part of the mandible is advanced gently to ensure that the split is complete and the mandibular body can be mobilized without interference with the position of the proximal segment/condyle.

5 Conclusion

The technique described here for splitting the mandible has proven itself in clinical practice worldwide and is also used with occasional variations in terms of instruments. The splitting procedure itself must be well prepared to be successful.

References

1. Bell HW, Proffit WR, White RP. Surgical correction of dentofacial deformities, vol. 1-3. Saunders; 1980.
2. Böckmann R, Schön P, Neuking K, Meyns J, Kessler P, Eggeler G. In vitro comparison of the sagittal split

osteotomy with and without inferior border osteotomy. J Oral Maxillofac Surg. 2015;73(2):316–23.
3. Dal Pont G. L'osteotomia retromolare per la correzione della progenia. Minerva Chir. 1958:1.
4. Epker BN. Modifications in the sagittal osteotomy of the mandible. J Oral Surg. 1977;35(2):157–9.
5. Epker BN, Stella JP, Fish LC. Dentofacial deformities. Integrated orthodontic and surgical correction, band 3. Mosby. 1998;
6. Escobar V, Greenberg AM, Schwimmer A. Mandibular Osteotomies and Considerations for rigid internal fixation. In: Greenberg AM, Prein J, editors. Craniomaxillofacial Reconstructive and Corrective Bone Surgery: Principles of internal fixation using AO/ASIF Technic. Springer; 2002.
7. Ghali GE, Patel S. Avoiding surgical complications in orthognathic surgery. In: Ghali GE, Woerner JE, Patel S, editors. Maxillofacial Surgery: Mandible (Third Edition). Livingstone: Churchill; 2017.
8. Hunsuck EE. A modified intraoral sagittal splitting technic for correction of mandibular prognathism. J Oral Surg. 1968;26(4):250–3.
9. Obwegeser H. Zur Operationstechnik bei der Progenie und anderen Unterkieferanomalien. Dtsch Zahn Mund Kieferheilk. 1955;23:1.
10. Spiessl B. Gesicht und Gesichtsschädel in Naumann HH: Gesicht- Kopf- und Hals-Chirurgie. Operations-Manual in 3 Bänden. Orthopädische Operationen am Kiefer , Bd.2/Teil 2. Thieme, Stuttgart 1974.
11. Spiessl B. New concepts in maxillofacial bone surgery. Berlin, Heidelberg: Springer; 1976.
12. Spiessl B Osteosynthese des Unterkiefers. Rekonstruktive Chirurgie, Teil III. Springer, Berlin, Heidelberg, New York, Tokyo, 1988.
13. Steinhäuser EW, Janson I. Kieferorthopädische Chirurgie Bd. I. Berlin, Chicago, London, Sao Paulo, Tokyo: Quintessenz; 1988.
14. Steinhäuser EW. Educational course on surgical methods in orthognatic surgery, vol. 8. Luzern, Switzerland; 1973. p. 4.
15. Wolford LM, Davis WM. The mandibular inferior border split: a modification in the sagittal split osteotomy. J Oral Maxillofac Surg. 1990;48:92–4.

Intraoperative Hazards and Risks 18

Peter Kessler and Nicolas Hardt

Contents

P. Kessler (✉)
Department of Cranio-Maxillofacial Surgery, Maastricht University Medical Center, Maastricht, The Netherlands
e-mail: peter.kessler@mumc.nl

N. Hardt (✉)
Kantonsspital Lucerne, Clinic and Policlinic of Cranio-Maxillofacial Surgery, Lucerne, Switzerland

P. Kessler et al. (eds.), *Illustrated Manual of Orthognathic Surgery*,
https://doi.org/10.1007/978-3-031-06978-9_18

Abstract

Intraoperative risks/complications include arterial and venous vessel injuries, direct and indirect nerve and soft tissue injuries and incomplete or irregular osteotomies (bad splits) (Kim J Korean Assoc Oral Maxillofac Surg 431:3–15, 2017; van Merkesteyn et al. Int J Oral and Maxillofacial Surg 166:665–670, 1987; Houppermans et al. J Craniomaxillofac Surg 449:1170–1180, 2016). For the sake of completeness, possible damage to neighboring teeth must also be mentioned.

Intraoperative hazards and risks:

- Vascular injury.
- Nerve injury.
- Undesirable fracture lines—bad split.
- Incorrect positioning of the proximal segments/condyle

Keywords

General rules in sagittal splitting · BSSO relevant clinical and topographic anatomy · Short lingual osteotomy · Mandibular canal · Avoidance of iatrogenic fractures · Split patterns · Bad split · Vascular injury · Bleeding · Nerve injury · Inferior alveolar nerve · Hazards in BSSO

1 Vascular Injuries

The vascular structures defined below are at greatest risk of being injured during orthognathic procedures in the mandible:

- Inferior alveolar artery.
- Intraossary course/mandibular and mental foramina.
- Maxillary artery.
- Facial artery.
- Masseteric artery.
- Retromandibular vein.

Disturbing and sometimes even severe bleedings can occur as a result of injuries to larger arterial vessels, such as the maxillary artery in the pterygomandibular fossa, the masseteric artery in the sigmoid region, and the facial artery at the lower edge of the mandible in the region of the submandibular notch. The inferior alveolar artery can be disrupted in the pterygomandibular space in the region of the lingula or in the sagittal fissure after or while splitting the mandible.

Fierce maneuvers can also lead to rupture of venous vessels. Venous hemorrhages can be attempted sublingually, e.g., after mandibular split by excessive movement of the segments or also through the retromandibular vein, but in this case it is more likely that chisels and osteotomes slip off. But also careless maneuvers with drills and saws can lead to unpleasant bleeding. The overall risk of intraoperative bleeding when splitting the lower jaw is stated at 9% [5, 10].

Smaller vascular bleedings can be stopped by pressure tamponade with absorbable hemostatic materials such as gauze strips impregnated with thrombin or adrenaline or by electrocoagulation, vascular occlusion or with vascular clips.

Bleeding from cancellous bone is stopped by applying pressure and bone wax, vascular bleeding in the osteotomy area—such as the inferior alveolar artery—is stopped by applying multiple-folded, resorbable hemostats, such as surgical Tabotamp™ or Surgicel™, e.g., as an adjunct measure. Short-term readjustment of the split bone segments and compression with a strong surgical clamp for a few minutes can also be used.

> **Note**
> *Tabotamp™—An absorbable hemostatic agent that promotes platelet aggregation and activates the intrinsic clotting cascade. Tabotamp™ is in vitro bactericidal against gram-positive and gram-negative bacteria as well as aerobic and anaerobic bacteria

In the event of bleeding of large arterial vessels that cannot be stopped immediately by vascular ligation/obstruction, an emergency embolization must be performed with the indication of a life-threatening and difficult-to-stop bleeding.

The extent of the intraoperative bleeding and the possibility of further bleeding complications varies from patient to patient. For this reason, it is important to measure the relative blood loss during the procedure continuously and patient specifically. The controlled lowering of blood pressure intraoperatively helps to prevent greater blood loss.

Extensive surgery and a reduced body mass index are associated with a relatively increased intraoperative blood loss [23].

> **Note**
> Significant blood loss after sagittal splitting of the ramus is usually the result of persistent oozing bleeding from severed muscles, such as the masseteric and/or medial pterygoid muscles and inadequate intraoperative blood pressure control.
>
> Minimal and strictly subperiosteal detachment of muscles and periosteum from the ramus reduces intraoperative and postoperative bleeding and swelling.

2 Prevention of Vascular Injuries in the Pterygomandibular Space

2.1 Inferior Alveolar Artery

By careful and clear positioning of the horizontal osteotomy line slightly superior of the lingula with corresponding vertical safety distance between the lingula/neurovascular bundle and the horizontal osteotomy line on the lingual side.

By using special retractors to protect the soft tissues and by careful positioning of the retractors superior and posterior to the lingula.

2.2 Maxillary Artery

The maxillary artery runs directly under the periosteum in front of or behind the lateral pterygoid muscle and ascends through the two heads of the lateral pterygoid muscle to the pterygopalatine fossa (Fig. 18.1).

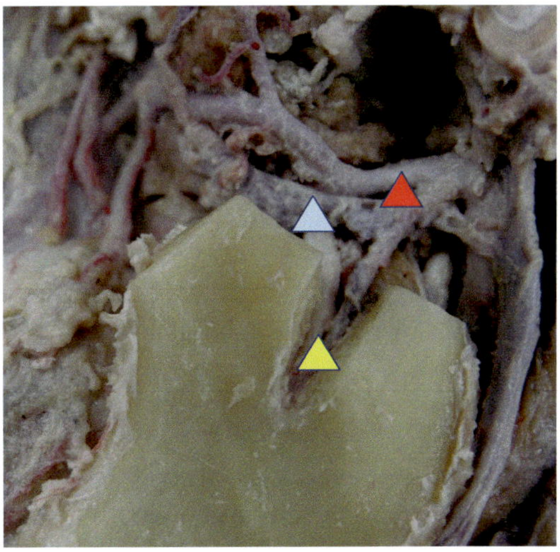

Fig. 18.1 Course of the maxillary artery in the profound region of the face. The maxillary artery is marked red triangle at the crossing with the lateral pterygoid muscle. Concomitant veins are marked with blue triangle. The neurovascular bundle entering the mandibular canal is marked with yellow triangle. The muscular (coronoid process) and condylar processes is resected.

Surgical trauma/tearing/rupture of the maxillary artery or its branches is usually the result of a non-conforming approach to the planned osteotomy site on the lingual side of the ascending mandibular ramus. Lack of exposure and visualization of the relevant structures in this not always clearly arranged region is the reason for loss of orientation. The leading structure is the neurovascular bundle of the inferior alveolar nerve, artery, and vein.

The direct cause is a laceration of the periosteum/the pterygoid muscle and the associated rupture of the maxillary artery or its branches running under the periosteum.

Careful subperiosteal dissection along the base of the muscular process (coronoid process) to the posterior edge of the mandibular ramus and subsequent careful widening of the lingual tunnel prevents injuries to the maxillary artery.

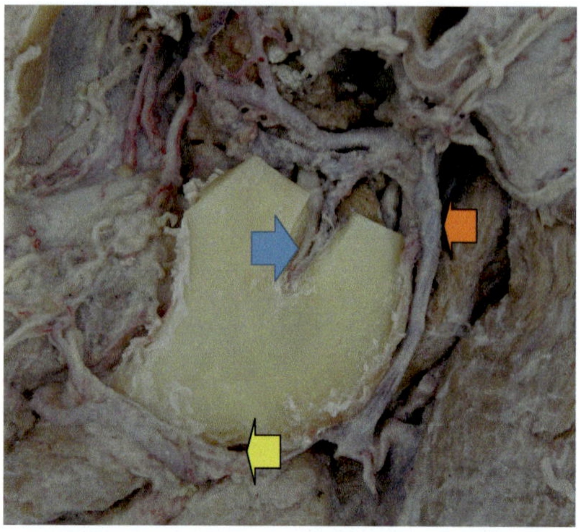

Fig. 18.2 The vascular environment of the region where the BSSO is performed. Lateral sagittal section—retromandibular region and temporomandibular joint (resected). Retromandibular venous plexus is dissected (orange arrow). Mandibular canal is opened (blue arrow). Facial artery and vein at the crossing point of the mandible (yellow arrow).©Copyright Department Anatomy and Embryology Maastricht University, 2021. All rights reserved

3 Prevention of Vascular Injuries in the Retromandibular Region

3.1 Retromandibular Vein/Retromandibular Venous Vascular Plexus

The posterior margin of the ascending mandibular ramus, which should be carefully prepared subperiosteally, must be clearly visible and protected if injury to the retromandibular venous vessels by the drill/instruments is to be avoided. Careful handling virtually eliminates the likelihood of retromandibular bleeding. Under certain circumstances, injuries to the retromolar vein can lead to life-threatening bleeding (Fig. 18.2).

Therapy: Hemostasis via the surgical access route, if unavoidable also via an extraoral access.

Note
Profuse venous bleeding due to injury to the retromandibular venous plexus is due to "blind stripping" of the periosteum and the muscles of the posterior margin of the ramus

4 Intraoperative Measures for Vascular Lesions

4.1 Inferior Alveolar Artery

Bleeding of the inferior alveolar artery and vein can usually be easily stopped with the bipolar forceps.

CAVE: Lesion of the inferior alveolar nerve—possibly also of the lingual nerve—when bleeding from the mandibular canal or tissue outside the osteotomy area.

4.2 Maxillary Artery

The maxillary artery runs directly under the periosteum in front of or behind the lateral pterygoid muscle and ascends through the two heads of the lateral pterygoid muscle to the pterygopalatine fossa (Rohen and Yokochi 1982, [6]).

If the injured artery cannot be visualized directly, the bleeding site should be temporarily compressed with gauzes. For serious bleeding digital pressure against the external or even common carotid artery can help to temporarily reduce excessive bleeding until the vessel is identified and vessel clips can be applied. Alternatively, in case of a threatening bleeding a minimally invasive embolizing vascular transcatheter closure may be considered.

4.3 Facial Artery

Precise detachment of the periosteum at the edge of the lower jaw in the area of the vertical osteotomy, if possible without tearing the periosteum, and the insertion of a protective, curved retractor prevents injuries to the facial artery.

Hemostasis through the surgical access, in extreme situations also through an extraoral access. There is an increased risk of inadvertently injuring the mandibular branch of the facial nerve due to poor visibility by coagulation through the transoral approach. The submandibular approach and preparation of the facial artery and its ligature can be performed by extraoral submandibular access, while protecting the mandibular branch of the facial nerve.

5 Nerve Injuries

- Inferior alveolar nerve—IAN.
  Course in the mandibular canal/mandibular foramen.
- Lingual nerve
  Lingual side /pterygomandibular space/floor of the mouth.
- Facial nerve
  Retro- and submandibular part

6 Paresthesia/Anesthesia

After osteotomies in the mandible, the risk of nerve injuries with long-term neurosensory deficits is higher than after upper jaw osteotomies. The combination of a BSSO with genioplasty increases the incidence of long-term neurosensory IAN deficits.

Paresthesia/anesthesia of the IAN is caused by a direct injury or contusion in the area of the lingula or by a split-related injury/contusion in the area of the sagittal split.

Functional deficits of the facial nerve result from a direct injury through instrumentation retromandibular (rare) and of the lingual nerve through pressure and stretching during mobilization of the mandibular segments or during osteosynthesis of the segments. The IAN can also be injured during screw and/or plate stabilization.

An operating age > 40 years, additional intraoperative manipulations, wide segment displacements and excessive segment manipulations as well as anatomical variations in the course of the nerves can lead to an increased incidence of neurosensory deficits after the operation [5].

7 Damage to the IAN

Surgical interventions of all kind are generally associated with the risk of injury to neural structures. Injuries to the IAN can generally occur during a BSSO, while splitting the mandible (osteotomy), during segment mobilization or segment fixation (osteosynthesis).

7.1 In Detail, Intraoperative Injuries of the IAN Occur:

- During the dissection of the lingual pterygomandibular tunnel and when the lingual horizontal osteotomy is performed.
- When performing the sagittal osteotomy, if the osteotomy line is not strictly laterally placed (buccal mandibular cortex).
- If the vertical osteotomy line is applied, if the bone cut is too deep or the basal mandibular cortex is incised too deeply (inferior mandibular rim). The buccal vertical osteotomy should be terminated when bleeding from cancellous bone indicates that the buccal cortex has been completely cut.

7.2 Injuries to the Inferior Alveolar Nerve Can Be Avoided by:

- Strictly subperiosteal tunneling of the medial side of the ascending ramus.
- Avoidance of stretching of the nerve by the tissue retractor on the lingual side.
- Rotating and oscillating instruments should exclusively and specifically be used for the separation of the cortical structures.
- Osteotomes must be guided during the split of the cortex on the lingual side.

The incidence of complete nerve transection in orthognathic surgery is low. The incidence of a complete transection of the IAN during a BSSO is reported as 1.3–7% [5, 25].

A neurosensory disturbance of the IAN occurs in most cases immediately after the BSSO. However, long-term deficits of the IAN (not all of which are symptomatic) occur in 10–15% of patients under 40 years of age. The overall risk of IAN deficits after BSSO was estimated of about 33% [5].

In order to reduce IAN injuries, it is important to evaluate the course of IAN preoperatively, if possible with three-dimensional imaging (CBCT, MSCT). At least an orthopantomogram must be performed preoperatively, since several variations of the course of IAN through the mandible are possible [1].

Note

Neurosensory disturbances of the inferior alveolar nerve occur in the vast majority of cases immediately after sagittal split osteotomy and cannot be entirely avoided.

Long-term deficits (not all of which are symptomatic) occur in 10–15% of patients younger than 40 years.

7.3 Treatment of IAN Injuries

7.3.1 Complete Transection of the Inferior Alveolar Nerve—IAN

If a complete IAN transection occurs—e.g., during a mandibular advancement procedure—the distal nerve segment should be released from the mandibular canal to gain sufficient length for the primary anastomosis of the nerve (Fig. 18.3) [22].

The use of a surgical microscope is extremely difficult, so magnifying glasses with magnifying optics must be used for a direct nerve suture.

Strategy: If the IAN is completely transected in the area of the mandibular foramen during a BSSO at the level of the lingula:

The proximal segment of the mandible is retracted laterally and the proximal nerve segment is carefully freed from the surrounding soft tissue. The distal nerve segment is prepared from the distal mandible.

The IAN lies on the lingual side of the distal segment if the split is correct. Nerve continuity can be restored by primary nerve anastomosis using epineural sutures, usually 7–0 Prolene. The proximal nerve end is grasped first, as the distal

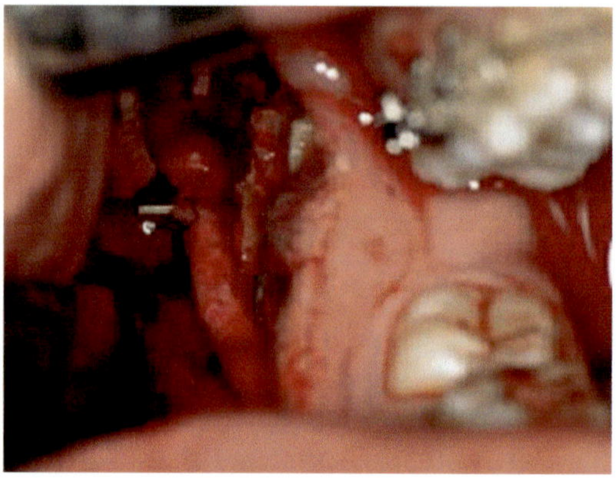

Fig. 18.3 Complete transection of the IAN in the region of the mandibular foramen during BSSO [5]

nerve end allows more freedom of movement. At least three circular sutures should be applied 6-0 or even 5-0 Prolene can be used as well.

8 Damage to the Lingual Nerve

Osteotomy-related sensitivity disorders of the lingual nerve are not common. Immediate postoperative tongue paresthesia due to an alteration of the lingual nerve occurs in less than 10% of patients.

The risk of long-term lingual nerve deficits after BSSO ranges from 1% to 12% [5, 24, 25].

> **Note**
> Lingual sensory nerve disturbances are not common.
>
> Immediate postoperative tongue paresthesia secondary to lingual nerve injury probably occurs in less than 10% of patients.
>
> Long-term deficit occurs in less than 1–12%.

8.1 Injuries to the Lingual Nerve can be avoided by:

- Appropriate placement of the retromolar mucosal incision.
- Careful subperiosteal preparation of the lingual tissues, especially in the area of the third molar.
- If bi-cortical screws are used: Due to the proximity of the lingual nerve to the lingual mandibular cortex, penetration of bi-cortical screws should be avoided as this may increase the risk of nerve injury.
- If bi-cortical screws are used: Placement of a retractor between the lingual cortex and lingual soft tissues prevents iatrogenic injury to the lingual nerve during placement of drill holes for screw fixation.
- After placement of bi-cortical screws, the lingual cortex should be palpated with a finger to feel protruding screws. These screws should be removed and replaced with shorter screws.

> **Note**
> The placement of a flexible retractor between the lingual mandibular cortex and lingual soft tissues during bi-cortical screw osteosynthesis is the best way to prevent iatrogenic injury to the lingual nerve.
>
> The use of bucco-laterally positioned mono-cortical osteosynthesis plates avoids the abovementioned risk.

8.2 Treatment of Lingual Nerve Injuries

8.2.1 Complete Transection of the Lingual Nerve

Two procedures exist:

The direct nerve suture can be performed immediately after the nerve rupture is detected. The nerve endings are carefully removed from the surrounding soft tissue—about two centimeters proximally and distally—and adapted with prolene 7x0 under suitable optical magnification. The nerve sheath must be grasped with the utmost care, it is extremely vulnerable.

Alternatively, there is the possibility of delayed nerve suturing about 6 weeks postoperatively. If the nerve endings cannot be adapted without problems, nerve interpositions, e.g., of the sural or posterior auricular nerve, must be lifted to be inserted between the nerve stumps. The delayed procedure has its justification in the generally poor functional regeneration of this nerve (Fig. 18.4).

The inserted nerve autograft can be wrapped with Axoguard® nerve protector as a tissue separator to prevent connective tissue from growing into the nerve anastomoses.

To avoid the morbidity caused by lifting a neural autograft, neural allografts can also be used.

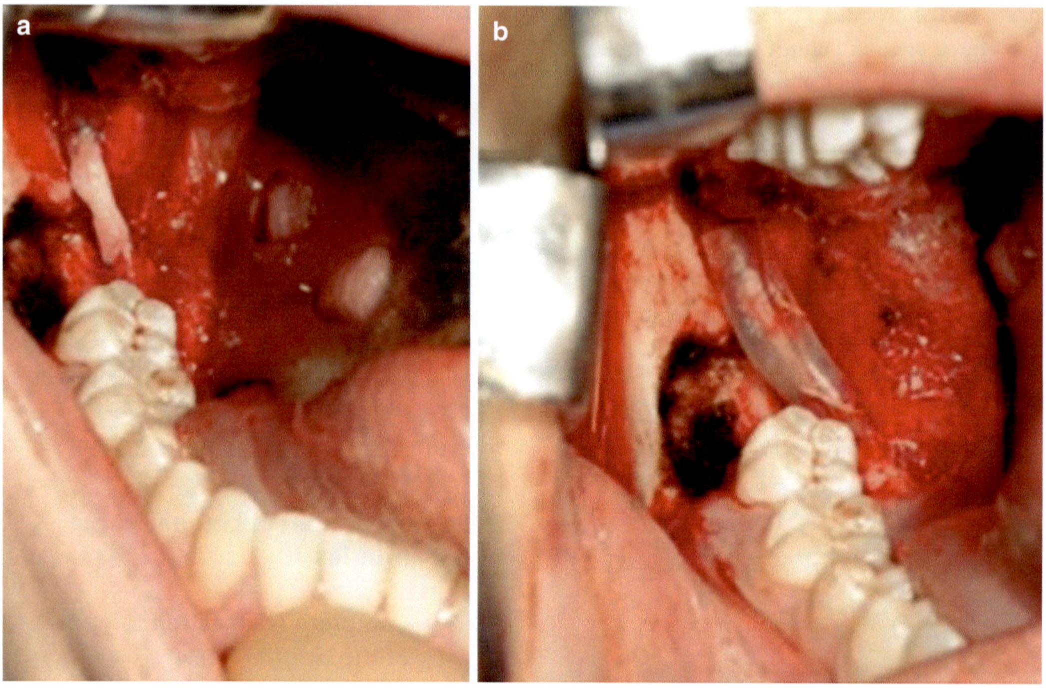

Fig. 18.4 (**a**) Nerve interposition for complete transection of the lingual nerve. (**b**) Protection of the interposition with Axoguard® nerve protector [5]

9 Damage to the Facial Nerve

Complete facial paralysis or partial paresis as a result of an injury to the facial nerve is extremely rare and is typically associated with surgery on a setback of the lower jaw and usually resolves spontaneously. Although rare, facial nerve injury leads to significant morbidity for the patient.

Facial nerve deficits after BSSO are reported in the literature with an incidence of 0.1–1% [5, 10].

Damage to the marginal branch of the facial nerve:

The marginal branch can be injured by very careless instrumentation when the bucco-lateral bone cut is made. Injuries due to pressure, tension and stretching, but also direct trauma from drills or chisels cannot be excluded. Nerve adaptation is technically almost impossible and can only be carried out via a submandibular approach.

Note

Facial paralysis or paresis secondary to facial nerve injury is extremely rare and typically is associated with mandibular setback procedures.

Facial nerve disturbances associated with sagittal split osteotomies have resolved spontaneously in all reported cases.

Note

Injuries to the facial nerve can be avoided by careful subperiosteal dissection and avoidance of periosteal injuries to the posterior margin of the ramus and by gentle tissue retraction. The same applies for the buccal osteotomy line.

10 Split Patterns during BSSO

10.1 Sagittal Split Variants

In general, only 0.5% of sagittal splits follow exactly the osteotomy lines according to Obwegeser and Dal Pont, while 40% follow the osteotomy lines of the Hunsuck-Epker modification.

After BSSO, different fracture patterns can be detected, especially in the lingual fracture line (Fig. 18.5) [2, 4, 8, 9, 14, 19].

The split pattern of type I was found in 60%, types II, III, and IV accounted for 11.2%, 16.2%, and 5.0%, respectively, and type V for 7.5%. Type VI represents a bad split.

According to the lingual split scale—Lingual Split Scale (LSS) [14], in 51% of cases the fracture line (LSS1) runs from the inferior mandibular rim (bucco-lateral bone cut end) in a vertical arc through the lingual cortex and reaches the mandibular foramen ("true Hunsuck"). LSS1 runs dorsally of the mandibular canal.

The LSS2 fracture line (14%) runs from the inferior mandibular rim along the dorsal rim of the mandibular angle and corresponds to the classic osteotomy through the posterior margin ("true Obwegeser").

The LSS3 fracture line (32.5%) runs from the inferior mandibular rim directly vertically through the lingual cortex and ends in the mandibular canal in the region of the lingula (Figs. 18.5 and 18.6)

The unfavorable splits occur mainly in the angular and supra-angular region (Fig. 18.7).

Experience has shown that regardless of the osteotomy technique used, only a minority of splits follow the fracture pattern indicated by Obwegeser and Dal Pont.

The vast majority of fracture lines follow the lingual side from the dorsal end of the lingual cut to the caudal end of the buccal osteotomy rather randomly [2, 3, 12, 19].

10.2 Bad Splits in BSSO

An unfavorable and unforeseen pattern of sagittal split osteotomy is commonly referred to as "bad split " [7, 11, 13, 15].

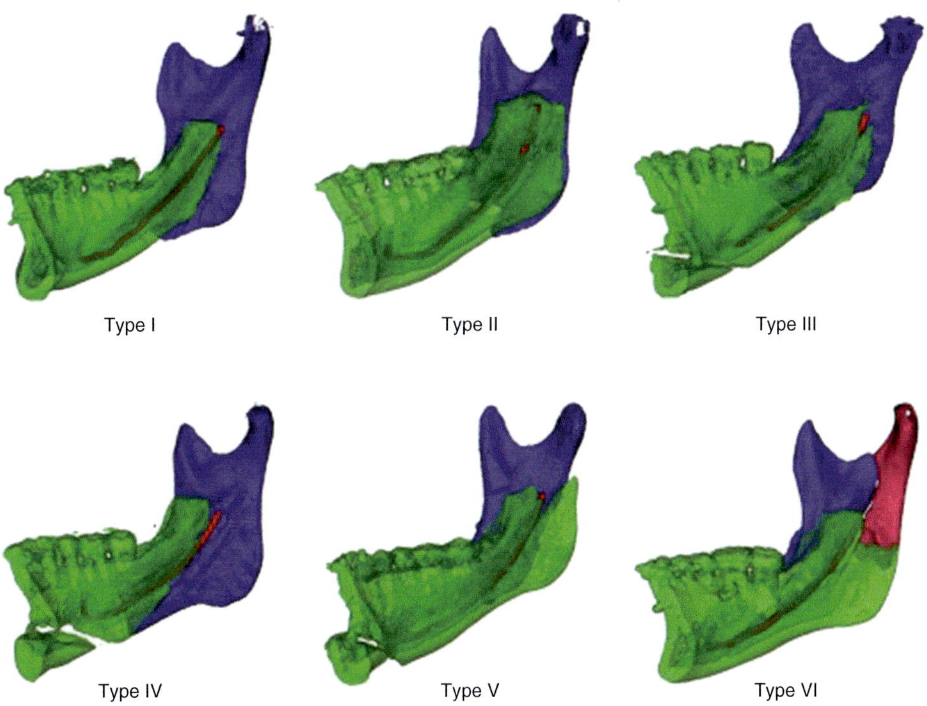

Fig. 18.5 Variations of the course of the fracture line after bilateral sagittal split osteotomy on the lingual side of the ramus (types I to VI) [14]

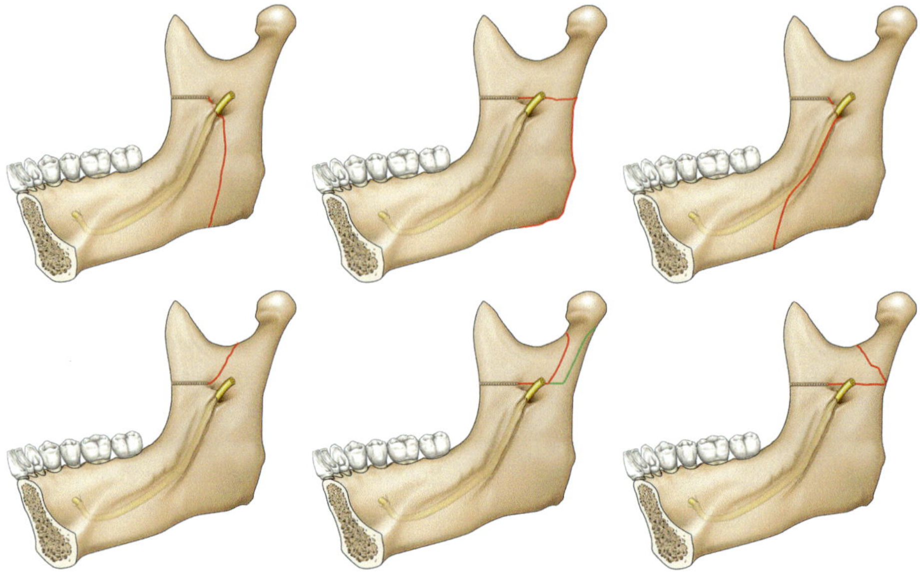

Fig. 18.6 Fracture patterns after sagittal split on the lingual side of the ramus. Upper row: Schematic drawing of the main types of lingual split LSS 1 to LSS 3 [14] Lower row: Variants of bad splits on the lingual side. ©Copyright Keisuke Koyama 2020. All rights reserved

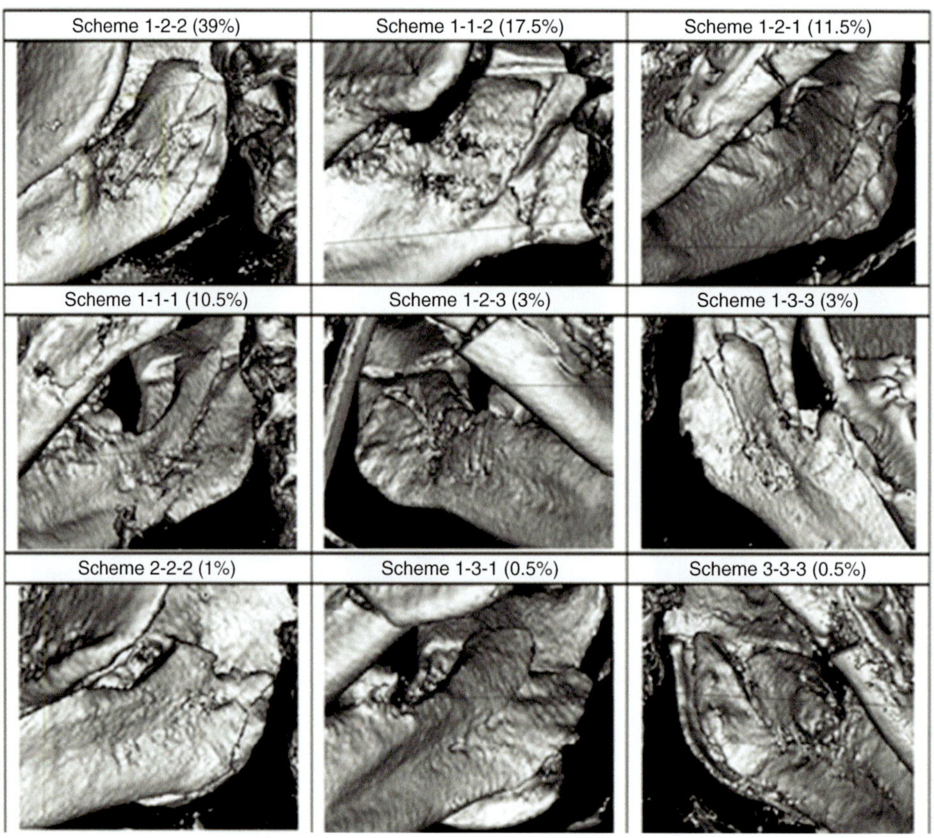

Fig. 18.7 Lingual views after 3D reconstruction of nine more frequent split patterns and their percentage distribution (based on 200 sagittal splits) [3]

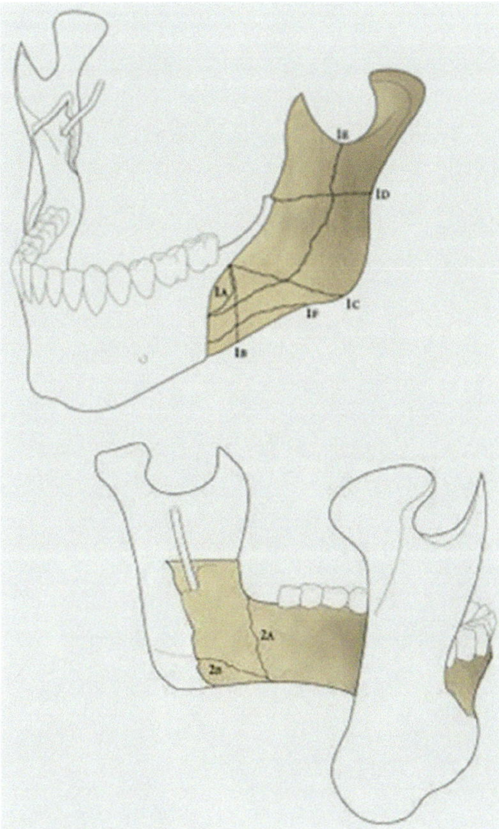

Fig. 18.8 Iatrogenic bad fractures of the proximal segment (Types 1A-1F) and of the distal segment (Types 2A und 2B) (postoperative—CBCT—Images) [20, 21]

The incidence of a bad split BSSO ranges from 2.3% [21] to 13.5%. The latter mainly affected the buccal surface of the proximal segment to a majority of 9% [3].

The most common iatrogenic and unwanted bad splits affect the cortex of the proximal segment (type's 1A-1F) and then the lingual cortex of the distal segment (types 2A and 2B) (Fig. 18.8) [21].

A significant correlation was found between undesirable fracture patterns in the lateral buccal segment and the course of splitting.

This is the case for horizontal sagittal osteotomies that ended in buccal position at the posterior margin of the ramus (P-0.001) as well as for vertical caudal osteotomies that did not split the mandibular margin but ended in a buccal position above the mandibular rim (P-0.001) [3].

This means that the horizontal lingual osteotomy should not cut too deeply and the buccolateral osteotomy should include the mandibular margin to avoid undesirable fracture patterns (Fig. 18.9).

10.3 Danger Points: Bad Split

1. Horizontal lingual osteotomy performed too high above the lingula or horizontal osteotomy incision too deep to the buccal cortex
   - wrong preparation with the burr/ultrasonic osteotome,
2. Course of the sagittal connecting osteotomy line on the external oblique line and not median of the line.
   - wrong preparation with the burr/saw/ultrasonic osteotome,
3. Incomplete or omitted osteotomy of the inferior mandibular margin/rim on the buccal side.

   The risk of fracture of the buccal cortex is particularly high if the osteotomy of both bone segments at the inferior rim of the mandible is incomplete. An incomplete split occurs, the buccal cortical bone breaks off, and post-osteotomy surgery is required, putting the IAN at risk [3].

- Incomplete preparation with the burr/ultrasonic osteotome.
- Incomplete osteotomy of the inferior rim of the mandible.

4. Excessive, forced separation of the bone segments with transverse bone loading by twisting/rotation using wide osteotomes when

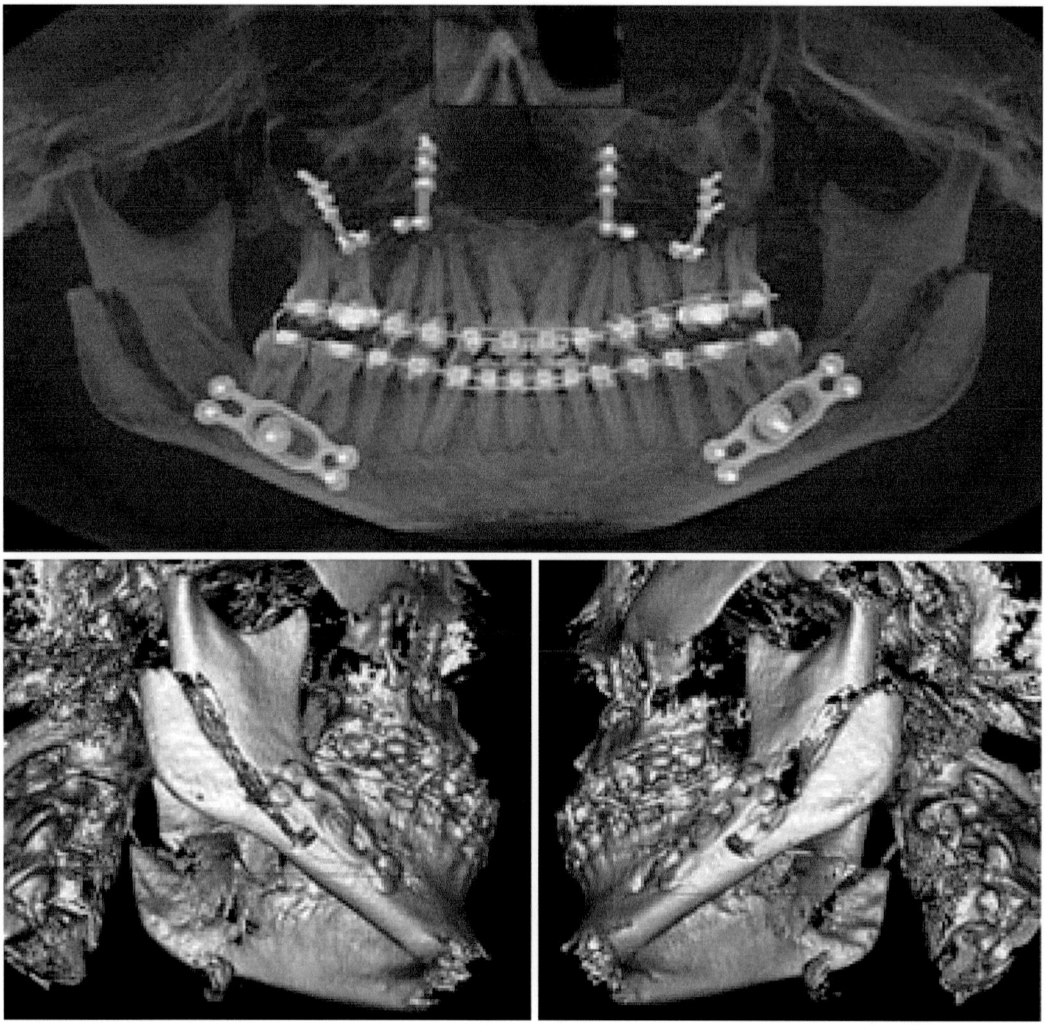

Fig. 18.9 Example of a bad split in the angular and supra-angular region. View from the lateral side after 3D reconstruction [3]

separating the proximal and distal segments (Fig. 18.10).
   - wrong splitting technique/wrong instrument,
5. Incomplete separation of the ramus posterior margin or the jaw angle with too early use of wide osteotomes.
   - wrong splitting technique/wrong instrument,
6. Use of chisels instead of finely ground osteotomes.
   - wrong instruments.

The extraction of the third molar teeth nine, six, or 3 months before BSSO or simultaneously with BSSO is controversially assessed with regard to its influence on the splitting quality [16–18].

The removal of afunctional or impacted third molars is generally recommended 6 months before a BSSO.

10.4 Avoidance of Bad Splits

Precise and step-by-step procedure of the splitting

- Horizontal lingual cut.

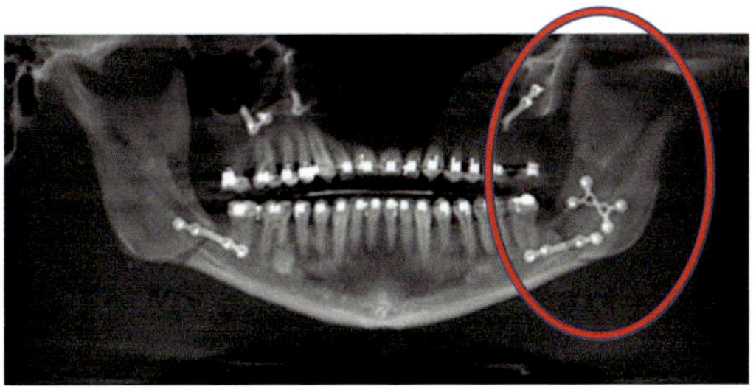

Fig. 18.10 Bad split on the left side with lingual split line running upward to the semilunar notch. Additional fixation plate. Compare with Fig. 18.6

Horizontal-medial osteotomy (complete) with fine osteotome (chisel) or Epker osteotome (chisel)

- Vertical buccal cut.

Vertical-buccal osteotomy (complete) with fine osteotome (chisel), or Epker osteotome (chisel) for entry and then a straight osteotomy

- Sagittal Cut.

Gradual, systematic deepening of the supra-IAN splitting zone, continuous splitting from distal to proximal with fine straight osteotomes (chisels) not wider than 10 mm

- Upon reaching the infra-IAN splitting zone.

Gradual splitting in constant alternation of fine osteotome (progressive split = use of the chisel) and wide osteotome (gap expansion, don't use chisels for this maneuver)

- Splitting of the mandibular margin/mandibular rim.

Starting from the lower part of the bucco-vertical osteotomy with a curved osteotome/chisel (Epker chisel e.g.)

- After advanced splitting of the infra-IAN fission zone.

Start of controlled rotation of the wide osteotome to expand the osteotomy gap and further splitting of the basal bony residual connections with a fine osteotome after identification of the mandibular canal under visual control.

Note

Working with the wide osteotome energetically and without feeling before completing all osteotomy steps leads to uncontrolled force and fracture lines.

Control of the complete split with fine osteotome. There must be no bony connections to be identified.

11 Complications during and Immediately after Extubation

- Greatest danger of suffocation is if the removal of the pharyngeal tamponade after extubation is forgotten with the jaw in intermaxillary fixation.
- Great danger exists if no wire cutter is provided when transporting the patient to the recovery room, so that in an emergency (e.g., vomiting) the intermaxillary fixation can be cut immediately.
- Great danger exists if there are fluctuations in blood pressure during the end of anesthesia leading to spontaneous bleeding from the wound area.
- Danger exists if the patient suffers from suffocation in the event of intermaxillary fixation and swelling of the nasal airways.
- If the lower jaw is repositioned, in unfavorable cases the tongue may be displaced dorsally and the upper respiratory tract may be obstructed, there is a risk of suffocation.
- Rare but dangerous are bleedings into the tongue, which can lead to massive swelling of the tongue with obstruction of the airways. Massive swelling of the tongue can also occur spontaneously without bleeding.

Note

The surgeon in charge should be present in the OR until spontaneous breathing has stabilized and, if necessary, accompany the patient to the recovery room.

12 Conclusion

There are no surgical interventions free of risks. Good anatomical knowledge, good case analysis, good education, and training are the prerequisites to recognize and avoid complications and also to manage complications.

References

1. Beukes J, Reyneke JP, Damstra J. Unilateral sagittal split mandibular ramus osteotomy: indications and geometry. Br J Oral Maxillofac Surg. 2016;54(2):219–23.
2. Böckmann R, Schön P, Neuking K, Meyns J, Kessler P, Eggeler G. In vitro comparison of the sagittal split osteotomy with and without inferior border osteotomy. J Oral Maxillofac Surg. 2015;73(2):316–23.
3. Dreiseidler TJJ, Bergmann GHM, Zirk M, Rothamel D, Zöller J, Kreppel M. Three-dimensional fracture pattern analysis of the Obwegeser and Dal Pont bilateral sagittal split osteotomy. Int J Oral Maxillofac Surg. 2016;45(11):1452–8.
4. Epker BN. Modifications in the sagittal osteotomy of the mandible. J Oral Surg. 1977;35(2):157–9.
5. Ghali GE, Patel S. Avoiding surgical complications in orthognathic surgery. In: Ghali GE, Woerner JE, Patel S, editors. Maxillofacial surgery: mandible. 3rd ed. Churchill Livingstone; 2017.
6. Hardt N, Kessler P. Surgical repair of craniofacial fractures. In: Hardt N, Kessler P, et al., editors. Craniofacial trauma. Diagnosis and management. Springer; 2010.
7. Hönig JF. Maxillomandibuläre Umstellungsosteotomien. Steinkopff; 2013.
8. Houppermans PNWJ, Verweij JP, Mensink G, Peter JJ, Gooris JP, van Merkesteyn R. Influence of inferior border cut on lingual fracture pattern during bilateral sagittal split osteotomy with splitter and separators: a prospective observational study. J Craniomaxillofac Surg. 2016;44(10):200.
9. Hu J, Song Y, Wang D, Yuan H, Jiang H, Cheng J. Patterns of lingual split and lateral bone cut end and their associations with neurosensory disturbance after bilateral sagittal split osteotomy. Int J Oral Maxillofac Surg. 2019;19(3):1311.
10. Kim YK. Complications associated with orthognathic surgery. J Korean Assoc Oral Maxillofac Surg. 2017;43(1):3–15.
11. Minde R, Schamsawary S. Mund-Kiefer-Gesichtschirurgie. Deutscher Ärzte-Verlag; 2008.
12. Muto T, Takahashi M, Akizuki K. Evaluation of the mandibular ramus fracture line after sagittal split ramus osteotomy using 3-dimensional computed tomography. J Oral Maxillofac Surg. 2012;70:e648–52.
13. O'Ryan F, Poor DB. Completing sagittal split osteotomy of the mandible after fracture of the buccal plate. J Oral Maxillofac Surg. 2004;62:1175–6.
14. Plooij JM, Naphausen MTP, Maal TJJ, Xi T, Rangel FA, Swennnen G, de Koning M, Borstlap WA, Berge S. 3D evaluation of the lingual fracture line after a bilateral sagittal split osteotomy of the mandible. Int J Oral Maxillofac Surg. 2009;38:1244–9.
15. Posnick JC, Choi E, Liu S. Occurrence of a 'bad' split and success of initial mandibular healing: a review of 524 sagittal ramus osteotomies in 262 patients. Int J Oral Maxillofac Surg. 2016;45:1187–94.
16. Precious DS, Lung KE, Pynn BR. Goodday RH presence of impacted teeth as a determining factor of unfavorable splits in 1256 sagittal-split osteotomies. Oral Surg Oral Med Oral Pathol Oral Radiol Endod. 1998;85:362–5.
17. Reyneke JP, Tsakiris P, Becker P. Age as a factor in the complication rate after removal of unerupted/impacted third molars. At the time of mandibular sagittal split osteotomy. J Oral Maxillofac Surg. 2002;60:654–9.
18. Schwartz HC. Simultaneous removal of third molars during sagittal split osteotomies: the case against. J Oral Maxillofac Surg. 2004;62:1147–9.
19. Song JM, Kim YD. Three-dimensional evaluation of lingual split line after bilateral sagittal split osteotomy in asymmetric prognathism. J Korean Assoc Oral Maxillofac Surg. 2014;40:11–6.
20. Steenen SA, van Wijk AJ, Becking AG. Bad splits in bilateral sagittal split osteotomy: systematic review and meta-analysis of reported risk factors. Int J Oral Maxillofac Surg. 2016;45:971–9.
21. Steenen SA, Becking AG. Bad splits in bilateral sagittal split osteotomy: systematic review of fracture patterns. Int J Oral Maxillofac Surg. 2016;45:887–97.
22. Stotland MA, Kawamoto HK. Plastic Surgery Secrets Plus. 2nd ed; 2010.
23. Thastum M, Andersen K, Rude K, Nørholt SE, Blomlöf J. Factors influencing intraoperative blood loss in orthognathic surgery. Int J Oral Maxillofac Surg. 2016;45:1070–3.
24. van Merkesteyn JPR, Groot RH, van Leeuwaarden R. Kroon FHM Intra-operative complications in sagittal and vertical ramus osteotomies. Int J Oral Maxillofac Surg. 1987;16(6):665–70.
25. Verweij JP, Houppermans PN, Mensink GP, van Merkesteyn JP. Risk factors for common complications associated with bilateral sagittal split osteotomy: a literature review and meta-analysis. J Craniomaxillofac Surg. 2016;44(9):1170–80.

Further Readings

Rohen J, Yokochi C. Anatomie des Menschen/Kopf, Hals. Schattauer: Rumpf-Band; 1982.

Surgical Tricks

19

Peter Kessler, Nicolas Hardt, and Suen An Nynke Lie

Contents

P. Kessler (✉) · S. A. N. Lie
Department of Cranio-Maxillofacial Surgery, Maastricht University Medical Center, Maastricht, The Netherlands
e-mail: peter.kessler@mumc.nl; suen.lie@mumc.nl

N. Hardt (✉)
Kantonsspital Lucerne, Clinic and Policlinic of Cranio-Maxillofacial Surgery, Lucerne, Switzerland

P. Kessler et al. (eds.), *Illustrated Manual of Orthognathic Surgery*,
https://doi.org/10.1007/978-3-031-06978-9_19

Abstract

Each surgical procedure becomes safer with increasing experience, and each surgeon will find his or her own style of successfully performing a sagittal split osteotomy of the mandible. At the same time, you develop your style, which may be alien to others. What is routine to one is new to another. The reference to surgical tricks and recommendations should help to close this gap.

Keywords

Anatomy of the mandible · Approach · Preparation for sagittal split · Lingula · Osteotomy lines · Osteotomy of the mandible · BSSO · Sagittal split ramus osteotomy (SSRO) · Osteotome

1 Display of Important Anatomical Points and Structures in BSSO

1.1 Mucoperiosteal Incision in Relation to the Nerve Branches near the Ramus, the Muscular and Vascular Structures

A vestibular placement of the mucosal incision in the posterior mandibular vestibule and in the retromolar region, clearly lateral to the marginal periodontium, prevents injury to the lingual nerve, which is located close to the ramus on the lingual side, and provides sufficient cuff tissue during subsequent wound closure. The buccal artery and vein cross the muco-periosteal incision and must be coagulated.

However, avoid lateral vestibular overextension of the incision, which can result in injury to the buccinator muscle and possible herniation of the buccal fat pad (corpus adiposum buccae) [1, 2]. The scalpel blade should always be in contact with underlying bone tissue to avoid straying into the layers of buccal soft tissue or even lingually located structures (Fig. 19.1).

Note

Creation of the mucosal incision

- Point of orientation: External oblique line.
- Surgical access: Lateral to the external oblique line.
- Cutting length: Continuous mucoperiosteal incision from the temporal/coronoid process to the crista buccinatoria in the region of the second molars.

Note

- Access to the sub-masseteric space.
  Subfascial space between the lateral surface of ascending mandibular ramus and fascia of the masseteric muscle.
- Surgical access: Anterior aspect of the ramus.
  External oblique line.
  Coronoid process.
- Landmarks: Base of the condylar process.
  Incisura semilunaris.
  Posterior aspect of the ascending ramus.
  Mandibular angle.

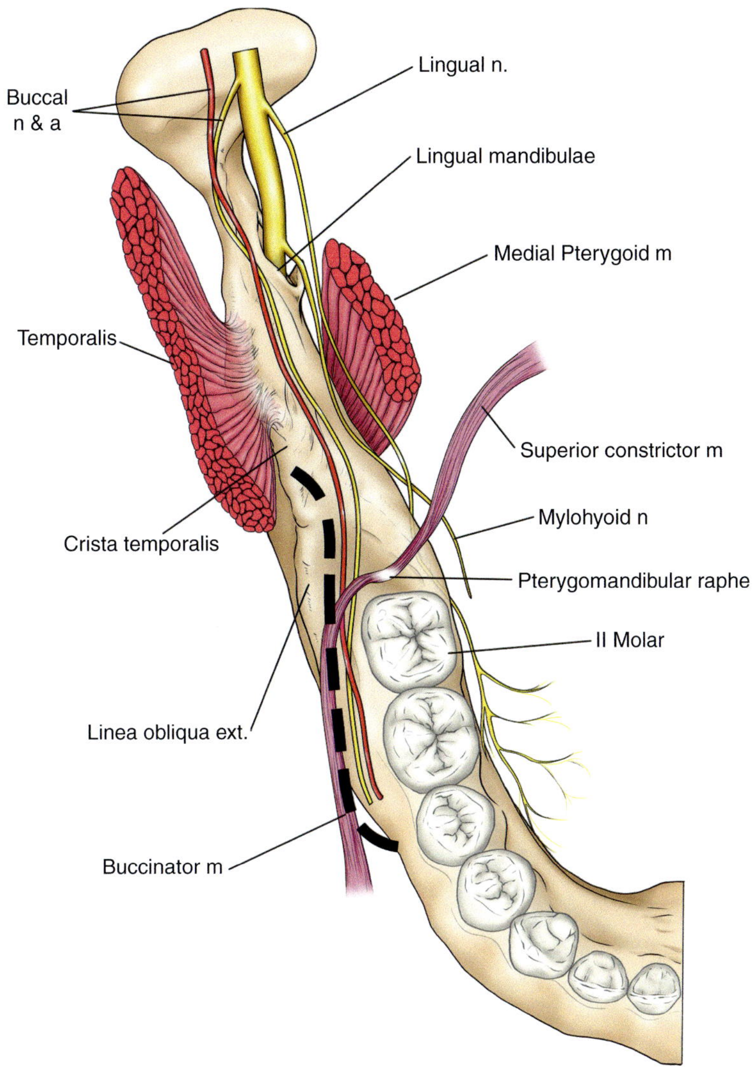

Fig. 19.1 Muco-periosteal incision (black-broken line). View of the retromolar region and the ascending ramus and the relationships of the buccal nerve, artery, and vein such as the lingual nerve to the medial border of the retromolar fossa.

2 Preparation of the Masseterico-mandibular and Pterygo-Mandibular Spaces

Strictly subperiosteal preparation of the masseterico-mandibular and the pterygo-mandibular spaces with identification of the respective anatomical lead structures (Fig. 19.2a, b; Fig. 19.3). Detachment of the neuro-vascular bundle on the lingual side and preparation to the posterior margin of the ramus.

The pterygo-mandibular periosteal deflection on the lingual side is then widened into a viewable subperiosteal tunnel and carried to the posterior margin of the ramus or immediately posterior to the neurovascular bundle at the mandibular foramen. The medial bone surface is visualized to the lingula and the neurovascular bundle can be identified (Fig. 19.4).

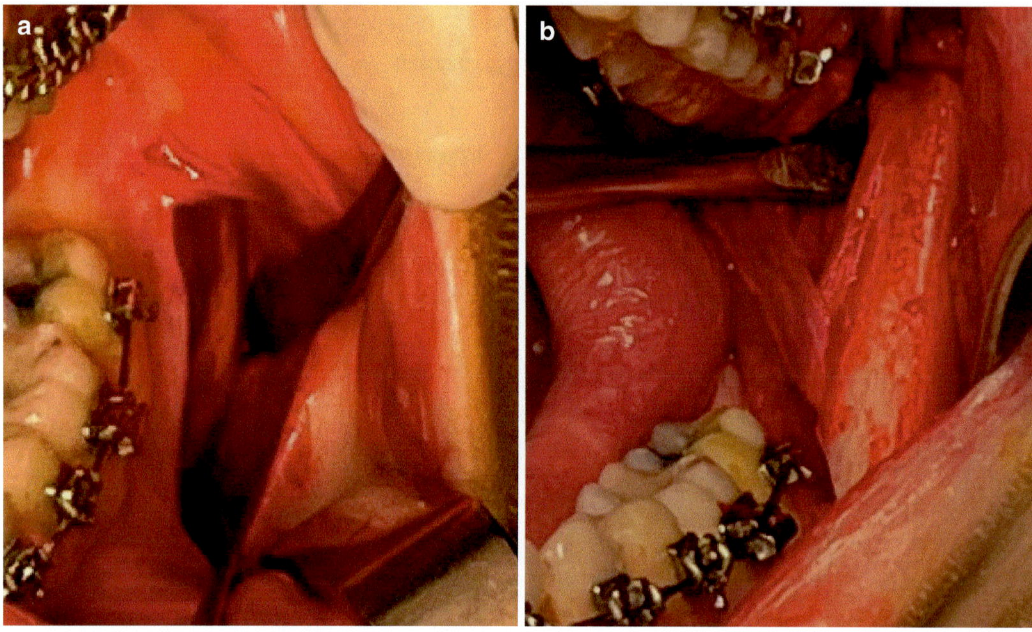

Fig. 19.2 (**a**) Preparation of the masseterico-mandibular space (**b**) Preparation of the ptergygo-mandibular space

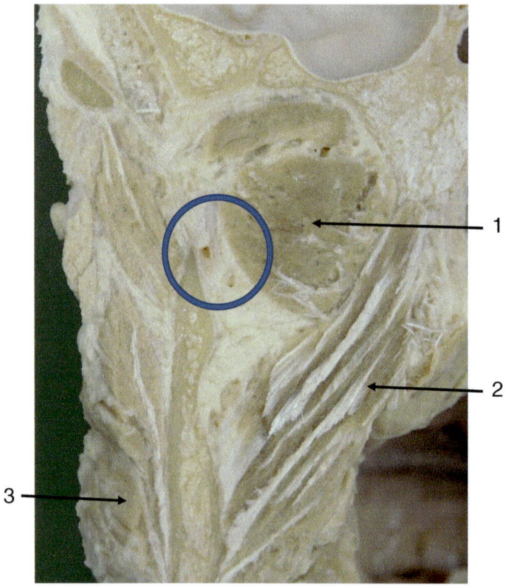

Fig. 19.3 Frontal section: Topographic situation in the pterygo-mandibular and masseterico-mandibular spaces. Vascular structures in pterygomandibular region are encircled: maxillary artery and vein 1 = lateral pterygoid muscle, 2 = medial pterygoid muscle, 3 = masseteric muscle

Note

- Access to the pterygo-mandibular space.
  Subfascial space between the medial surface of ramus and fascia of the medial pterygoid muscle.
- Surgical approach.
  Base of the coronoid process.
- Landmarks.
  Oblique external and internal line.
  Semilunar notch.
  Mandibular foramen.
  Lingula.
  Neuro-vascular bundle.
  Base of the condylar process.
  Posterior border of the ascending ramus on the medial side.

Note

The more generous the detachment of the soft tissues on the lingual side—containing the neuro-vascular bundle—the more safely the vessels and nerves (maxillary artery and inferior alveolar nerve) woven into the tendon-muscle plate can be spared.

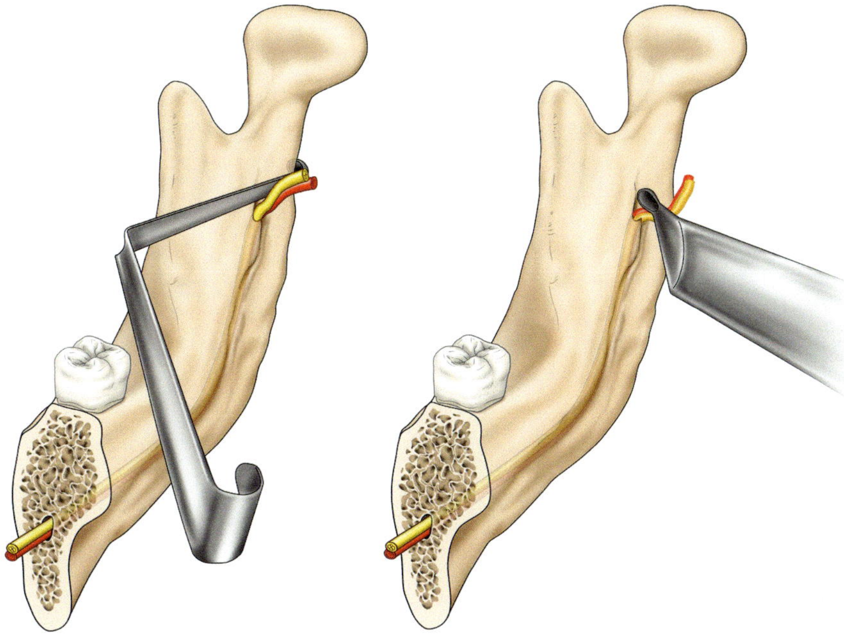

Fig. 19.4 Two possible positions of the retractor on the lingual side

3 Identification of the Mandibular Foramen and the Neurovascular Bundle

A retractor (Seldin retractor, e.g.) is inserted superior to the lingula into the lingual subperiosteal tunnel and tilted 45° so that the periosteum is tented in the area of the foramen.

Under direct visualization, the entrance to the foramen is identified and a blunt nerve probe is placed in the foramen entrance. The nerve probe is thus located at the upper edge of the foramen—corresponding to the position of the lingula (Fig. 19.5).

This procedure allows the bony distance between the lingula and the lingually planned osteotomy line to be estimated slightly above this level.

Prior to osteotomy, the retractor is then tilted 45° to the opposite direction to protect the inferior alveolar neurovascular bundle and create space for the medial osteotomy [3].

The horizontal bone cut should be made as low as possible, close to and above (approx. 4–5 mm) the lingula. In this region, there is still enough cancellous bone between the external and internal cortices, which facilitates the split.

Note

The lingual osteotomy should be slightly above the lingula—corresponding to the position of the inserted nerve probe.

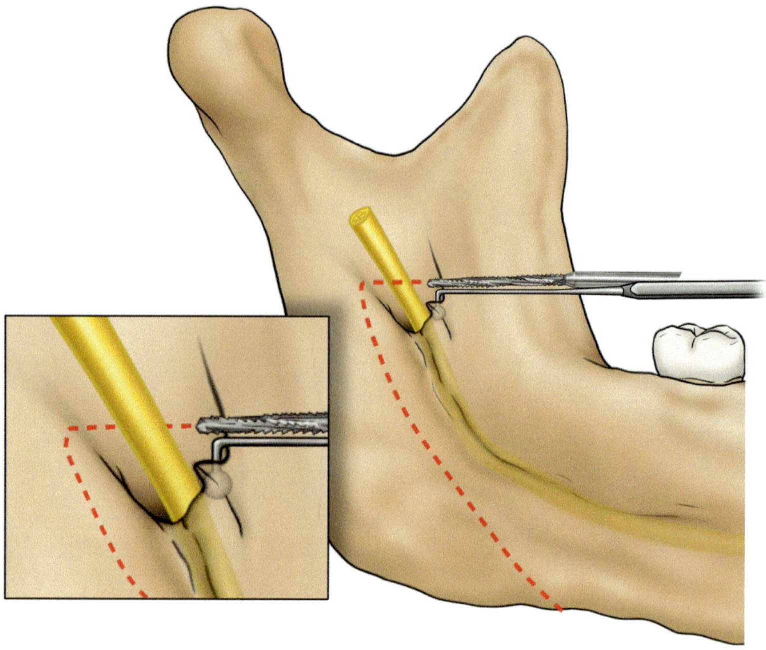

Fig. 19.5 Lateral view of the nerve probe placement in the mandibular foramen and the determination of the position of the osteotomy line.

4 Creation of Bone Cuts in Preparation of the Sagittal Split (SSRO/BSSO)

4.1 The Sagittal Osteotomy Line

The sagittal osteotomy runs medially and along the external oblique line. The creation of the preparatory drill holes for the sagittal osteotomy is difficult because of the rigidity of the thick and oblique bone surface.

Note
Creation of the sagittal osteotomy incision

- Osteotomy about 5 mm medial and parallel to the externa oblique line
- Length: From the intersection point of the lingual-horizontal cut to the point of intersection with the vertical-buccal cut.

A corticotomy of the narrow edge of the external oblique line to the visible boundary between cancellous bone and lateral cortex greatly facilitates the marking and creation of the sagittal osteotomy line with a small Lindemann burr [1, 2, 4]. Direction and path for the subsequent sagittal split are thus established (Fig. 19.6).

Note
The width of the osteotomy facilitates insertion and freedom of movement of the osteotome and avoids pressure loading and splintering of the ramus edge and allows a good guidance of the osteotome for the sagittal split.

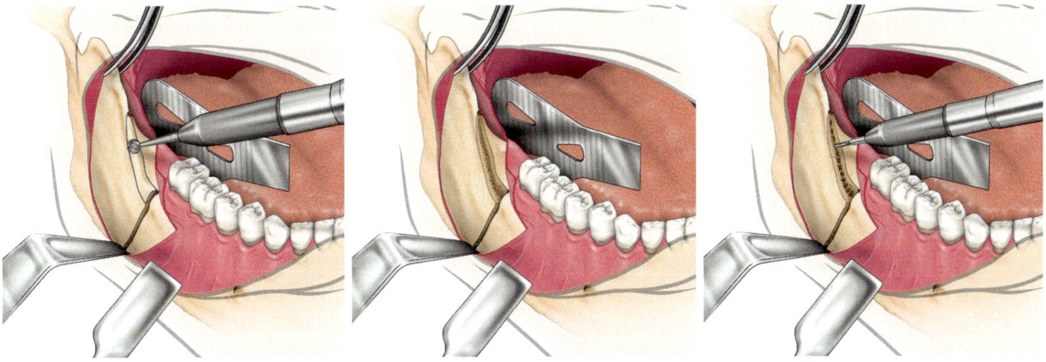

Fig. 19.6 Corticotomy of the edge of the external oblique line to the visible boundary between spongiosa and lateral cortex ([1, 2, 4]

5 Creation of the Horizontal Osteotomy Line (Fig. 19.7)

Note

Creation of the upper horizontal osteotomy incision

- Landmarks: about 10 mm inferior to the semilunar notch, 4–5 mm above the lingula.
- Position of the bone cut: horizontal and parallel the occlusal plane of the mandible.
- Length of the bone cut: Anterior margin of the ramus—internal oblique line to a point anterior to the posterior margin of the ascending ramus, but posterior to the *CEC* = crista endocoronoidea in the region of the coronoid sulcus—modification according to Hunsuck.

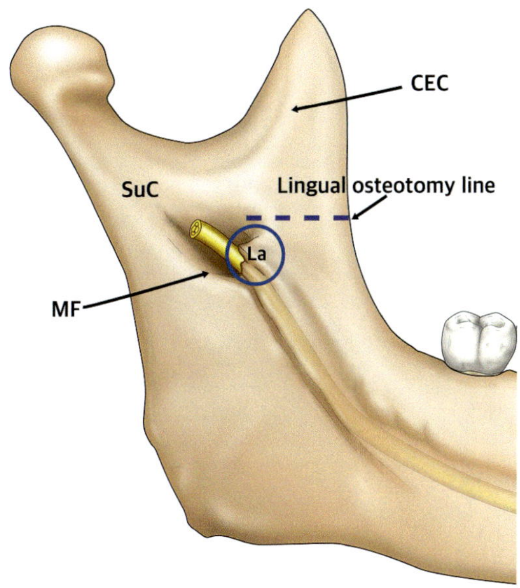

Fig. 19.7 Position of the lingual osteotomy line: *MF* mandibular foramen, *SuC* sulcus colli, *CEC* crista endocoronoidea, *La* lingula

Note

- Keep an eye on the outer surface of the ramus to estimate the depth of the lingual cut.
- Take into account that the inner cortical layer is concave on the inside.

6 Creation of the Vertical/Buccal Osteotomy Line

Note

Creation of the lower vertical osteotomy section

- Landmarks: second molar buccal aspect and end point of the external oblique line.
- Osteotomy straight downward to the region of the submandibular notch according to Dal Pont.
- Or oblique placement of the bone cut in direction to the attachment of the masseteric muscle—short osteotomy.

Note

In addition to transecting the buccal cortex, the inferior basal cortex is also transected down to the cancellous bone layer.

7 Correct Transitions and Pre-splitting of the Osteotomy Sections

After the horizontal, vertical, and sagittal bone cuts have been made, the transitions from the horizontal to the sagittal cut as well as the transition from the vertical to the sagittal bone cut—the so-called Steinhäuser Points—should be prepared deeply with the incremental drill so that there is good guidance for the splitting direction of the fine osteotomes. Both the horizontal and vertical bone cuts should then be carefully pre-split with fine osteotomes or chisels ([1, 2, 4] (Fig. 19.8).

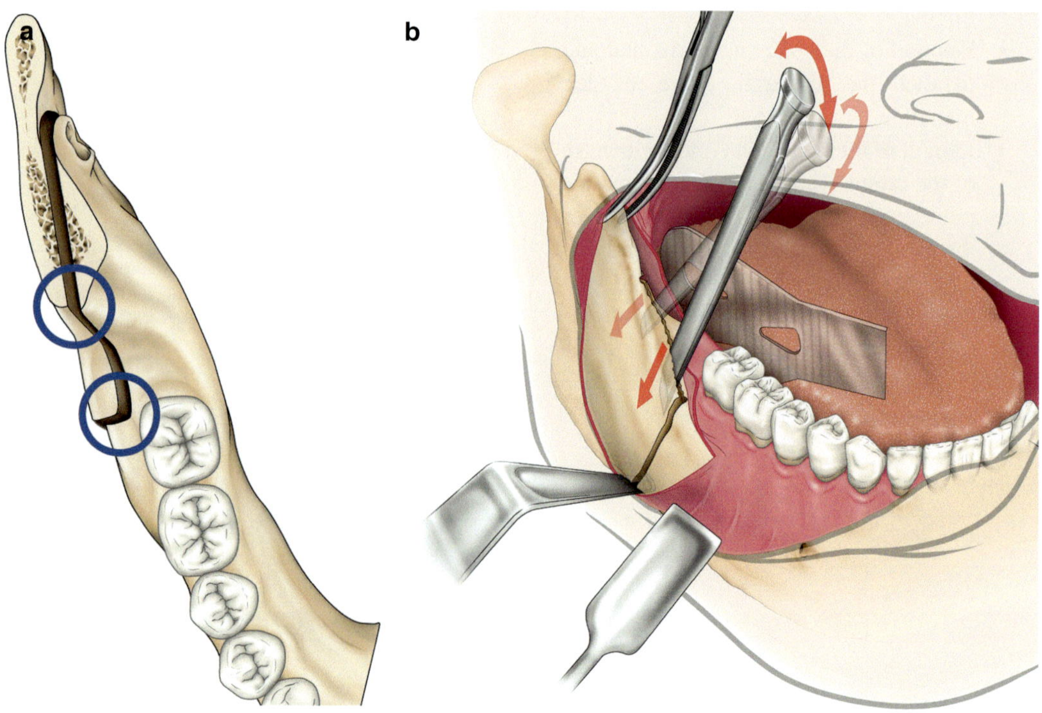

Fig. 19.8 (**a**) Careful and deep preparation of the connecting points—marked with circles—of the three basic osteotomy lines: lingual—sagittal—buccal (Steinhäuser Points) (**b**) Then careful beginning of the splitting procedure with fine chisels

8 Correct Mandibular Split

8.1 Technique of the Pre-angular Split

The mandibular canal runs in the pre-angular region near the lingual margin. Between the buccal cortex and the lateral canal wall there is a cancellous bone layer which is as wide as the adjacent lateral cortex (Fig. 19.9).

Split in the pre-angular section is successive and takes into account the surface curvature up to and including the jaw angle. This split region represents the "safe" zone in which the nerve or mandibular canal can be injured the least (Fig. 19.9b).

Note
Be consistent!

If you consequently stick to the inner side of buccal cortical layer while splitting the mandible the risk of injury to the IAN is minimal.

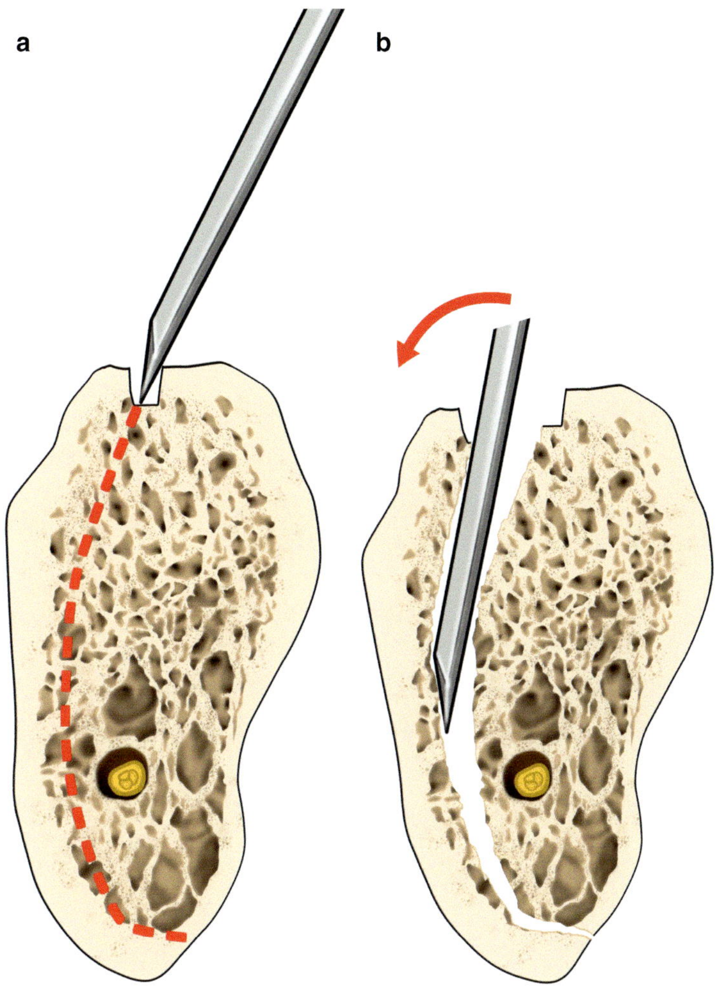

Fig. 19.9 Topography of the pre-angular region (**a**) The width of the lateral cancellous layer corresponds to the width of the lateral cortex (**b**) Successive splitting to the inferior mandibular rim ©Copyright Keisuke Koyama 2020. All rights reserved

8.2 Technique of Angular and Post-Angular Split

In the angular and post-angular sections, there is little to very little cancellous bone layer between the canal wall and the lateral cortex.

The most difficult part of the splitting is in the post-angular section. The split starts directly at the entrance to the lingual bone cut.

Basic direction of the osteotome: Lingula

Junction line of mandibular midline—oblique line (Fig. 19.10).

> **Note**
> Sagittal split in the post-angular section on the lingual side
>
> - Insert the chisel directly at the cranially located lingual bone cut:
>   30° to the outer surface of the ascending ramus (Fig. 19.10). Direction lingula.
>   The osteotome crosses the center of the anterior arch.
> - After a penetration depth of about 15 mm, slowly pivot the chisel in an oral direction. Under light, short hammer blows, the osteotome penetrates to the interface of the cortical bone slightly above or in the lingula.
> - Then the chisel is swiveled in the sagittal direction (parallel to the outer surface of the ascending ramus). The posterior section is split cranially of the mandibular angle. You can tell by the tapping sound when you have come through the bone.

> **Note**
> Sagittal split in the angular region
>
> After the split procedure has progressed to the point where the course of the mandibular canal is visible, one osteotome is left cranial to the canal and a second osteotome is used to continue the osteotomy along the outer cortex lateral to the canal to the mandibular angle.
>
> The last bony connections are carefully detached by spreader movements with an osteotome/spreader.

8.3 Avoidance of Iatrogenic Fractures during Splitting in the Proximal Segment: Lingual Split

The horizontal lingual osteotomy should not run too deep to the lateral cortex and not too high, but should be made just above the mandibular foramen.

In the original Obwegeser technique, the posterior margin of the ascending ramus must be included in the bone incision. Splitting is performed with finely ground straight chisels of 5 mm width.

For short split according to Hunsuck-Epker, the curved 5 mm Epker-chisel can serve well, with the curvature following the concave shape of the inner side of the ascending mandibular ramus.

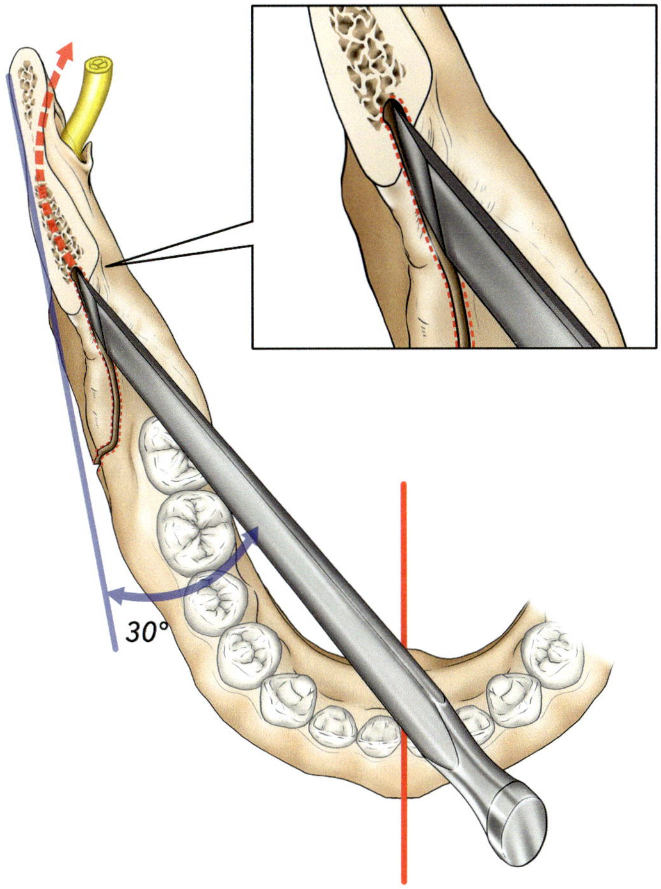

Fig. 19.10 Sagittal split in the post-angular section [5] ©Copyright Keisuke Koyama 2020. All rights reserved

8.4 Avoidance of Iatrogenic Fractures during Splitting in the Angular Region below the Mandibular Canal

To prevent undesirable fractures in the angular region below the course of the mandibular canal, the separation of the mandibular rim at the vertical buccal cut should be completed. The osteotome is inserted horizontally between the partially split bone segments in the region of the lower vertical bone cut. When separating the mandibular margin, the osteotome is pressed lightly against the distal segment to direct the splitting pressure against the inner surface of the proximal segment and the mandibular margin is pre-split (Figs. 19.11, 19.12).

Note
The sagittal split of the mandibular rim is performed before the splitting is completed in the region of the mandibular angle below the mandibular canal.

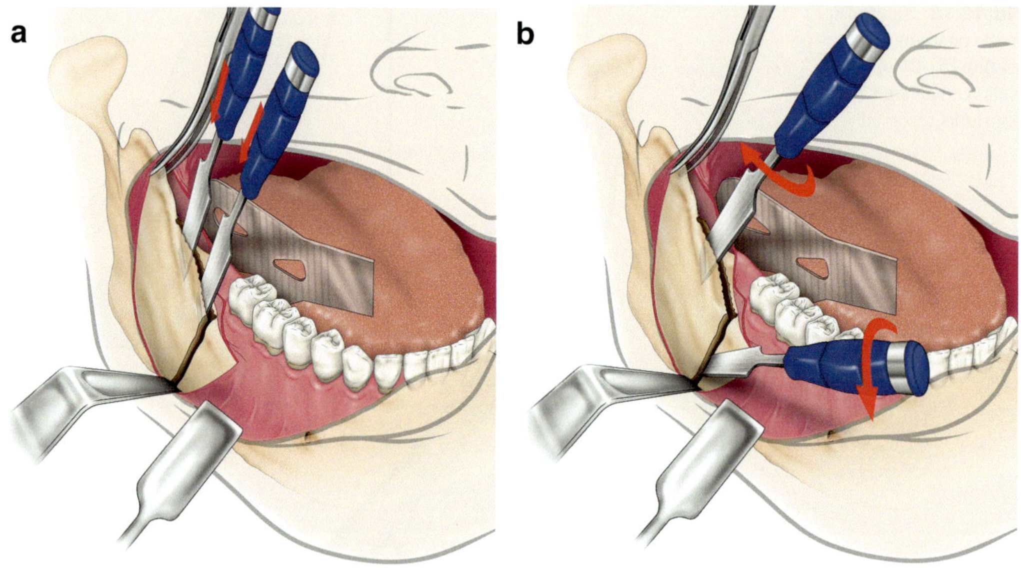

Fig. 19.11 Technique of the mandibular rim splitting (**a**) First the area above the mandibular canal is widened until the course of the IAN can be assumed (**b**) The osteotome is inserted horizontally in the region of the lower vertical bone cut. When separating the mandibular rim, the osteotome is pressed lightly against the distal segment to direct the splitting pressure against the inner surface of the proximal segment

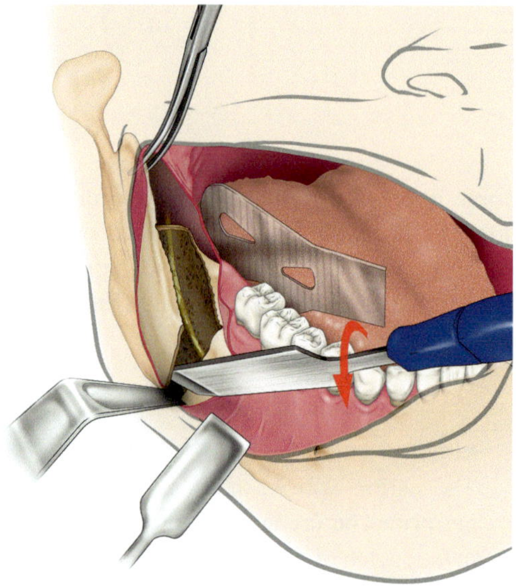

Fig. 19.12 After the split area can be controlled visually the remaining bone bridges below the mandibular canal can be separated to complete the split

9 Piezosurgical Splitting of the Inferior Mandibular Rim

Instead of the curved osteotome for splitting the caudal mandibular rim, the inferior mandibular rim can be split precisely, atraumatically and—without the splitting pressure of the osteotome—piezosurgically, thus increasing the certainty of a proper segment split in the infranerval caudal splitting area (Fig. 19.13) [6].

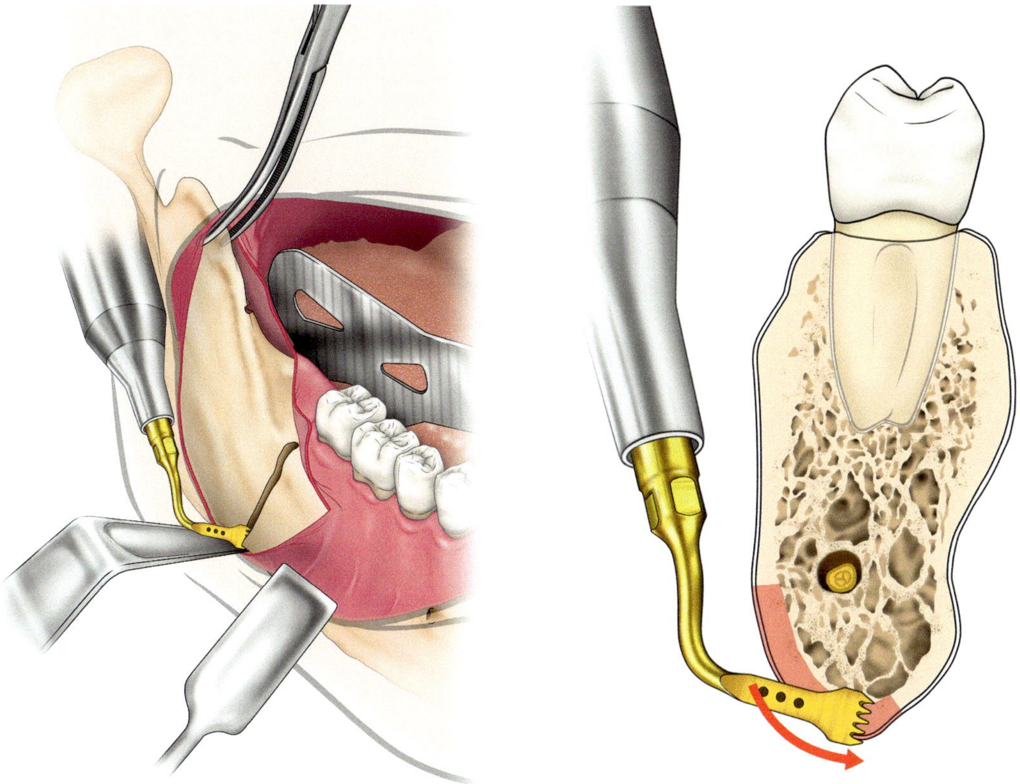

Fig. 19.13 Alternative piezosurgical splitting of the lateral and medial segment in the basal mandibular rim area, starting from the inferior vertical osteotomy [6].

10 Avoidance of Caudal-Basal Step formation in the Area of the Vertical Split

One problem with vertical bone splitting in BSSO, especially with extensive mandibular advancement, is the bony defect (gap) created at the inferior mandibular margin with undesirable step formation. This can happen if the basal osteotomy has cut through the buccal to the lingual cortex. A precautionary measure is to bevel the sharp osteotomy margins (Fig. 19.14) [6]. Another alternative is an additional groove at the inferior rim as described extensively by Böckmann and Wolford [7, 8].

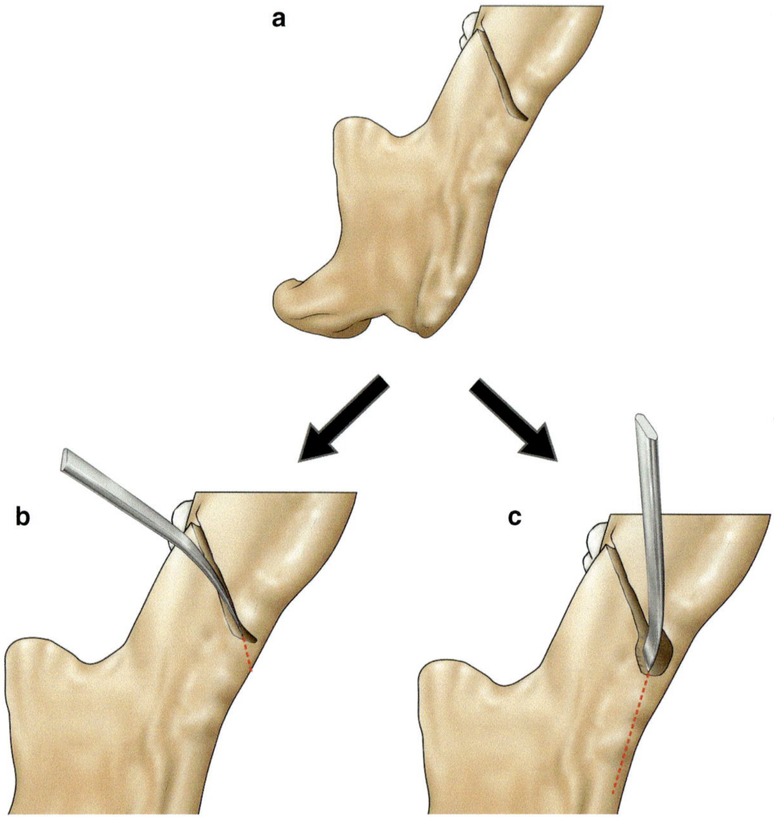

Fig. 19.14 (**a**) Without beveling (**b**) Prophylactic beveling of the inferior osteotomy margins (**c**) The Wolford-Böckmann osteotomy at the lower mandibular margin

11 Conclusion

There is no substitute for personal experience. This chapter is intended for the exchange of experience and to help identify unforeseeable difficulties in good time in order to avoid undesirable results.

References

1. Steinhäuser EW, Janson J. Kieferorthopädische Chirurgie. Berlin, Chicago, Sao Paulo, Tokio: Quintessenz-Verlag; 1988.
2. Steinhäuser EW. Educational course on surgical methods in orthognathic surgery. Luzern, Switzerland; 1973.
3. Ghali GE, Patel S. Avoiding Surgical Complications in Orthognathic Surgery. In: Ghali GE, Woerner JE, Patel S, editors. Maxillofacial Surgery: Mandible. 3rd ed. London: Churchill-Livingstone; 2017.
4. Bell WH, Proffit WR, White RP. Surgical correction of dentofacial deformities, band, vol. 1–3. Saunders; 1980.
5. Spiessl B.Chirurgie der Kiefer. In: Naumann HH Kopf-und Hals-Chirurgie. Indikation, Technik, Fehler und Gefahren. Operations-Manual. 3 Bdn. /Bd.2 Thieme, Stuttgart 1974.
6. Houppermans PNWJ, Verweij JP, Mensink G, Gooris PJJ, van Merkesteyn JPR. Influence of inferior border cut on lingual fracture pattern during bilateral sagittal split osteotomy with splitter and separators: a prospective observational study. J Cranio-Maxillofac Surg. 2016;44(10):1592–8.
7. Böckmann R, Schön P, Neuking K, Meyns J, Kessler P, Eggeler G. In vitro comparison of the sagittal split osteotomy with and without inferior border mosteotomy. J Oral Maxillofac Surg. 2015;73:316–23.
8. Wolford LM, Davis WM. The mandibular inferior border split: a modification in the sagittal split osteotomy. J Oral Maxillofac Surg. 1990;48:92–4.

Further Reading

Rohen J, Yokochi C. Anatomie des Menschen/Kopf, Hals. Schattauer: Rumpf-Band; 1982.

Post-Surgical Complications and Care

20

Peter Kessler, Nicolas Hardt, and Suen An Nynke Lie

Contents

P. Kessler (✉) · S. A. N. Lie
Department of Cranio-Maxillofacial Surgery,
Maastricht University Medical Center,
Maastricht, The Netherlands
e-mail: peter.kessler@mumc.nl; suen.lie@mumc.nl

N. Hardt (✉)
Kantonsspital Lucerne, Clinic and Policlinic of Cranio-Maxillofacial Surgery, Lucerne, Switzerland

P. Kessler et al. (eds.), *Illustrated Manual of Orthognathic Surgery*,
https://doi.org/10.1007/978-3-031-06978-9_20

Abstract

Postoperative complications can be divided into immediate complications during the termination of the anesthesia and the first 3 h thereafter (emergence), as well as complications that can occur in the first 12–24 h after the end of the operation, when the patient is usually on the normal ward or at home. The most serious complications affect the functions of the lungs, heart, and all forms of weaning disorders, in which the patient becomes a danger to himself/herself (Van Merkesteyn et al. Int J Oral and Maxillofacial Surg 16:665–670, 1987).

After orthognathic surgery various complications can occur and cause serious situations. To avoid postoperative respiratory complications, all patients in this treatment group require critical and professional support in the immediate postoperative phase.

Complications related to the respiratory system include airway obstruction, hypoventilation, tachypnea, tracheal swelling, bronchospasm, aspiration, and rarely spontaneous atelectasis or even a pneumothorax (Ogle Oral Maxillofacial Surg Clin N Am 18:49–58, 2006).

It should not be forgotten that repositioning of the lower jaw can lead to a narrowing of the posterior airway. Especially in class III patients, the preoperative assessment of the airway space requires interdisciplinary cooperation between surgeons and anesthesiologists to avoid unpleasant and almost unresolvable airway constrictions at the end of a mandibular setback. In extreme situations, the planned mandibular setback must be reduced and, if necessary, solved by a bimaxillary intervention. Checklists will help to avoid these complications (Choi et al. Maxillofac Plast Reconstr Surg 36:185–191, 2014; Soydan et al. Int J Oral Maxillofac Surg 44:1351–1354, 2015).

Keywords

Complications in BSSO · Early and late complications · Airway obstruction · Bleeding · Edema · Aspiration · Infection · Pain · PONV · Instability of osteosynthesis · Relapse · Bone healing · Bone necrosis · Pseudarthrosis

1 Immediate Complications after Orthognathic Surgery

1.1 Mechanical Airway Obstruction

- Pharyngeal tamponades.
- Residual fluids.
- Epistaxis.

Pharyngeal tamponades, if forgotten, represent a life-threatening problem by suffocation, especially after rigid intermaxillary fixation. Surgical protocols, checklists, time-out procedures, and memo-tapes on the patient/tube help to avoid this.

Any patient receiving a rigid intermaxillary fixation (IMF) must be provided with wire scissors for transport to the recovery department and for the time thereafter, which must always remain within reach of the patient to release the IMF in an emergency. The best protection is to avoid the rigid IMF.

Residual fluids Have to be suctioned carefully after end of surgery and again during extubation.

Epistaxis Generally occurs due to damage of the Kiesselbach's plexus in the anterior part of the nasal septum where branches from several arteries, including branches of the ophthalmic, maxillary, and facial arteries, anastomose to form a vascular plexus. To avoid this complication, the tracheal tube should be inserted into the nasal cavity such that its bevel tip comes to the lateral side of the nostril. However, if the bleeding occurs on insertion of the tube, the nasotracheal intubation should be completed to chiefly protect the airway and also to tamponade the bleeding point. If bleeding occurs after extubation, the nasal airway has to be tamponaded with gauzes (Merocel™, e.g.).

1.2 Functional Respiratory Insufficiency

Functional respiratory abnormalities such as:

- Asthma.
- Chronic obstructive pulmonary disease (COPD).
- Pneumonia.

or other etiological factors related to abnormalities of the trachea or bronchi can cause breathing disorders with hypo-oxygenation at the end of an operation. But also anxiety, panic attacks, and a drug overdose may be the reason for that.

The Esmarch maneuver, placement of a laryngeal tube (e.g., Guedel tube), and mask oxygenation help to control the situation until a stable breathing condition is reached again. If indicated, the patient must be re-intubated.

Other rare but life-threatening respiratory complications should be mentioned for completeness, but are not specifically associated with orthognathic surgery.

1.3 Bronchospasm

Bronchospasm is often related to asthmatic diseases, with obstruction of the airway. The key to an uncomplicated peri and postoperative course are the meticulous attention to detail in preoperative assessment and the maintenance of anti-swelling and bronchodilator management during the perioperative phase. Potential triggers should be identified and avoided. Many routinely used anesthetics have an alleviating effect on airway constriction.

Nevertheless, acute bronchospasms can occur, especially during induction, and should be treated immediately and methodically with medication (glucocorticoids).

1.4 Tracheal Edema

Respiratory insufficiency can also be caused by intubation due to damage to the vocal cords, swelling of the trachea caused by incorrect tube position and manipulation during intubation. The commonly used nasal intubation can lead to bleeding from the upper airways. Aspiration of blood and secretions due to damage to the nasal mucosa can be the result.

Possible edema of the perioral soft tissues and the floor of the mouth require careful airway management. This swelling may not fully manifest until about 12 h postoperatively and may continue to increase 48 h after surgery. Bleeding into the floor of the mouth can also lead to critical airway situations.

1.5 Tachypnea and Shortness of Breath

Mostly painful and reinforced by IMF and/or tight bandages that constrict the floor of the mouth or larynx. Also think of swelling of the tongue and, in the case of repositioning of the lower jaw, constriction of the posterior airway. Shortness of breath and tachypnea can often be resolved by adjusting bandages, opening intermaxillary fixation and appropriate pain therapy.

1.6 Aspiration

Aspiration dyspnea may occur as a result of extubation without adequate suction or incorrect positioning after extubation, especially after severe intraoperative bleeding or severe secretion accumulation. Aspiration pneumonia can occur as a complication when food, saliva or nasal secretions enter the bronchial tree. The rate of aspiration pneumonia after orthognathic interventions is about 0.01–0.03% (Kim et al. 2010, [1]).

Complication: Aspiration	
Symptoms	• Aspiration pneumonia: Dyspnea, cyanosis, rales, tachycardia, • Blood pressure drop, until cardiac arrest, • Cough.
Reasons	• Vomiting in case of not observed preop fasting, • Disorders of the gastrointestinal passage with simultaneous insufficiently existing protective reflexes, • Extubation without suction of the oral cavity, • Incorrect patient positioning after extubation.
First measures	• Clear the airway and suction of the surgical field, • Oxygen application by mask ventilation, • Airway support by intubation.

1.7 Postoperative Nausea and Vomiting (PONV)

PONV is a common, distressful, and debilitating occurrence that many patients describe as the most distressing part of their anesthetic experience. In a hospital-based surgery report, the incidence of PONV is in 14% after general anesthesia or IV sedation [2].

1.8 Reasons

Female gender, increased intravenous fluid supplementation (overfilling), longer duration of anesthesia, and the use of nitrous oxide are factors that promote postoperative nausea.

Favoring factors for postoperative vomiting are ethnic origin and individual disposition: the risk of vomiting among non-Caucasians is 2.49 times higher than among Caucasians. Additional risk factors are obesity, age less than 16 years, additional surgical procedures, and the use of opioids [1, 3].

The first measure is to calm the patient. If this is not sufficient, the treatment of PONV consists of mainly by using drugs from the antiemetic group such as serotonin receptor antagonists, dimenhydrinate, droperidol, glucocorticoids, or metoclopramide. If there is an increased risk of PONV, an antiemetic is administered as a preventive measure during the operation and anesthesia. Nitrous oxide should not belong to the selection of anesthetic drugs. The intravenous anesthetic propofol is currently the least emetogenic general anesthetic.

Complication: Nausea and Vomiting	
Symptoms	• Deep-set eyes, • Wide pupils, • Dry, brittle tongue, • Fear, pain, sweating, • Pale face, • Feeling of pressure in the stomach,
Reasons	• Anesthetic drugs side effects, • Severe pain, hypotension, • Patient was not fasting, • Gastrointestinal atony, • Side effects of other medication, • Elevated intracranial pressure.
First measures	• Position of patient's upper body high, • Emesis basin, • Substitution of saline solution and electrolytes, • Antiemetics and sufficient pain medication, • Check gastric tube for patency, • Prolongation of fasting.

2 Pain Management

Pain is uncomfortable and unnecessary, and its control must be a primary goal in postoperative care.

Pain interferes with oxygenation, delays healing, affects patient attitudes, and is a source of dissatisfaction with surgical and medical care. Since there are no identifiable behavioral or clinical signs that can be reliably used to determine the actual degree of subjectively felt postoperative pain, it is best to trust patients' assessment of their own pain. Pain scores are reliable tools for this purpose.

The pain experienced by different patients during the same surgical procedure varies from person to person, and responses to the same level of pain are expressed differently by different people. The best measure of adequate analgesia is therefore the patients' own perceptions.

A scoring system should be used to assess the level of pain and monitor the effectiveness of treatment.

2.1 Algorithms for Pain Therapy

Postoperative pain can be managed well with patient-controlled analgesia techniques (PCA) and modern pain therapy combinations. Numerical rating scales (NRS) and pain scale diagrams have proven to be useful for assessing the severity of pain. In addition, the age of the patient and his cognitive ability must be taken into account in the assessment.

Pain treatment is classified as either preventive or on demand. On-demand pain medications typically include either opioid or non-steroidal anti-inflammatory drugs (NSAID) or use ketamine. On-demand drugs can be administered by a clinician or by the patient using PCA. PCA has been shown to provide slightly better pain control and higher patient satisfaction compared to conventional methods [4].

2.2 Expected Pain Level

- Mild pain (NRS 1–3): non-opioid analgesics, e.g., metamizole, ibuprofen, and paracetamol.
- Moderate to severe pain (NRS ≥4–10): Highly potent opioid in combination with a non-opioid drugs.

2.3 Pain Therapy on the Ward

- Regular evaluation of pain intensity (NRS) at rest and under stress, e.g., movement of the lower jaw.
- Pain therapy primarily according to pain intensity.
- Pain therapy in consultation with the pain team.

Non-opioid analgesics are a heterogeneous group of pharmaceuticals that all have in common their use in pain therapy. In addition, they are used in the treatment to reduce fever. Some of them inhibit platelet aggregation and may not be used in post-surgical pain therapy.

They mainly unfold their effect by inhibiting cyclooxygenases, but they also have other central effects in isolated cases. The respective side effects depend on the drug subgroup used. Above all, non-steroidal anti-inflammatory drugs are often underestimated with regard to their risks for the stomach and kidneys.

Overview analgesics (exemplary)		
NSAID	Low-potency opioids	High-potency opioids
• Diclofenac. • Ibuprofen. • Paracetamol. • Metamizol.	• Tramadol. • Tilidine/naloxone.	• Morphine. • Oxycodone. • Fentanyl. • Piritramide (PCA).

Note

Immediate postoperative treatment with low-potency analgesics is generally not advisable, since intraoperatively, usually high-potency opioids are used.

A common "mistake" in pain therapy is the implementation of an analgesic therapy using only one opioid.

In order to achieve effective and balanced analgesia, the (additional) administration of a non-opioid analgesic and, if necessary, a coanalgesic should be carried out in each treatment stage

2.4 Postoperative Pain Therapy—Pain Score and Basic Medication

2.4.1 Mild Pain (NRS 1–3)

Basic medication: Non-opioid analgesic—NSAID, e.g., ibuprofen.

Adaptation in case of insufficient effect:

Combination with low-potency opioid, e.g., tramadol, or combination with highly potent opioid, e.g., oxycodone.

2.4.2 Moderate Pain (NRS 4–6)

Basic medication: Primary low potent opioid, e.g., tramadol.

Adaptation in case of insufficient effect:

Combination with a non-opioid analgesic, e.g., ibuprofen.

2.4.3 Severe Pain (NRS 7–10)

Basic medication: Primary highly potent opioid, e.g., oxycodone.

Adaptation in case of insufficient effect:

Combination with a non-opioid analgesic such as ibuprofen.

The World Health Organization (WHO) publishes stage schemes for pain therapy. The combination of different pain medications in one effect group should be entrusted to experienced pain specialists in order to avoid endangering the patient's health by combining highly effective medications. Especially the accumulation of side effects can lead to unexpected complications.

Pain is felt subjectively. A good preparation of the patient for the postoperative phase, including the expected pain, helps to reduce the use of pain medication. Rules of conduct also contribute to this. After orthognathic surgery, mild to moderate pain can be expected. Credible severe pain should be the reason for excluding a surgical or infectious cause.

The above recommendations are based on the WHO stage scheme. It should not be forgotten that after selection of the pain medications, the dosage must also be appropriate to the patient's age and weight, general state of health, and type of surgery.

2.5 Postoperative Facial Swelling

Postoperative edematous facial swelling usually persists for 2–3 weeks, which then subsides to residual edema after 3–4 weeks after surgery. This can persist for up to 6 months and occasionally increase. Of course, cooling measures in the operating area also help to prevent swelling.

Pre and perioperative swelling prophylaxis based on glucocorticoids helps to reduce edematous swelling. See also Chap. 2.

2.6 Postoperative Fever

Non-infectious causes of postoperative temperature rise can be different events. These can overlap, complement, and reinforce each other:
Temperature rise:

- Surgical trauma: Day 1–2.
- Drug fever: Day 1–8.
- Hematoma: Day 2–4.
- Rarely: Thromboembolism: Day 4–10.

Infectious causes:

- Aspiration pneumonia: Day 1–2.
- Various infections: pneumonia, urinary tract infection: Day 3–8.
- Wound infection with abscess formation: Day 5–10.

> **Note**
> The "rule of 5W" for postoperative fever:
> Wind → Lung (pneumonia).
> Water → Urinary tract (cystitis).
> Walking → Thrombosis/pulmonary embolism.
> Wound → Wound infection.
> Watt → Myocardial infarction

3 Indirect Complications after Orthognathic Surgery

These include (Kim et al. 2010, [1, 5])

- Soft tissue and/or bone infections.
- Neurological deficits due to intraoperative nerve injury.
- Secondary occlusional or articular disorders, mandibular relapse.
- Bone malunion due to incorrect or missing bony stabilization.

> **Note**
> The overall rate of postoperative complications after orthognathic surgery is between 9.7% and 24.5%.

The individual surgical risks are distributed as follows [1, 6]:

- 50% Nerve injury and sensory disorders
- 14% Temporomandibular joint disorders (TMJ dysfunction)
- 4–7% Infections
- 4.5% Bone non-union in the mandibular split
- 4% Mandibular relapse
- 2.5% Fractures of osteosynthesis material
- 2% Direct trauma to the IAN
- 0,3% Nerve injury to the facial nerve.

3.1 Wound Infections

Postoperative infections such as soft tissue infections and/or osteomyelitis of the mandibular bone are rare events. Aseptic working methods, less traumatizing surgical techniques, a generally good blood supply of the operation field, usually young and healthy patients, and targeted intra- and postoperative prophylactic antibiotic shielding make orthognathic surgery a safe surgical intervention.

The infection rate in osteotomies of the lower jaw is between 1 and 8% [1, 7, 8].

3.2 Postoperative Soft Tissue Infections

Soft tissue infections can usually be treated easily by local measures—suture removal, wound spreading, drainage—and antibiotic therapy after wound swab.

3.3 Postoperative Bone Infections

Historically, the rate of wound infections with bone involvement was higher at the beginning of rigid osteosynthesis than with wire ligatures. The enormous advancement of osteosynthesis materials and technical procedures, the reduction of surgical time through improved preoperative planning and targeted antibiotic support make osteomyelitic infections a rare complication. Nevertheless, basic surgical principles, such as the most economical denudation of the mandible, must be observed. Great importance is also attached to preoperative patient selection, in which patients with an increased risk of infection, e.g., type I diabetes, must be identified.

Peri-implant infections are typically caused by biofilm-forming microorganisms [9].

Early Infections are usually caused by virulent pathogens such as Staphylococcus aureus or gram-negative bacteria, whereas delayed and late infections are caused by low virulent pathogens such as coagulase-negative Staphylococci.

Among the pathogens of serious importance are those which might be present in the biotome of the oral cavity of an individual for which there are no effective antibiotics, if these pathogens are the cause of an infection in an adjacent wound area.

"Difficult-to-treat"-pathogens [9]:

- Rifampicin-resistant gram-positive staphylococci.
- Ciprofloxacin-resistant gram-negative bacteria.
- Enterococci.
- Fungi (Candida).

Patients who wish to undergo orthognathic surgery must be prepared for the procedure with the utmost care. This includes the restoration of all carious defects, the removal of all suspected pathological findings, and periodontal restoration prior to surgery. Only in this way can the risk of infection be considered low [9, 10].

3.4 Delayed Bone Union or Bone Non-union

Delayed bony consolidation of an osteotomy can occur as a result of compromised healing of hard and soft tissue.

The risk of bone non-union is high when inadequate segment fixation is performed with nonrigid materials such as wires, and when the anterior displacement of the distal segment is very large, resulting in insufficient bone contact. This may be due to planning errors which must be absolutely avoided with the planning options available today.

Postoperative occlusal pre-contacts, an unbalanced occlusion, and improperly designed splints may also interfere with the healing of bony segments, if the mandible is not sufficiently functionally relieved.

A delayed bone healing of osteotomized segments may also occur in patients with systemic disease, which in turn may interfere with wound healing. This must be avoided by careful anamnesis and patient selection.

3.5 Mandibular Relapse

Relapse and changes of occlusion after orthognathic surgery in the mandible are mostly the result of [1, 11, 12].

- Improperly performed segmental fixation at the osteotomy sites.
- Insufficient occlusal stability during osteosynthesis.
- Deficits in rigidity of osteosynthetic plates with insufficient bending strength.
- Occlusal displacements during fixation.
- Incorrect positioning of the condyles.

3.6 Factors that Can Lead to a Relapse after Mandibular Split are

- Muscle-related physiological effects on the jaw position despite correct mandibular positioning.
- Changes in the physiological balance of the pterygo-masseteric muscular loop. The changes in muscle insertion (length) and function (contractability) tend to cranialize the proximal segment. Changes in position of the horizontal branch of the mandible could result in leverage changes of muscle contractability.
- Increased muscular tension in the suprahyoidal muscles can produce an open bite, especially during mandibular anti-clockwise rotation and advancement with insufficient stabilization. Changes in the mandibular plane.
- Asymmetric mandibular position between the left and right side.
- Incorrect positioning of the temporomandibular joint/joints.
- Excessive segment inclination.
- Insufficient segment fixation, improperly produced splints.
- Orthodontic misalignment of the dentitions of upper and lower jaw, insufficient orthodontic preparation for surgery.
- Changes in tooth position, loss of teeth.

Large mandibular advancements of more than 7 mm can lead to an increased risk of relapse. To prevent this, increased attention should be paid to

- TMJ positioning.
- Avoidance of rotational mandibular movements.
- Adequate osteosynthetic stabilization with two parallel placed 2.0 mm plates, if necessary.
- Extended intermaxillary fixation with elastics for 1–2 weeks.
- Suprahyoid myotomy/Botox-injections.
- Orthodontic overcorrection to anticipate a slight relapse.

3.7 Mandibular Relapse and Rotation

The stability of the surgical result obtained by BSSO decreases as counterclockwise rotation of the distal segment increases. This is true even with mandibular setback corrections. This is presumably due to a muscular-neurophysiological imbalance between the muscle groups that close the jaw and those that open the mouth.

The relapse tendency also increases, if the proximal segment, which was previously rotated clockwise, is activated counterclockwise after the operation [13–15].

> **Note**
> Postoperative relapse can be prevented by minimizing rotation of the proximal segment

3.8 Mandibular Relapse and Intersegmental Distance

The occurrence of intersegmental interferences between the distal and the two proximal segments after BSSO is unavoidable. Interference between bony segments, combined with rigid segment fixation, can force changes in the position of the condyles, leading to positional relapse of the mandible, condylar resorption and, causally, to the loss of the targeted result.

See also Chap. 9.

The application of osteosynthesis in the distal segment posterior to the last molar, interposition of a bone graft in a wide segment gap to prevent changes of position and a functionally stable plate osteosynthesis without compression is advisable.

3.9 Malocclusion

Postoperative occlusion disorders after BSSO can manifest clinically as frontal or lateral or combined fronto-lateral open bite and/or lateral mandibular shifting. Mandibular misalignment in the frontal plane may result from occlusal interferences.

Anterior and lateral open bite:

- Inadequate osteosynthetic fixation.
- Posterior open bite during fixation due to insufficient splint.
- Insufficient orthodontic presurgical treatment, e.g., imbalance of curve of Spee.
- Insufficient anterior overbite, missing curve of Spee.
- Too early functional load by chewing.

Lateral mandibular displacement:

- Different sagittal mandibular repositioning with right/left disbalance.
- Symmetric sagittal mandibular repositioning with loss of the midline.
- Twisting of the proximal segment(s).
- Inadequate transverse width between mandible and maxilla.

Treatment of mild postoperative malocclusion:

- Vertical traction with elastics when there is no anterior-posterior disharmony for 2–3 weeks.
- In case of anterior-posterior discrepancies reenter, explore the situation and correct the discrepancy.

Note

The use of vertical forces by elastics can have detrimental effects on teeth

3.10 Bone Necrosis

Bone necrosis of the ascending ramus may occur as a result of local ischemia following excessive soft tissue ablation and hematoma formation, such as after complete buccal and lingual denudation. There is also an increased risk in excessive manipulations of the proximal segment during joint positioning and osteosynthesis. Especially when using the transbuccal approach for screw fixation an uncontrolled soft tissue stripping on the buccal side can happen. This maneuver also increases the risk of hematoma formation between bone and cheek soft tissues.

3.11 Prophylaxis

The best prophylaxis is the careful handling of the covering soft tissues. However, an economical exposure that provides sufficient visibility is sometimes difficult to achieve. In very rare extreme cases it may be necessary to remove necrotic bone areas, often together with the osteosynthesis material.

3.12 Pseudarthrosis

Pseudarthrosis is rare and usually caused by infection and instability in the osteotomy area due to inadequate stabilization. Even a too early onset of excessive mastication can lead to pseudarthrosis due to premature material loosening despite sufficient osteosynthesis.

Therapy: Adequate osteosynthesis and IMF.

4 Conclusion

Any surgical procedure presents a challenge to the patient's biology, which must allow the iatrogenically inflicted wound to heal. The surgeon, through his careful and cautious approach, must ensure that the conditions for recovery are ideal. The special feature of orthognathic surgery is the combination of soft tissue and bone tissue surgery in the region of the oral cavity, which is always potentially at risk of infection, with transoral access. The risks of the procedures lie between the known risks of orthopedic and oral surgery. The desire for early mandibular movement and keeping the airway open must also be given much consideration [16–19].

After unsatisfactory experiences with various osteotomy techniques, the bilateral sagittal split according to Obwegeser–Dal Pont, as refined by Hunsuck and Epker, has prevailed since the 1950s and is considered the standard procedure for relocating the mandible to correct the jaw position. In addition to the technique of splitting, the intraoral approach has since become firmly established. The technique is elegant, but it always presents even the experienced surgeon with the challenge of adjusting this technique individually, which can be associated with complications. The increasing demand for facial corrections for aesthetic indications puts pressure on the surgeon to perform the operation flawlessly. However, this can never be guaranteed, as unexpected events can always occur in the course of a split jaw, mainly due to the fact that in the end the fracture of the lower jaw occurs spontaneously.

References

1. Kim YK. Complications associated with orthognathic surgery. J Korean Assoc Oral Maxillofac Surg. 2017;43(1):3–15.
2. Chye EP, Young IG, Osborne GA, et al. Outcomes after same-day oral surgery: a review of 1180 case at a major teaching hospital. J Oral Maxillofac Surg. 1993;51:846.
3. Phillips C, Brookes CD, Rich J, Arbon J, Turvey TA. Postoperative nausea and vomiting following orthognathic surgery. Int J Oral Maxillofac Surg. 2015;44:745–51.
4. Gélinas C, Fillion L, Puntillo KA, Viens C, Fortier M. Validation of the critical-care pain observation tool in adult patients. Am J Crit Care. 2006;15(4):420–7.
5. Jędrzejewski M, Smektała T, Sporniak-Tutak K, Olszewski R. Preoperative, intraoperative, and postoperative complications in orthognathic surgery: a systematic review. Clin Oral Investig. 2015;19:969–77.
6. Te Veldhuis EC, Te Veldhuis AH, Bramer WM, Wolvius EB, Koudstaal MJ. The effect of orthognathic surgery on the temporomandibular joint and oral function: a systematic review. Int J Oral Maxillofac Surg. 2017;46(5):554–63.
7. Davis CM, Gregoire CE, Steeves TW, Demsey A. Prevalence of surgical site infections following orthognathic surgery: a retrospective cohort analysis. J Oral Maxillofac Surg. 2016;74:1199–206.
8. Posnick JC, Choi E, Liu S. Occurrence of a 'bad' split and success of initial mandibular healing: a review of 524 sagittal ramus osteotomies in 262 patients. Int J Oral Maxillofac Surg. 2016;45:1187–94.
9. Kleber C, Schaser KD, Trampuz A. Komplikationsmanagement bei infizierter Osteosynthese : Therapiealgorithmus bei periimplantären Infektionen [Complication management of infected osteosynthesis: therapy algorithm for periimplant infections]. Chirurg. 2015;86(10):925–34.
10. Trampuz A, Zimmerli W. Diagnosis and treatment of infections associated with fracture-fixation devices. Injury. 2006;37(Suppl 2):S59–66.
11. Lee JH, Lee IW, Seo BM. Clinical analysis of early reoperation cases after orthognathic surgery. J Korean Assoc Oral Maxillofac Surg. 2010;36:28–38.
12. Van Sickels JE, Richardson DA. Stability of orthognathic surgery: a review of rigid fixation. Br J Oral Maxillofac Surg. 1996;34(4):279–85.
13. Han JJ, Yang HJ, Lee SJ, Hwang SJ. Relapse after SSRO for mandibular setback movement in relation to the amount of mandibular setback and intraoperative clockwise rotation of the proximal segment. J Craniomaxillofac Surg. 2014;42(6):811–5.
14. Proffit WR, Phillips C, Dann C 4th, Turvey TA. Stability after surgical-orthodontic correction of skeletal class III malocclusion. I. mandibular setback. Int J Adult Orthodon Orthognath Surg. 1991;6(1):7–18.
15. Yang HJ, Hwang SJ. Bone mineral density and mandibular advancement as contributing factors for postoperative relapse after orthognathic surgery in patients with preoperative idiopathic condylar resorption: a prospective study with preliminary 1-year follow-up. Oral Surg Oral Med Oral Pathol Oral Radiol. 2015;120(2):112–8.
16. Choi SK, Yoon JE, Cho JW, Kim JW, Kim SJ, Kim MR. Changes of the airway space and the position of hyoid bone after mandibular set back surgery using bilateral sagittal split ramus osteotomy technique. Maxillofac Plast Reconstr Surg. 2014;36:185–91.
17. Ogle OE. Postoperative care of oral and maxillofacial surgery patients. Oral Maxillofacial Surg Clin N Am. 2006;18:49–58.
18. Soydan SS, Bayram B, Akdeniz BS, Kayhan Z, Uckan S. Changes in difficult airway predictors following mandibular setback surgery. Int J Oral Maxillofac Surg. 2015;44:1351–4.
19. Van Merkesteyn JPR, Groot RH, van Leeuwaarden R, Kroon FH. Intra-operative complications in sagittal and vertical ramus osteotomies. Int J Oral Maxillofac Surg. 1987;16(6):665–70.

Part IV

Mandibular Deficiency - Surgical Technique - BSSO

Indications for Mandibular Advancement

21

Peter Kessler and Suen An Nynke Lie

Contents

Abstract

The word retrognathism—class II dysgnathia, mandibular retrognathism—is derived from Latin retro ("backward") and the Greek word γνάθος (gnáthos, "jaw"). Clinical symptoms can be very diverse. They include negative anterior steps in the dentition, a volumetrically small lower third of the face up to the receding chin in conjunction with a symmetrical or asymmetrical mandibular growth deficiency of various degrees. A narrow upper jaw with crowding and retrusion of the central/lateral incisors is typical in class II/2 dysgnathias, but also compensatory extraverted upper jaw fronts as well as compensatory protruded lower incisors (class II/1). Furthermore, it must be differentiated whether the respective class II is a forward displacement of the maxilla or a horizontal or combined horizontal and vertical growth deficit in the mandible. A combination of both symptoms is possible.

Mandibular retrognathism can be treated at different ages and stages of development. In most cases, pure orthodontic treatment with functional orthodontic appliances is sufficient. However, if growth induction by orthodontics is insufficient or when the growth deficit is too pronounced, different surgical means can be used. Common to all these means of treatment is that they are perceived as esthetically positive by the patients. Often, in combination with mandibular advancement, there is also a need/possibility for correction of the chin position (genioplasty)

P. Kessler (✉) · S. A. N. Lie
Department of Cranio-Maxillofacial Surgery, Maastricht University Medical Center, Maastricht, The Netherlands
e-mail: peter.kessler@mumc.nl; suen.lie@mumc.nl

P. Kessler et al. (eds.), *Illustrated Manual of Orthognathic Surgery*,
https://doi.org/10.1007/978-3-031-06978-9_21

Keywords

Class II relation/malocclusion · Mandibular retrognathism · Mandibular retrognathia · Maxillary protrusion · Dental crowding · Tongue function · Indications for mandibular advancement · Sagittal splitting · BSSO · Mandibular advancement · Special surgical aspects · Mandibular segment osteotomy · Modifications and surgical alternatives · Distraction osteogenesis · Genioplasty

The typical patient with a class II malocclusion, proclination, or crowding of the mandibular anterior teeth, and a moderate-to-low mandibular plane angle is a planning and treatment challenge. The following points must be considered before or at the start of treatment, because class II patients have a smaller effective mandibular base length:

- Crowding—extraction of teeth or decompensation without extraction: extraction versus non-extraction cases.
- Is there an asymmetry of the number of teeth in the upper and lower jaw.
- Tongue function and lip habits—forced lip closure.
- Presence of wisdom teeth.
- In case of a deep bite: is the correction in one jaw (mandible) sufficient? How is the vertical problem approached: Segment or bimaxillary correction.
- A large pretreatment mandibular plane angle leads to unfavorable results.

The initial task in most patients with mandibular deficiency is to eliminate dental compensation by retrusion of the lower front and protrusion of the upper front as well as by bucco-lingual correction of the inclination of the posterior teeth, in the maxilla to the vestibular side, in the lower jaw to lingual. If extreme vertical overbite is present at the same time, additional orthodontic means are necessary to successfully level the occlusion. These remarks are intended to make it clear that, especially in class II malocclusion, interdisciplinary contact and cooperation with the orthodontist are crucial for success [1]

1 Morphological and Dental Criteria

Dental class II is the most common form of treatment in orthodontics and orthognathic surgery. It is precisely for this reason that assessment, planning, and treatment require attention, circumspection, and experience, since this form of dysgnathia can occur in all conceivable combinations and configurations.

The morphological characteristics of mandibular retrognathism are responsible for a typical patient appearance, which is judged subjectively as less disturbing than a mandibular prognathia. Patients with class II position of the lower jaw are less dissatisfied with their appearance since the receding mandibular position can be compensated by conscious or unconscious protrusion of the mandible. In contrast, in cases of pronounced mandibular retrognathism or even mandibular micrognathia, the three-dimensional loss of volume in the lower third of the face is perceived as very disturbing.

The extraoral facial profile is often harmonious, with a negative lip line with the lower lip receding dorsally and a pronounced lip red may be present. A pronounced retracted sublabial fold is noticeable in forms of dentoalveolar retrognathia, whereby the nose position, and also the chin position, can be correct.

In a fully developed class II mandibular retrognathia the receding of the lower jaw, chin, and lower lip can be seen in both lateral and en-face views. Nevertheless, mild forms are often perceived by patients as not very disturbing (Fig. 21.1). Pronounced forms, however, lead to increased suffering, since a "receding" chin causes the esthetically significant chin prominence to disappear, resulting in a very disturbing transitionless chin-neck area.

Intraorally, in addition to a class II occlusion in the first molar region, an enlarged positive dental anterior overjet is usually noticeable, which may be pronounced by lingual tilting of the lower and labial tilting of the upper front teeth (Fig. 21.2).

On the other hand, the clinical situation of a class II jaw relationship can be camouflaged by a palatal tilting of the upper and labial tilting of the

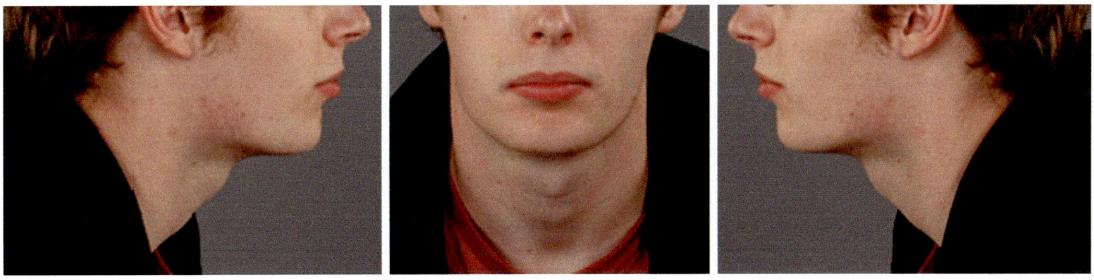

Fig. 21.1 Lower facial third: Typical facial appearance in Class II occlusion with mandibular deficiency

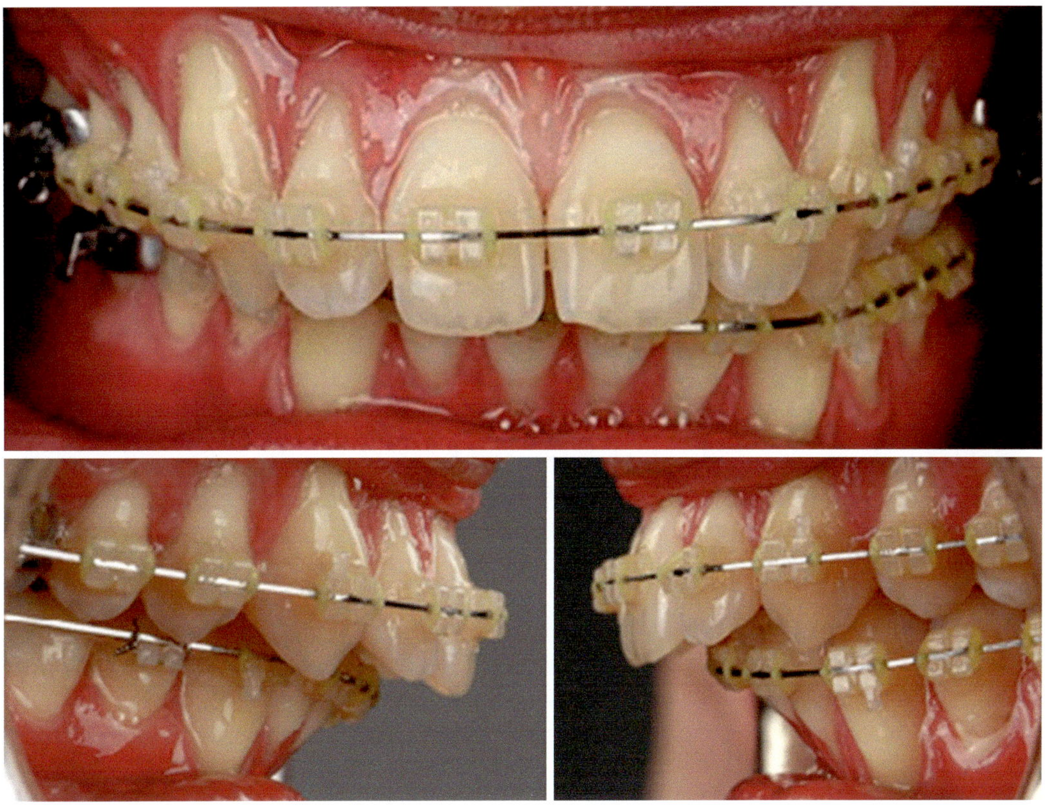

Fig. 21.2 Bite relation of the patient in Fig. 21.1 with positive dental anterior overjet

lower front teeth. The anterior tooth relationship also depends on the individual activity of the lip muscles. A narrow frontal overbite position can therefore also be present with a class II occlusion findings in the molar region.

However, there may also be a dental compensation with protrusion position of the mandibular and retrusion position of the upper front teeth and thus a reduction of the overjet. In addition to the characteristic class II occlusion, the dentoalveolar relation often shows crowding of the lower anterior and posterior teeth. This protrusion is caused by the sagittal underdevelopment of the tooth-bearing alveolar process. Often there may also be non-development of teeth in the premolar region, which should not be overlooked.

The clinical image of mandibular retrognathism in non-syndromal cases can be assigned to a dentoalveolar or skeletal class II with cause in the mandible only.

Clinical, radiological, and technical analyses (cephalometry), especially in the sagittal plane, are used to determine which diagnosis is applicable. These analyses must provide information about the position and size of the mandibular skeletal structures with respect to the degree of mandibular retrognathism within the respective facial growth pattern and clarify the extent of dentoalveolar and/or skeletal involvement in class II occlusion.

Special attention must be paid to the overall length of the face and the relative proportion of the lower third of the face in order not to overlook a vertical excess of growth in the middle and lower third of the face, which often requires bimaxillary correction (Fig. 21.4).

If patients complain of a gummy smile, extra attention has to be paid, if the malocclusion can be solved in a mono-maxillary surgical approach to the mandible.

In cephalometric analysis the simple class II cases show a jaw base harmony except for the mandibular retrognathism (SNB-angle). The sagittal interbasal relation (ANB-angle) is found to be increased (enlarged positive ANB-angle).

If the pogonion prominence is in harmony with the face, it indicates an alveolar mandibular underdevelopment. If the position of the pogonion is also in disharmony—sagittal retropositioning of the pogonion—the situation fulfills the criteria of a skeletal mandibular retrognathism (Fig. 21.3).

Vertical and mostly transversal disharmonies or discrepancies may be present in the planning of the procedure, which complicate planning and lead to rotational moments—mostly anticlockwise—in the correction of the mandibular malposition, which must be observed without fail while avoiding relapse or transverse disharmony.

The distinction between an orthognathic, retrognathic, and retrognathic-elongated facial type helps to avoid errors in planning and can occa-

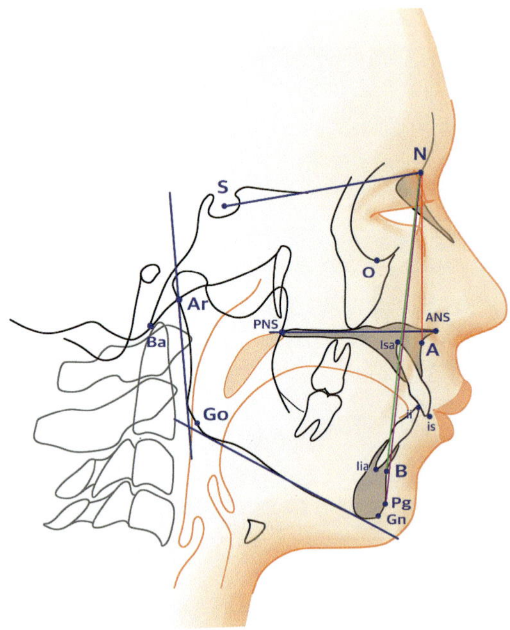

Fig. 21.3 Typical cephalometry for class II occlusion with mandibular retrognathism. ©Copyright Keisuke Koyama 2020. All rights reserved

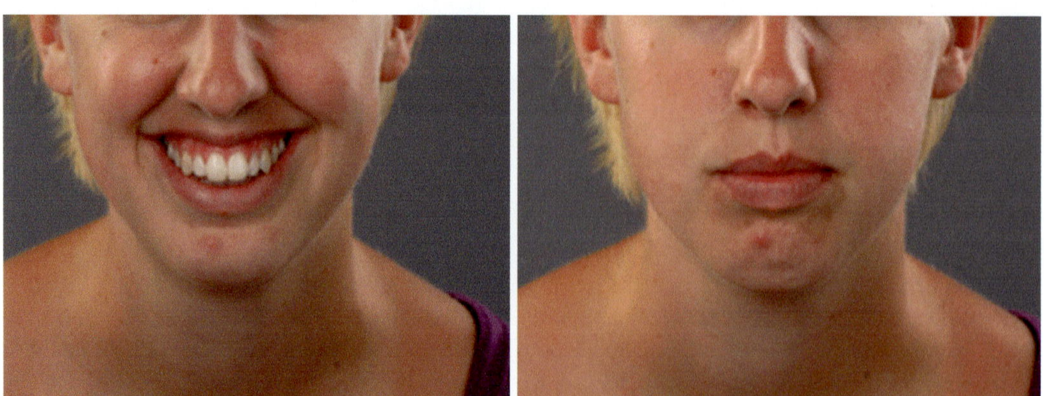

Fig. 21.4 Lower facial third: Typical facial appearance in class II occlusion with mandibular deficiency and vertical overgrowth of the maxilla. Retrognathic elongated facial type with forced lip closure

sionally lead to the decision to recommend bimaxillary correction in the case of retrognathic facial type with vertical elongation (dolichofacial type, long face).

Special attention must be paid to the relationship of the mandibular base to the skull base plane (ML-NSL) to avoid errors that may lead to an acceptable functional but unsatisfactory esthetic result.

The position of the chin (pogonion-gnathion) requires special attention in order to achieve a good esthetic result.

Note
In class II jaw relations the dysgnathic jaw position must made clear to patients.

- Dental compensation is a common clinical finding in class II dysgnathias.
- The indication for correction can be functional and/or esthetic.
- In planning, attention must be paid to the vertical sagittal position of the mandibular base—ML-NSL—and the position of the pogonion.

1.1 Skeletal Relation—Possible Conditions

- Disharmonious profile of the face.
- Lower lip incompetence and retrusion.
- Flattened sublabial fold.
- Receding chin.
- Open mouth posture with balanced, reduced, or increased vertical face height.
- Fibrillary muscle twitches in the chin area—m. mentalis—with compulsive lip/mouth closure.
- Voluminous lip red area of the lower lip.
- Class II relation in the molar region, increased overjet with protruded upper front teeth (class II division 1, class II/1).
- In adults, dental compensation without pronounced sagittal overjet.
- Protrusion position of the upper incisors.

1.2 Dentobasal Relation—Possible Conditions

- Dental compensation, protrusion of lower anterior teeth in case of retruded or normally positioned upper anterior teeth.
- Retroclined upper front teeth and retrusion and elongation of the lower front teeth (class II division 2, class II/2).
- Deep bite with reduced height of the lower third of the face and small vertical interbasal angle ML-NL.
- Deep bite with extruded lower front teeth, protruded upper front teeth, and harmonious facial height.
- Combination forms with exclusively retroclined central incisors with vertically harmonious jaw relation.

Note
The dentoalveolar relation with characteristic retrognathic mandibular base realignment may include all known tooth misalignments in the sagittal, vertical, and transverse directions.

2 Cephalometry in Skeletal Mandibular Retrognathia:

- SNB and SNPg reduced.
- SNA harmonious.
- ANB enlarged.
- ML-NL can show all variants.
- Transversal dysharmonies with a narrowed upper jaw base.

For completeness it must be mentioned that mandibular retrognathia can also occur in combination with maxillary retrognathia. On the other hand, mandibular retrognathia can also occur in maxillary prognathia or can be relatively masked by maxillary prognathia and an orthognathic mandible.

3 Indications

A class II mandibular growth deficiency must be regarded as risk factor for functional disorders of the stomatognathic system:

- Speech development.
- Speech disorders.
- Mouth breathing.
- Disturbed chewing function.
- TMJ dysfunctions.
- Impossibility of prosthetic-implantological rehabilitation, especially at an advanced age.

4 Conclusion

The dentoalveolar class II relation is the domain of orthodontics in growth age starting with the eruption of permanent teeth. But mandibular deficiency or skeletal mandibular retrognathia is also the domain of combined orthodontic and surgical treatment. During the assessment and cephalometric measurement in class II patients, the maxilla must never be disregarded in order to exclude incorrect treatment.

Reference

1. Vaden JL, Williams RA, Goforth RL. Class II correction. Extraction or nonextraction? Am J Orthod Dentofac Orthop. 2018;154(6):860–76.

Sagittal Split and Mandibular Advancement

22

Peter Kessler and Suen An Nynke Lie

Contents

Abstract

Corrections of mandibular position are the domain of bilateral sagittal splitting osteotomy—BSSO. The Obwegeser-Dal Pont technique is considered the overall standard technique for mandibular advancement.

The importance of alveolar segmental osteotomies has greatly decreased due to the differentiated orthodontic treatment options. The known risks of alveolar segmental osteotomies—loss of bone, teeth, fractures, and long-term damage to adjacent teeth—are not prevalent with today's surgical correction of the jaw bases.

Nevertheless, segment osteotomies can play a role, especially in extreme Class II/2 occlusal situations, to impact severely vertically exaggerated anterior segments and also to modify them in anteroposterior inclination. Negative occlusal curves (curve of Spee) can also be corrected by raising the anterior segment. Segment osteotomies can be combined with corrections of the mandibular base.

P. Kessler (✉) · S. A. N. Lie
Department of Cranio-Maxillofacial Surgery, Maastricht University Medical Center, Maastricht, The Netherlands
e-mail: peter.kessler@mumc.nl; suen.lie@mumc.nl

P. Kessler et al. (eds.), *Illustrated Manual of Orthognathic Surgery*,
https://doi.org/10.1007/978-3-031-06978-9_22

Keywords

Mandibular retrognathism · Indications for mandibular advancement · Sagittal splitting · BSSO - SSRO · Mandibular advancement · Segmental osteotomy · Special surgical aspects · Short lingual osteotomy—SLO · Modifications and surgical alternatives · Distraction osteogenesis

The total mandibular alveolar process osteotomy, as described by MacIntosh [1], has never been able to assert itself, because of the known risks especially for the inferior alveolar nerve similar to the stepwise osteotomy in the jaw body according to Pichler and Berg [2] for advancement of the mandible.

Correction of the mandibular deficiency is the domain of bilateral sagittal split osteotomy as described by *Dal Pont* [3]. The main argument is the largest possible bone attachment area between the distal and proximal bone segments (Fig. 22.1).

However, with the establishment of distraction osteoneogenesis as an additional therapeutic option in cranio-maxillofacial (CMF) surgery, osteotomy techniques have experienced a renaissance. There will always be patients with a class II mandibular deficiency in whom the desired result in the sagittal direction cannot be achieved during the course of orthodontic treatment in the growth age. If the transverse mandibular width in the molar region is favorable, these cases can alternatively be treated with Intermolar Mandibular Distraction Osteoneogenesis (IMDO). See Chap. 24.

In class II patients with extreme vertical growth excess or in the anterior segment of both the mandible and maxilla, segmental osteotomies may still be necessary.

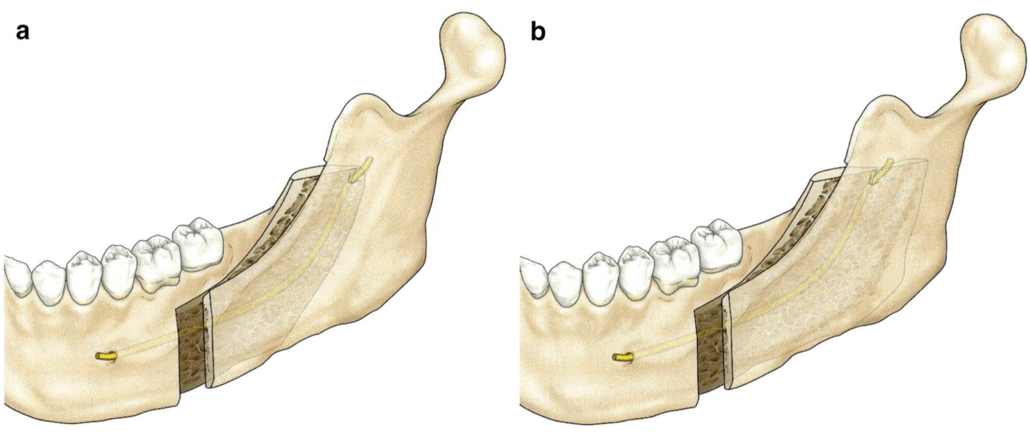

Fig. 22.1 Sagittal splitting according to Dal Pont: (**a**) SLO according to Hunsuck (**b**) Osteotomy on the lingual side according to Obwegeser ©Copyright Keisuke Koyama 2020. All rights reserved

1 Mandibular Advancement: BSSO

Chapter 17 describes the surgical procedure of the sagittal split in detail.

Of all the techniques and variations described in literature, two are still used regularly today: The osteotomy in the area of the jaw angle and in the area of the ascending mandibular ramus.

The main method, which is used in many places in the mandibular angle area, is the sagittal splitting, which was originally published by Obwegeser [4] in the ascending branch clearly above the jaw angle.

In *1958, Dal Pont* then placed the buccal cut in the horizontal mandibular body at the level of the second molar, resulting in extremely wide bone contact surfaces after sagittal splitting (Fig. 22.2) [3]. The masseteric muscle remains on the proximal segment, which is important for its blood supply.

Sagittal mandibular splitting, especially in the *Dal Pont* modification, is the standard procedure today (SSRO/BSSO/SLO). Many suggestions for modifying this successful method have been published. These modifications deal with the creation of osteotomy lines, the instruments for tissue retraction, splitting, and especially the fixation of the fragments. Only the most important ones are mentioned here [5–8].

In the case of a class II retrognathism, the lower jaw must be shifted forward—mandibular advancement—in order to achieve a regular dental occlusion in class I. Depending on the splitting technique, there will be a greater or lesser overlap of bone. The two most common osteotomy techniques used are SSRO/BSSO and IVRO. Even with a short lingual osteotomy (SLO) according to *Hunsuck* and *Epker*, an overlap must be assured [6, 7, 9].

If the SLO is applied the placement of the buccal osteotomy is absolutely relevant to achieve a good bone overlap between the proximal and distal segments. The buccal vertical osteotomy should deliberately be placed at the height of the second molar region or even further anteriorly (Fig. 22.2). Impacted third molars should have been removed at least 6 months before surgery.

Chapter 17 describes the surgical approach in detail:

Under nasal intubation anesthesia and after infiltration of the lingual and buccal jaw angle region with local anesthetics containing vasoconstrictors, the mucosal incision is made slightly lateral to the external oblique line from the distal aspect of the second premolar to the ascending mandible, but without cutting through the bucco-temporal fascia. To guarantee this the scalpel should always maintain a perpendicular

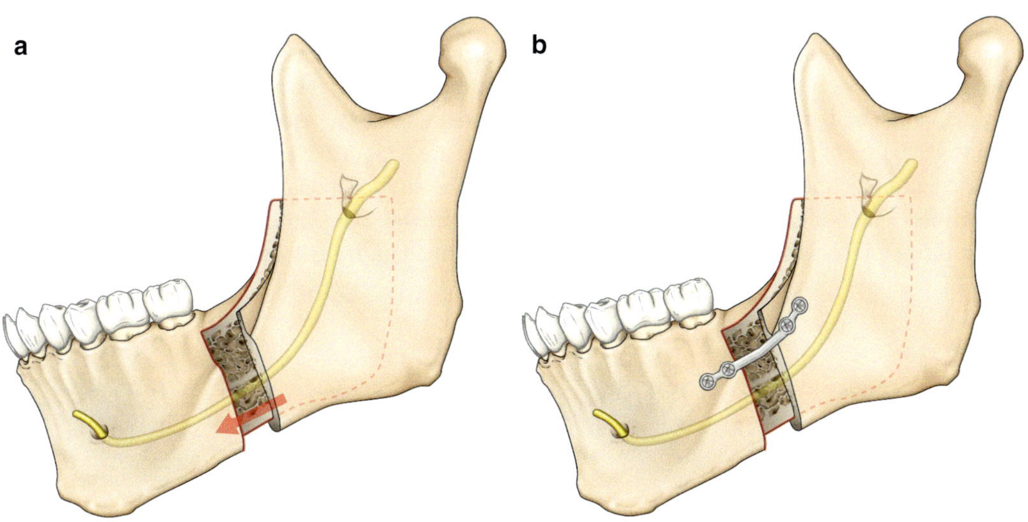

Fig. 22.2 (**a**) Obwegeser–Dal Pont procedure for mandibular advancement (Hunsuck–Epker modification) (**b**) Osteosynthesis using a 4-hole mini plate with bar (2.0 mm)

position towards the bony surface from the point where the external oblique line starts at the lateral aspect of the ascending ramus.

This avoids prolapse of the cheek fat body. The periosteum can now be easily pushed away from the mandibular body to the jaw angle by blunt dissection until the distal insertion of the masseteric muscle in the region of the mandibular angle is reached. The masseteric muscle must not be detached. A useful instrument for this preparation is the Minnesota retractor. The periosteum should be injured as little as possible. The attachment of the coronoid process is dissected, whereby the connective tissue attachment of the temporal muscle fibers should be dissected meticulously. Care is taken not to completely detach the periosteum on the lateral side, so as not to endanger the blood supply to the proximal fragment carrying the joint. A notched ramus hook is used to retain the soft tissues from the muscular/coronoid process.

The fibrous periosteum is now carefully detached lingually at the level of the base of the muscular/coronoid process caudally towards the point where the alveolar process is bulging out to the lingual aspect—undercut. Be sure to remain in the subperiosteal plane to avoid disrupting the soft tissue layers on the lingual side with the risks of bleeding and injuring the lingual nerve. After having achieved this a horizontal tunnel is made to the posterior edge of the ascending ramus above the lingula.

The lingula with the nerve and vessel exit remains caudally of the periosteal tunnel. For safe orientation the incisura semilunaris can now be identified with a blunt curved elevator, raspatory or dissector according to Freer. This is an optional procedure to ensure that the tunnel is prepared at the correct level.

Now a specially formed ramus clamp can be inserted, e.g., Satinsky clamp or DeBakey aortic clamp, above the lingual tunnel at the origin of the coronoid process to replace the notched ramus hook. Clamps are easier to handle to retain and protect the soft tissues cranially and lingually (Fig. 22.3a, b).

Next, the more or less prominent edge above the lingula, which represents an offshoot of the mylohyoid line/internal oblique line, can be ablated with a round burr. Especially in class II mandibles this bone excess at the entrance to the lingual tunnel is only rarely there. In most cases is due to the mandibular growth deficiency the coronoid process thin. The view to the dorsal edge of the ascending ramus is usually good.

Before the lingual osteotomy is performed, a channel retractor, which can surround the posterior edge, is inserted to prevent injury to the lingually located nerves and vessels. A blunt, 90° curved nerve hook can be used for reliable identification of the lingula before the channel retractor is inserted. The channel retractor should lie in contact with the lingual side of the ascending mandibular branch in such a way that it is turned 45° caudally.

Anatomically the channel retractor is positioned in the sulcus colli groove behind the crista endocoronoidea. In this position, the lingula as entrance port for the neurovascular bundle is protected and at the same time the lingual soft tissues are kept out (Fig. 22.4).

The lingual bone cut is made with the long Lindemann burr at a depth of 1.5–2 mm as described by *Hunsuck and Epker* (SLO). Caution

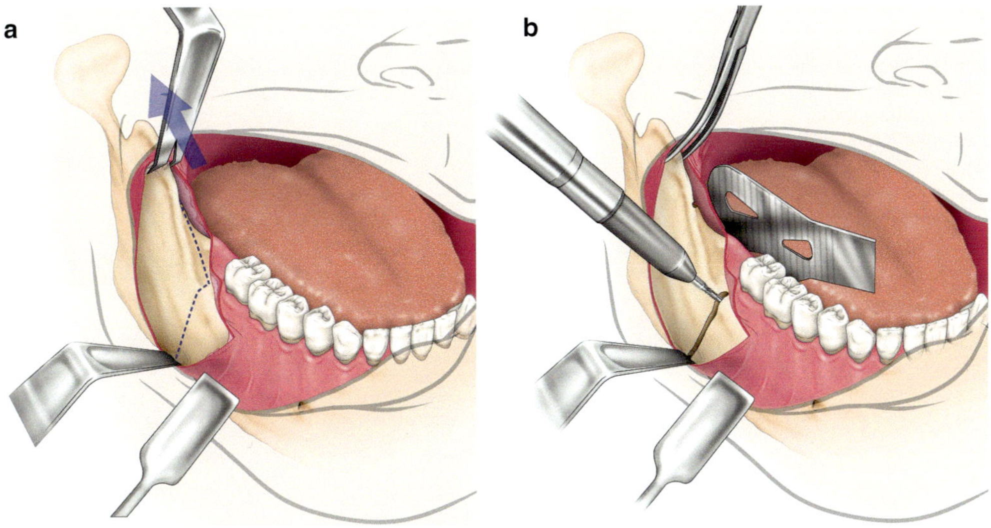

Fig. 22.3 (**a**) The surgical site is sufficiently prepared for a safe osteotomy. Osteotomy line is indicated. (**b**) Safe approach to the retromolar region for splitting the mandible

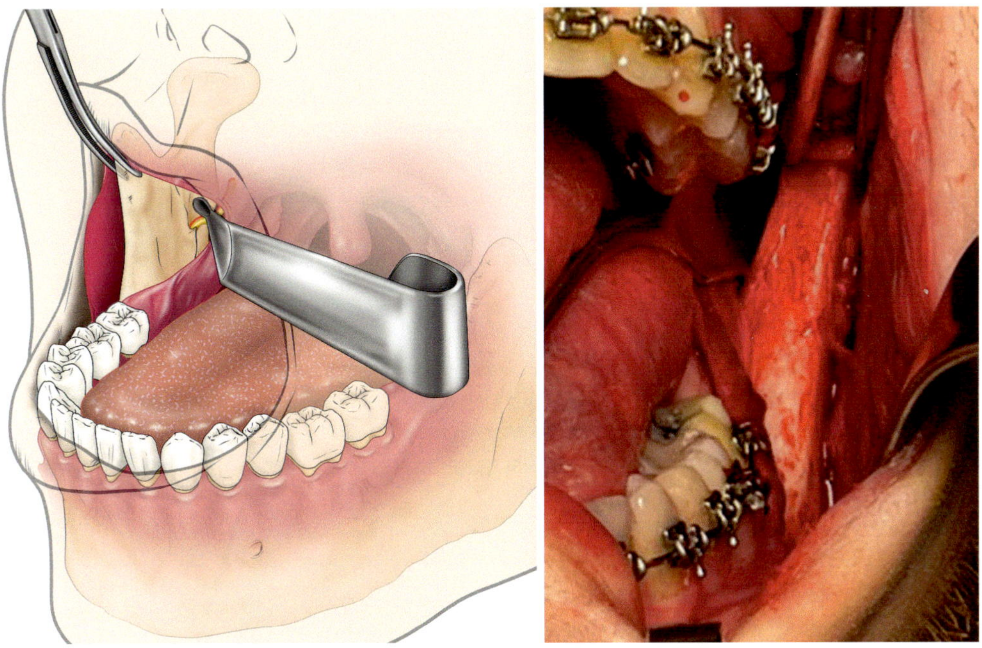

Fig. 22.4 Channel retractor placement on the lingual side for protection of the soft tissues and the IAN, clinical situation for safe access

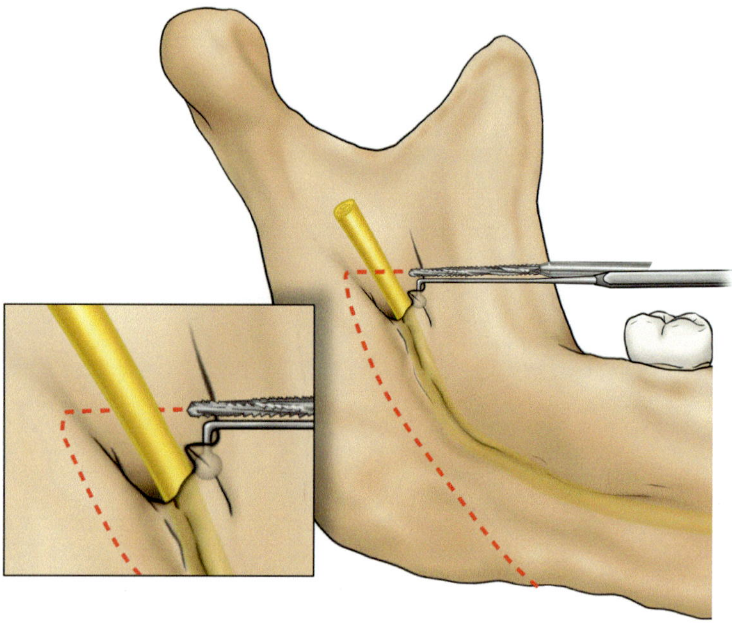

Fig. 22.5 The lingual osteotomy should run parallel to the occlusion of the lower jaw. Nerve probe as guiding tool

is required in the middle part of the ascending ramus, where the bone can be very thin; it is essential to avoid separating the condylar process from the proximal segment. The inclination of the Lindemann burr is decisive.

It is recommended to align the drilling plane parallel to the occlusal plane of the mandible and if possible parallel to the lingual retractor which can be used as a guiding tool (Figs. 22.5, 22.6, 22.7).

As second osteotomy the buccal cortical cut is made, which is usually placed in the region of the second molar or even anteriorly as classical Dal Pont osteotomy. Here, the cortical bone should be completely cut through to ensure easy splitting.

A connection between the two cortical incisions is then marked with an excavator drill, which is completed with a short Lindemann or fissure burr. This bone cut can also be made without predrilling in soft bone types and should safely cut through the cortex along the internal aspect of the buccal cortex. The two cortical cuts can also be connected directly with the saw.

Special attention must be paid to the complete osteotomy with the drill at the transition of the horizontal and buccal osteotomy to the connecting line (Figs. 22.8, 22.9). No cortical bridges

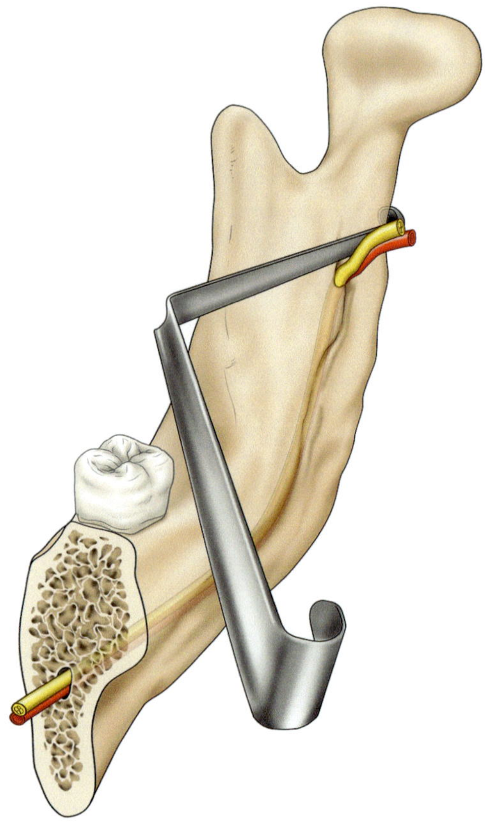

Fig. 22.6 Channel retractor placement for protection of the IAN and as guiding tool for the lingual osteotomy

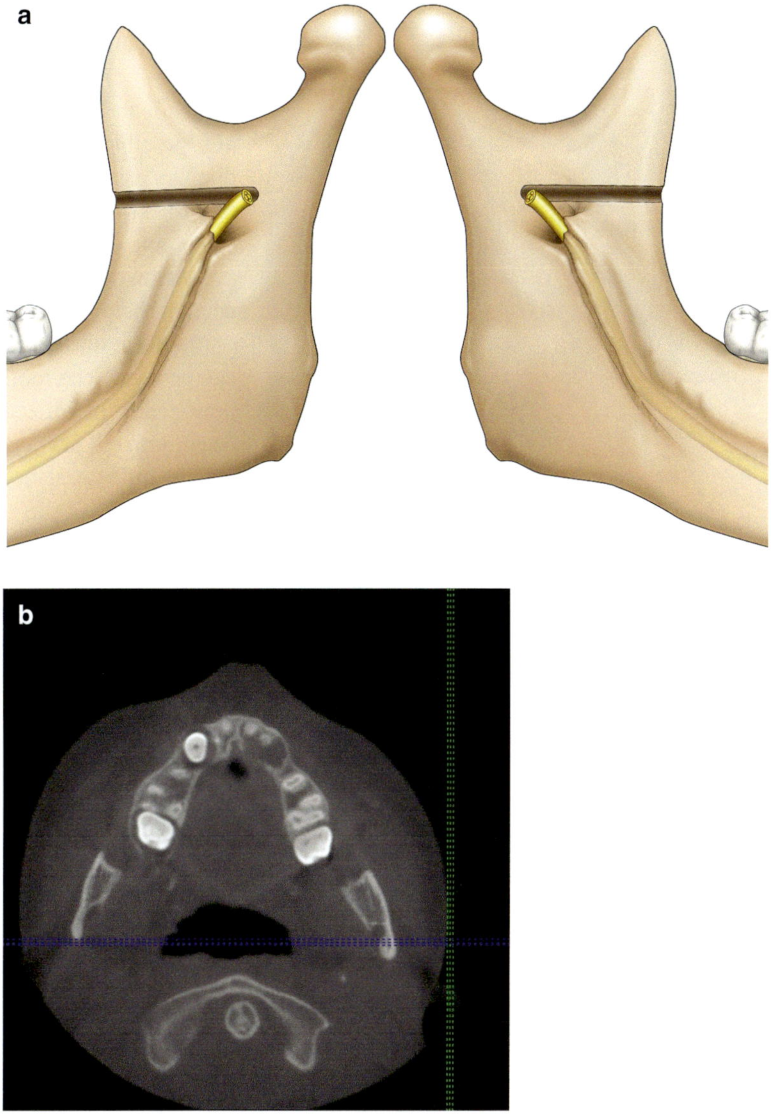

Fig. 22.7 (**a**) Short lingual osteotomy—SLO—on the lingual side according to *Hunsuck–Epker* (**b**) CBCT horizontal scan: on the right mandibular side only the SLO can be applied

must remain here. It is also recommended to carefully weaken the solid mandibular base at the lower edge of the buccal osteotomy as recommended by Böckman et al. and Wolford and Davis [5, 8] (Fig. 22.8).

To avoid problems during the sagittal split it is advisable to start the osteotomy on the lingual side at the lingual cut where solid cortical bone structures prevail. When using the Epker osteotome one feels the resistance of the bone against splitting which suddenly recedes after having reached the groove inferiorly of the condylar process (*sulcus colli*) where the SLO usually ends. After having weakened the bone here with a 5 mm Epker osteotome or a straight chisel it is easier to continue with the splitting procedure in an ascending manner from the buccal osteotomy to the lingual.

After the buccal edge of the lower jaw is also protected towards the cheek by a channel retractor we then split the mandible with thin, slightly laterally bent chisels (5 mm Epker osteotome) first to about the middle, then if possible towards the caudal end of the osteotomy (Figs. 22.10, 22.11).

This depends on the form of the mandible at the buccal osteotomy site: The lateral side of the mandible can be straight but is mostly curved

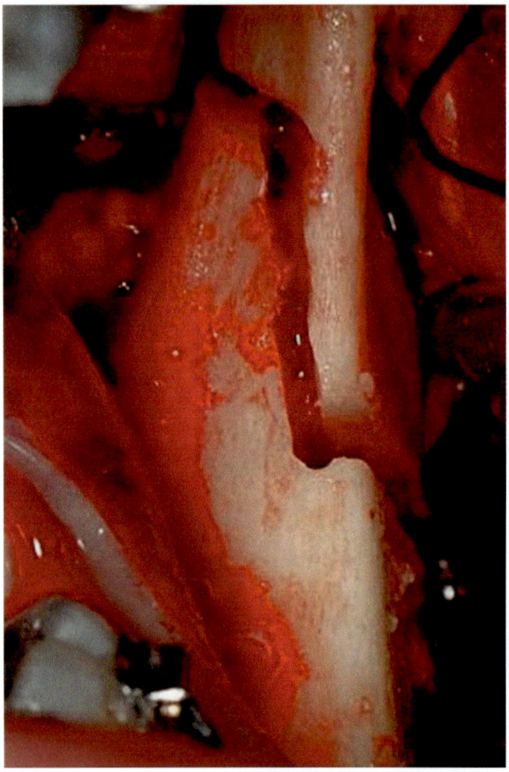

Fig. 22.8 Sagittal split completed with the burr

which makes chiseling more difficult. Alternatively straight 5 mm chisels can be used to deepen the buccal osteotomy in a vertical and slightly dorsal direction to create a gap between the cortical buccal plate and the remaining mandibular body. Make sure that the solid lower mandibular rim is fully osteotomized (Figs. 22.11, 22.12).

Straight 10 mm chisels can be used to deepen the connecting osteotomy line. While doing so experienced surgeons learn to differentiate between "harder" and "softer" bone substance which provides valuable information for the later splitting. Then wide osteotomes can be used with the help of the spreader to widen the gap and finally break the remaining bony connections.

As mentioned above

It is advisable to start the splitting procedure from anterior to posterior, which means from the buccal osteotomy towards the lingual osteotomy. During this process keep an eye on what is happening at the lingual osteotomy side.

While the osteotomy gap is widened, it is usually possible to identify the course of the mandibular canal. This lies mostly in the distal tooth-bearing segment. If this is successful, the osteotome can also be inserted deeper under the protection of the IAN in order to split bony connections below the course of the canal. Depending on the form of the mandible also straight chisels can be used. The tooth-bearing distal segment is now gently mobilized and freely movable. The osteotomized jaw can be relocated anteriorly against little resistance.

Detaching the masseterico-pterygoidal muscle loop is not recommended in mandibular advancement, but soft tissues/fibrous/muscular attachments at the lower border of the distal segment have to be removed for sufficient mobilization. This maneuver, which can be carried out with a strongly curved dissector, removes the remaining attachment of the medial pterygoid muscle from the tooth-bearing distal segment, but not from the proximal segment. This segment is now only fixed to the suprahyoidal muscles and the muscles of the floor of the mouth and tongue and can be moved ventrally against little resistance.

The instruments used to split the jaw angle, or the ascending ramus of the lower jaw, are chosen differently by each surgeon (Figs. 22.13, 22.14, 22.15). After making the connecting osteotomy between the lingual and buccal osteotomy, chisels and osteotomes are preferred. The order of the instruments mentioned seems to be more in keeping with habit.

Freihofer [10] recommended laterally curved chisels that can slide along the buccal cortex to deepen the connecting incision. In many operation theaters this instrument is called Epker osteotome.

The splitting itself can be performed with straight osteotomes (size 8, 10, and 12) or a bone spreader or a combination of both. Which instrument is used also has to do with the length of the connecting osteotomy line (Figs. 22.13, 22.14, 22.15).

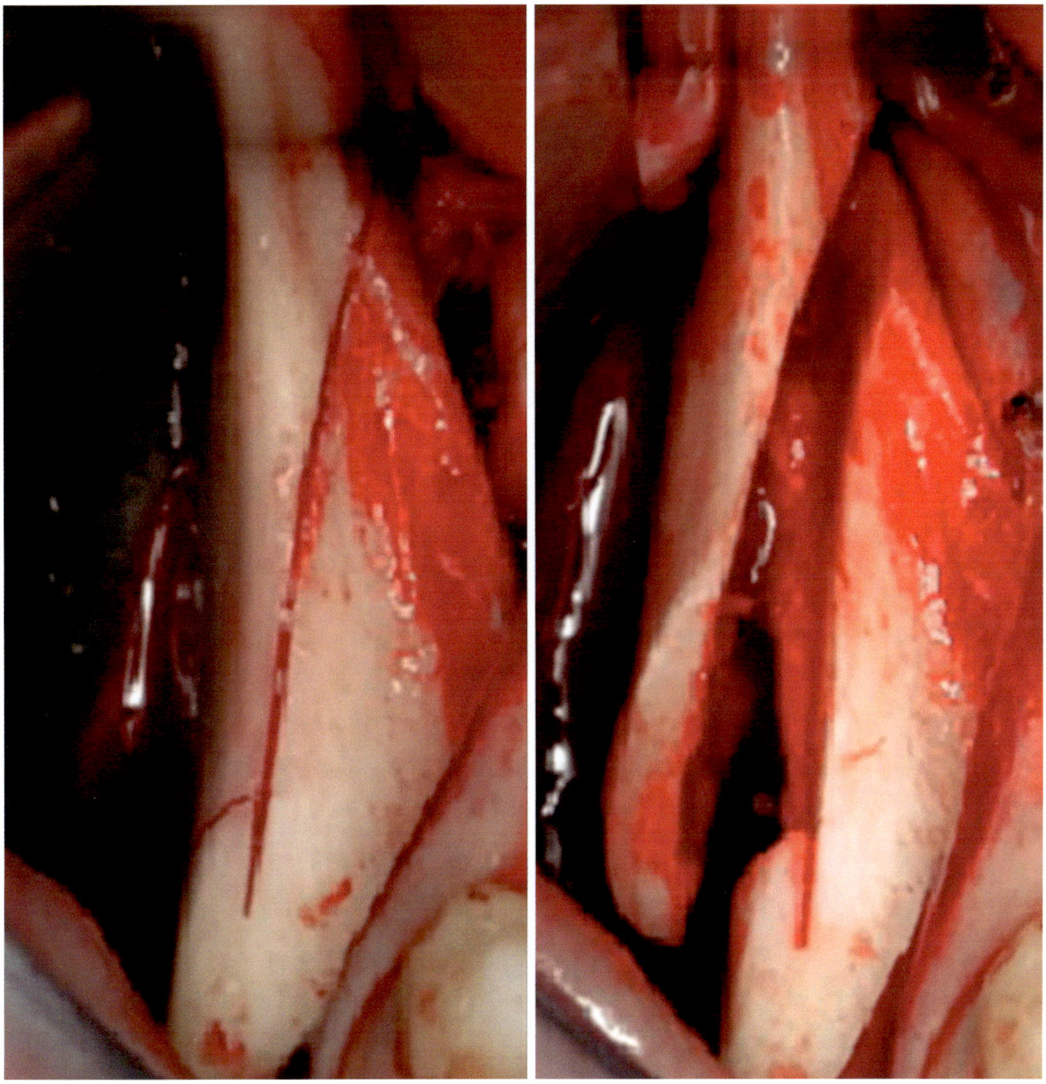

Fig. 22.9 Sagittal split completed with the saw

In the classic situation of sagittal splitting according to *Dal Pont* [3] the spreader can be inserted close to the buccal osteotomy from above and anteriorly, and then the osteotomes can be used to complete the splitting first buccally and then lingually after identification of the course of the IAN.

The split can also be performed by a combination of spreader and the Smith separator which is inserted in the buccal osteotomy. Spreader and Smith separator have to be activated simultaneously to split the mandible (Figs. 22.15, 22.16).

If the connecting osteotomy line between the lingual and buccal osteotomy is short, chisels and osteotomes are more likely to be used, as the spreader is less able to expand compact bone. In this case, more energy is required for splitting.

The Figs. 22.17 and 22.18 illustrate possible lingual splits in theory and reality.

Wire loops of 0.4 or 0.5 mm thick steel wire are used for intermaxillary fixation. These are looped over existing Kobayashi ligature hooks, crimpable hooks, or IMF screws (Figs. 22.19, 22.20). In any case, a safe and stable IMF must

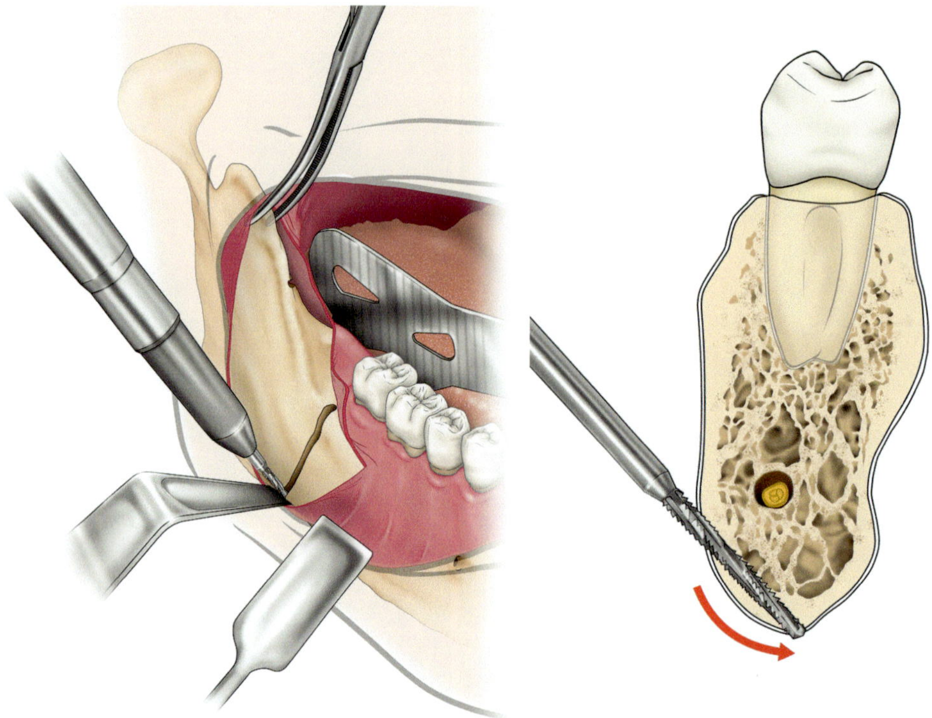

Fig. 22.10 Weakening the inferior mandibular rim for safe splitting

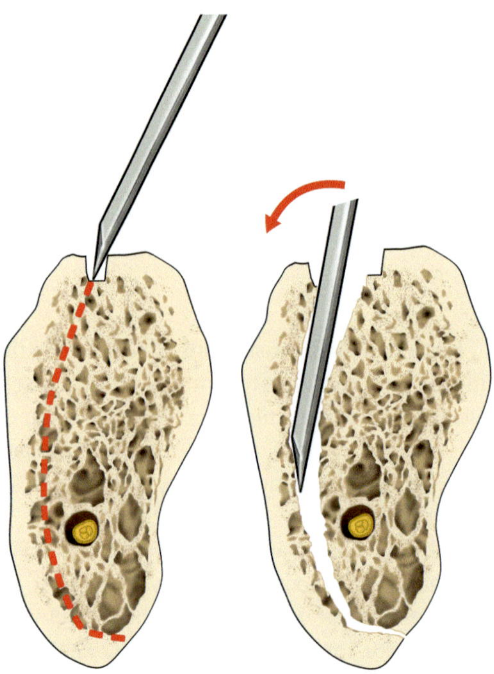

Fig. 22.11 Careful osteotomy along the inner side of the buccal cortex with the 5 mm chisel

be ensured to avoid displacement of the occlusion during osteosynthesis.

Even with symmetrical initial conditions, disturbing influences on the proximal segment—flaring, rotation, dislocation—must be expected [11].

- If rotational movements are added to the sagittal movement of the mandible, this can lead to a forced displacement of the temporomandibular joint (proximal segment), mostly on the contralateral side of the asymmetry.
- If the mandible is shifted for correction of asymmetry without rotation, the ipsilateral proximal segment can be affected.

Both movements can lead to temporomandibular joint diseases and functional restrictions of the lower jaw movements.

A special chapter is devoted to the procedures for asymmetrically shaped mandibles in detail.

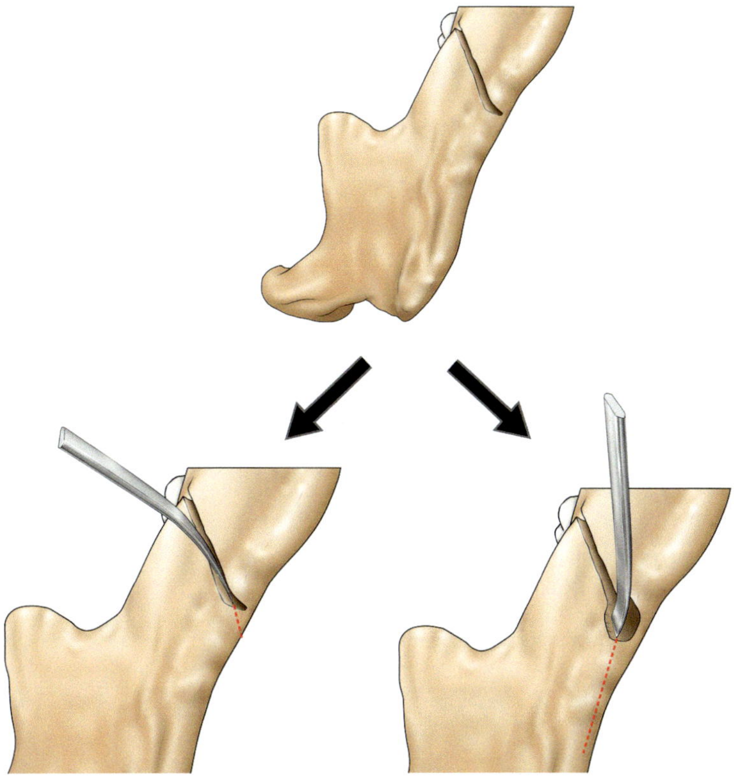

Fig. 22.12 Inferior mandibular rim osteotomy with special attention to split the mandible as described by Böckmann et al. and Wolford and Davis [5, 8] ©Copyright Keisuke Koyama 2020. All rights reserved

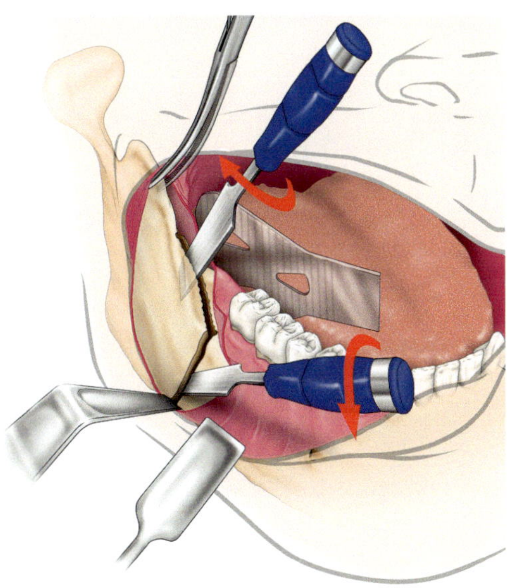

Fig. 22.13 Careful splitting using two osteotomes ©Copyright Keisuke Koyama 2020. All rights reserved

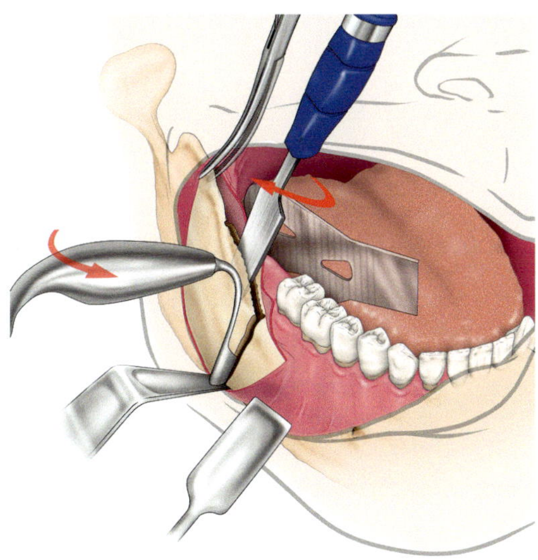

Fig. 22.14 Careful splitting using one osteotome and the Smith separator ©Copyright Keisuke Koyama 2020. All rights reserved

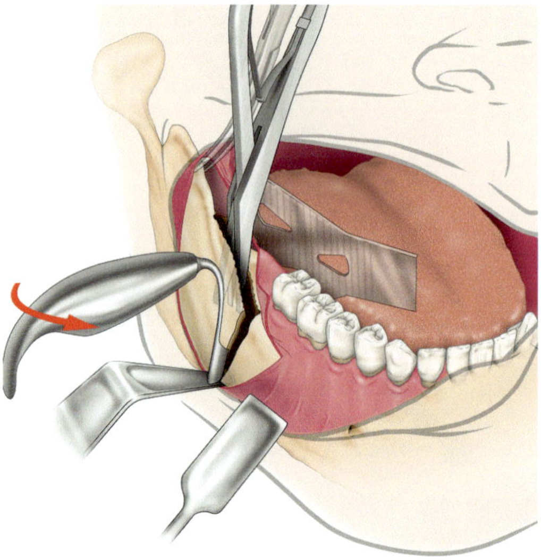

Fig. 22.15 Careful splitting using the spreader and the Smith separator ©Copyright Keisuke Koyama 2020. All rights reserved

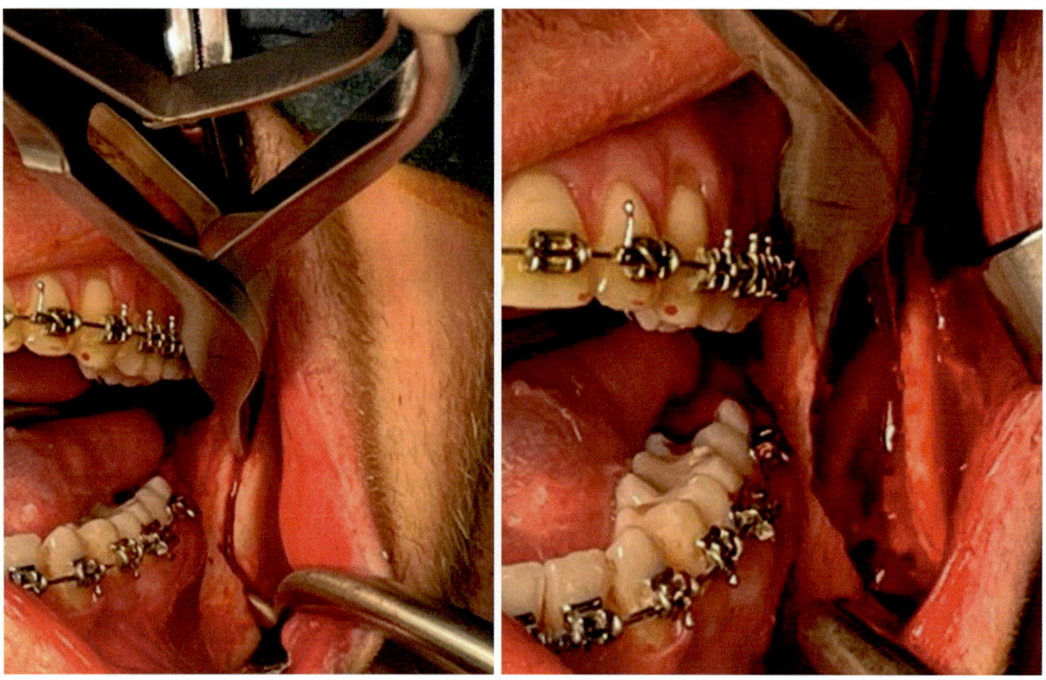

Fig. 22.16 Clinical situation: Sagittal split using the spreader and the Smith separator, identification of the IAN

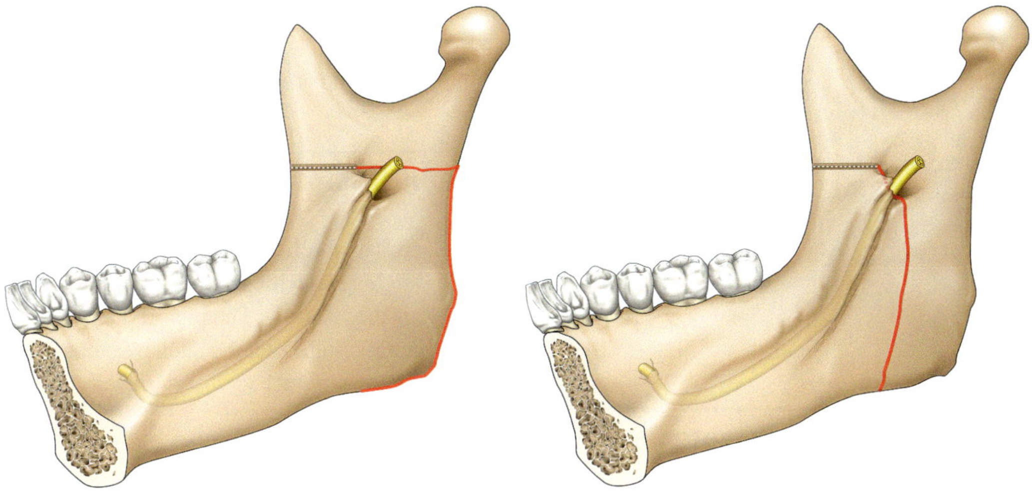

Fig. 22.17 Two possible variants of the lingual split ©Copyright Keisuke Koyama 2020. All rights reserved

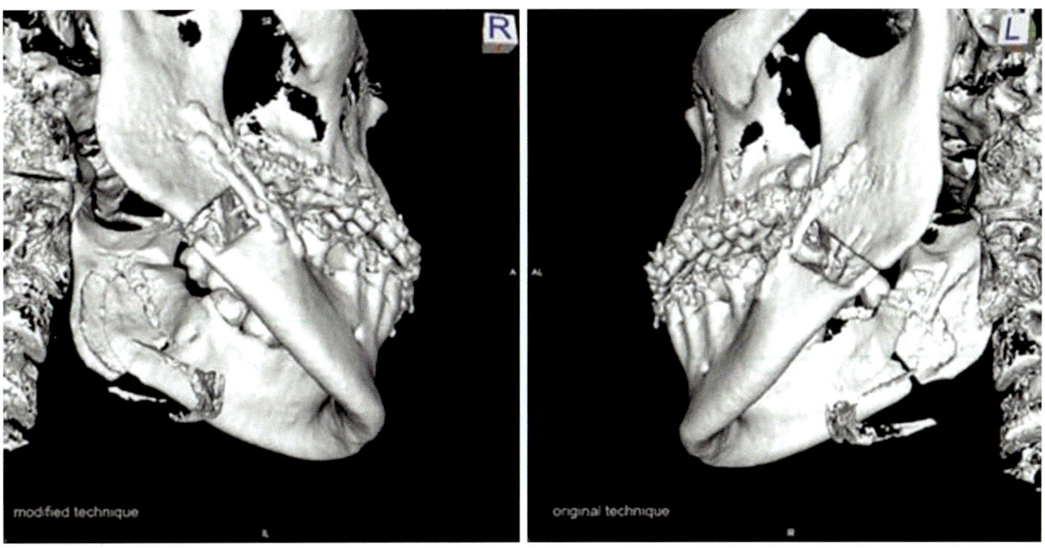

Fig. 22.18 BSSO: Focus on the lingual split which conforms to the schematic drawings of Fig. 22.17

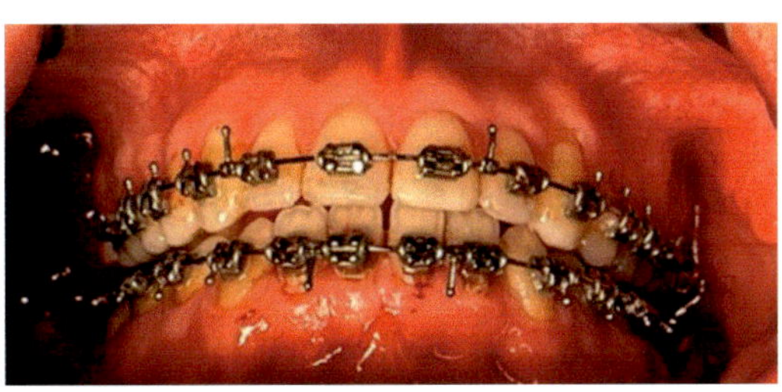

Fig. 22.19 Preparing for IMF with crimpable hooks, perfect midline

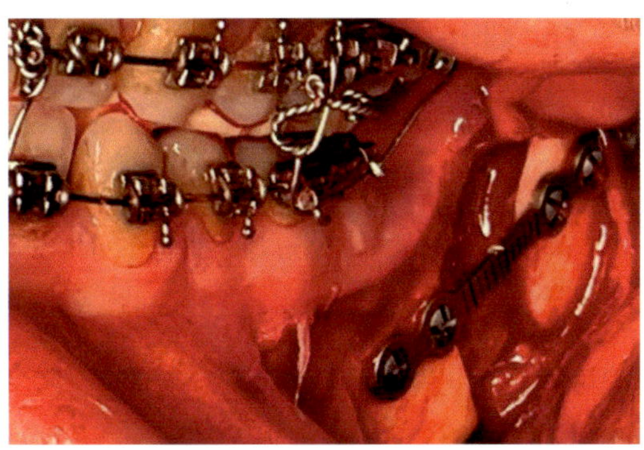

Fig. 22.20 IMF and rigid osteosynthesis with 2.0 mm 4-hole miniplate with bar

Note
The three moments of BSSO where nerve damage can occur are:

- Preparation of the lingual tunnel
- Splitting the lower jaw
- Crushing or direct nerve injury during osteosynthesis, especially when compression or positional screws are used

2 Combination of Osteotomies

2.1 Segment Osteotomies

In class II occlusal positions, there may be an extreme extrusion of the mandibular front, which cannot always be sufficiently levelled preoperatively by levelling the Spee curve.

In some cases there is an indication to correct the mandibular misalignment before orthodontic treatment (surgery first). In the classic approach, a combination of BSSO and anterior segment osteotomy can be performed, whereby the anterior segment is impacted first and then the BSSO is performed as described above.

Also, the final fixation of the anterior segment should only be performed at the end of the entire procedure to ensure that the occlusion is set as planned preoperatively. The combination of both osteotomies is technically difficult and lengthy. Particular attention must be paid to ensuring adequate perfusion of the anterior segment through the lingual soft tissue attachment.

3 The Chin

Another typical combination osteotomy in conjunction with advancement of the mandible is the chin osteotomy. The positioning of the chin can have a decisive influence on facial aesthetics and contribute more to the overall aesthetic assessment of the surgical result than mandibular advancement. For this reason, we have devoted a separate chapter to the possibilities of chin relocation. The techniques described there can be combined with BSSO and mandibular advancement.

4 Conclusion

The BSSO as a splitting technique in the mandibular angle region must be understood in order to apply it successfully. The pictorial and graphic representation points out the decisive steps of this outstanding technique.

References

1. MacIntosh RB. Total mandibular alveolar osteotomy. Encouraging experiences with an infrequently indicated procedure. J Maxillofac Surg. 1974;
2. Pichler H, Berg A. Kieferosteotomie als Korrekturverfahren bei hochgradiger Fehlokklusion und äusserer Entstellung im Kieferbereich. Fortschr Zahnheilk. 1933;IX:1. Teil
3. DalPont G. L' osteotomia retromolare per la correzione della progenia. Minerva Chir. 1958:1.
4. Obwegeser H. Zur Operationstechnik bei der Progenie und anderen Unterkieferanomalien. Dtsch Zahn Mund Kieferheilk. 1955;23:1.
5. Böckmann R, Schön P, Neuking K, Meyns J, Kessler P, Eggeler G. In vitro comparison of the sagittal split osteotomy with and without inferior border osteotomy. J Oral Maxillofac Surg. 2015;73(2):316–23.
6. Epker BN. Modification in the sagittal osteotomy of the mandible. J Oral Surg. 1977;35:157–9.
7. Epker B, Fish L. The surgical orthodontic correction of mandibular deficiency. Part I. Am J Orthod. 1983;84:408. Part II Am J Orthodont 1983; 84, 491
8. Wolford LM, Davis WM. The mandibular inferior border split: a modification in the sagittal split ramus osteotomy associated with the presence or absence of third molars. J Oral Maxillofac Surg. 2001;59(8):92–4.
9. Hunsuck EE. A modified intraoral sagittal splitting technic for correction of mandibular prognathism. J Oral Surg. 1968;26(4):250–3.
10. Freihofer HP. Proleme der Behandlung der Progenie durch sagittale Spaltung der aufsteigenden Unterkieferäste. Schweiz Mschr Zahnheilk. 1976;86:679.
11. Severt TR, Proffit WF. The prevalence of facial asymmetry in the dentofacial deformities population at the University of North Carolina. Int J Adult Orthodon Orthoganthic Surg. 1997;12:171–6.

Special Surgical Aspects in Mandibular Advancement - Flaring

23

Peter Kessler and Suen An Nynke Lie

Contents

Abstract

Due to the parabolic shape of the mandibular base, mandibular advancement by BSSO can lead to lateral or medial dislocation, or rotation about a vertical or also horizontal axis by the temporomandibular joint (TMJ) in the proximal segment, depending on the replacement distance and the fracture behavior in the region of the mandibular split. Combinations of all three movements are possible, and they can occur unilaterally or bilaterally. Careful preoperative 3D planning provides valuable information to address this fact.

P. Kessler (✉) · S. A. N. Lie
Department of Cranio-Maxillofacial Surgery, Maastricht University Medical Center, Maastricht, The Netherlands
e-mail: peter.kessler@mumc.nl; suen.lie@mumc.nl

Keywords

Mandibular split · BSSO · Mandibular advancement · Mandibular anatomy · Rotational movement · Osteosynthesis · Flaring · TMJ · 3D planning

1 Anatomical Surgical Background

After advancement of the mandible and adjusting the occlusion, the mandible is usually stabilized with functionally stable 2.0 mm osteosynthesis plates. For detailed description see *Osteosynthesis for Sagittal Splitting*. These plates must be long and strong enough to bridge the sagittal gap between the proximal and distal segments. If the long Dal Pont split leads to a wide bony overlap, which is desirable because of healing, and if the advancement of the distal segment is approximately 5–7 mm or more, the forward movement will inevitably impact the proximal segments due to the parabolic form of the mandibular base (Fig. 23.1).

P. Kessler et al. (eds.), *Illustrated Manual of Orthognathic Surgery*,
https://doi.org/10.1007/978-3-031-06978-9_23

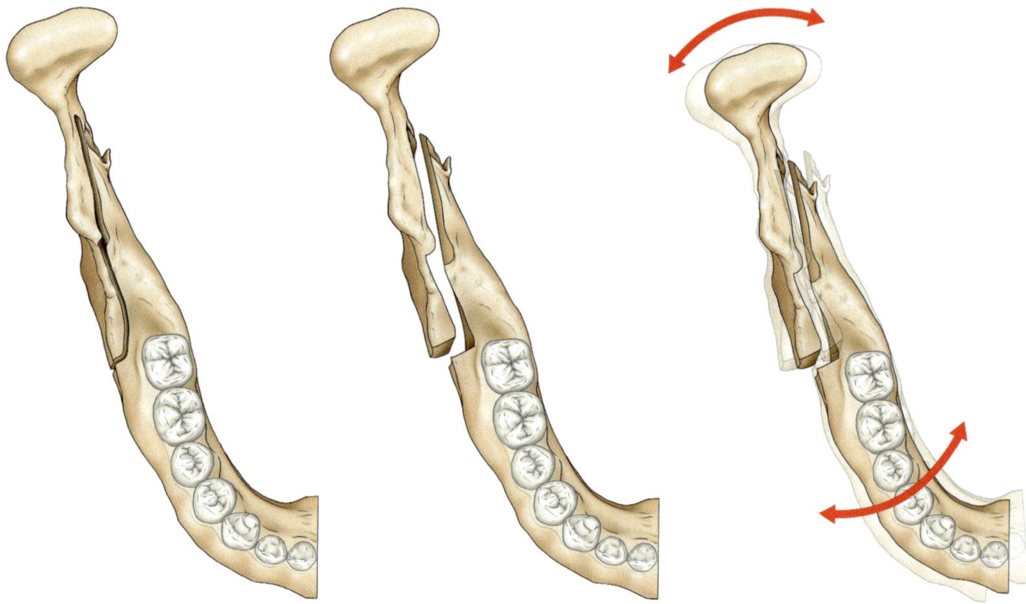

Fig. 23.1 The long bone overlap in the Dal Pont split may lead to rotational effects on the proximal segment: flaring.

Rigid screw fixation is more difficult because the mandibular forward displacement can result in an unfavorable position for screw fixation in the distal segment. Preference should be given to plate osteosynthesis.

> **Note**
> - The base of the mandible has the shape of a parabola.
> - If the mandible is split according to Dal Pont in the region of the jaw angle, i.e., at the base of the parabola, rotation of the TMJ-bearing proximal segments will occur when the mandible is moved forward and the split mandibular segments are superimposed.
> - This effect, known as flaring, depends on the length of the overlay in the split region, the transverse width of the mandible in the region of the gonion angle, and the advancement distance.

To avoid this, a correction must be made to relieve the TMJ. In most situations, a moderate correction of the excess bone in the gap area of the distal segment is sufficient to adjust the two segments so that the bone overlap is still sufficient to ensure direct bone regeneration.

Depending on the width and size of this lingual bone surplus, either the bone forceps (Liston forceps) or the burr must be used for this maneuver. All surrounding soft tissues must be carefully protected and the distal mandibular segment must be manually stabilized to allow a safe procedure. In 3D planning, the problem of flaring can be well represented and, if necessary, corrected by adjusting the buccal osteotomy depending on the planned advancement. The actual course of the split as well as the width of the connecting osteotomy line, the so-called third osteotomy, also plays a role in the evaluation of flaring.

Transfacial-transbuccal approaches to the surgical site in orthognathic surgery should be avoided. The use of angulated drill handpieces allows preparation and osteosynthetic stabilization of the proximal segment while bypassing a transbuccal approach. The angulated handpieces can also be used for manual screw fixation.

The TMJ should be pushed gently into the fossa articularis when the lower jaw is repositioned.

After the split and sufficient mobilization of the segments, the proximal segments can be pushed back- and upward under manual-digital control preauricularly to prevent unintentional dislocation of the TMJ during osteosynthesis or while positioning the mandible in intermaxillary fixation.

In class II cases with large mandibular advancement, the temporomandibular joint should be set in the position that corresponds to slight sagittal overcorrection. This means that gentle forces should act on the TMJ during the osteosynthetic stabilization when correcting class II mandibles.

The pre-fixation of the TMJ is certainly sensible for functional reasons, but clinically it does not meet the expectations placed on it, since the guaranteed precision and stability are not sufficient and the technical solution limits the overview. This is a classic indication for 3D planning in order to recognize the risk of flaring preoperatively, to search for alternative solutions and to judge them virtually.

Note

- Flaring with negative effects on the function of TMJ should be avoided.
- 3D planning enables the preoperative detection and correction of this problem.
- Intraoperative corrections are technically not easy to perform, their effect can hardly be verified.

2 Modifications and Surgical Alternatives

Computer-based planning is of great help when planning symmetrical or asymmetrical advancement operations in mandibular retrognathism, as it clearly shows the sagittal and rotational movements of the distal tooth-bearing mandibular segment in relation to the proximal mandibular segment (TMJ) and provides very useful information when selecting the appropriate splitting technique and defining the position of the buccal osteotomy.

In addition, individually manufactured osteosynthesis plates can transmit the preoperatively determined optimal surgical solution to the operating room. Laser-melted titanium plates are extremely hard and guarantee form and function stability at low volume.

Ultimately, stable osteosynthesis could also be dispensed with in order to give the proximal segment more freedom to rotate back into a functionally physiological position. However, this requires a long IMF, which in turn requires intensive cooperation of the patient [1].

This, however, means that the decisive advantage of rigid internal fixation, namely the ability to dispense with a long-term IMF, is abandoned. Further, instability of the proximal segment can lead to unwanted cranial rotation of the proximal segment due to muscle contraction, which can hardly be corrected at a later stage.

Real alternatives are the vertical osteotomy in the area of the ascending mandibular, which is described in Part VII. The oblique, inverted L- and C-shaped osteotomy can be considered. A second alternative to mandibular advancement is horizontal mandibular distraction. Both alternatives are discussed in separate chapters.

3 Conclusion

SSRO/BSSO with a short lingual osteotomy—SLO—acc. to *Hunsuck/Epker* is the standard technique in correction of symmetric/asymmetric mandibular retrognathism. Use 3D planning to avoid negative effects on the TMJ structures due to flaring and excessive TMJ rotation. Asymmetric mandibular retrognathism is challenging and needs more attention during planning and surgery.

The mandibular split technique by means of BSSO per se and the shape of the mandibular base must be placed in relation to the TMJ whenever the mandible is replaced. 3D planning provides a significant contribution to avoid intraoperative problems in functional terms, but also with a view to a stable result and a non-compromised TMJ function. As a safe technique, the advantages of the BSSO outweigh any possible consequences or technique-related functional limitations.

Reference

1. Ohba S, Nakao N, Kawasaki T, Miura K, Minamizato T, Koga T, et al. Skeletal stability after sagittal spit ramus osteotomy with physiological positioning in patients with skeletal mandibula prognathism and facial asymmetry. Br J Oral Maxillofac Surg. 2016;54:920–6.

Intermolar Mandibular Distraction Osteogenesis IMDO

24

Suen An Nynke Lie and Peter Kessler

Contents

Abstract

Lengthening the human mandible by distraction osteogenesis (DOG) has become an accepted treatment to correct severe mandibular hypoplasia (Kessler et al. Mund Kiefer Gesichtschir 4(3):178–182, 2000a; Wiltfang et.al. Br J Oral Maxillofac Surg 40:473–479, 2002). Mandibular distraction osteogenesis is especially used for neonates and infants with upper airway obstruction secondary to micrognathia. In infants extraoral appliances and in young adults intraoral distraction devices are used.

As described in this chapter, there is a very different genetic distribution of growth patterns in the viscerocranium. In some regions, class II jaw relations predominate up to 60% of all treatment cases, while in Asian countries class III or relative class III jaw relations are more common. The success of distraction treatments, especially in newborns and patients with syndromal growth disorders

S. A. N. Lie · P. Kessler (✉)
Department of Cranio-Maxillofacial Surgery, Maastricht University Medical Center Maastricht, Maastricht, The Netherlands
e-mail: suen.lie@mumc.nl; peter.kessler@mumc.nl

P. Kessler et al. (eds.), *Illustrated Manual of Orthognathic Surgery*,
https://doi.org/10.1007/978-3-031-06978-9_24

affecting the jaws, has led to DOG also being used in classic orthodontic treatments (Kessler et al. Mund Kiefer Gesichtschir 4(6):373–376, 2000b; Breik et al. Int J Oral Maxillofac Surg 45(6):769–782, 2016).

The structure that stays behind in growth in the mandible is usually the lower jaw body. For special indications or treatment courses, intermolar osteotomy and DOG treatment in the mandible represents an additional surgical treatment option during growth (Garcia-Piña and Coceancig Int J Oral Maxillofac Surg 481:118, 2019).

Keywords

Class II relation · Mandibular retrognathism · Mandibular retrognathia · Indications for mandibular advancement · Mandibular advancement · Special surgical aspects · Modifications and surgical alternatives · Root damage · Distraction osteogenesis—DOG · Intermolar osteotomy · IMDO · Pubertal growth spurt · Patient satisfaction

1 Indication

Orthodontic treatment starts when the first premolars erupt at an average age of 10–12 years. Patient cooperation and sufficient growth are prerequisites for success [1–3].

1.1 Indications for Intermolar Osteotomy and DOG are

- Class II/1 or class II/2 occlusion (Fig. 24.1).
- Lack of growth of the mandible during orthodontic treatment.
- Treatment with functional appliances is not effective.
- Lack of patient compliance at young age.
- Desire to complete the treatment successfully and quickly.

It is not recommended to perform an early mandibular DOG if the maxillary/midface complex is also retrusive. In this case a bimaxillary advancement at a later age is indicated.

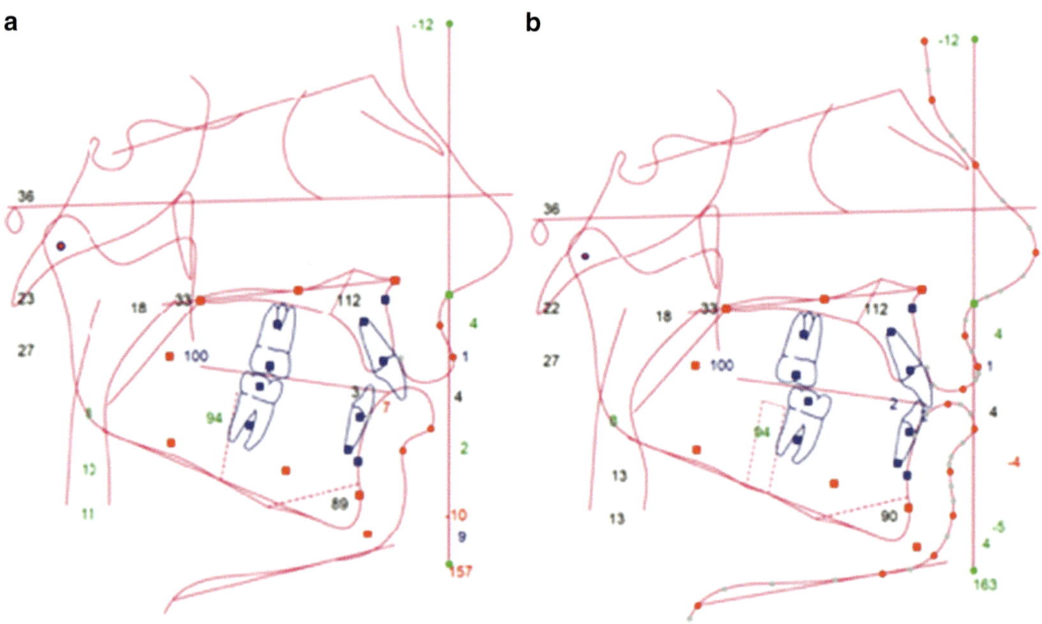

Fig. 24.1 Cephalometric analysis before distraction treatment (**a**) class II/1 occlusion (**b**) Desired mandibular advancement distal to the first mandibular molar

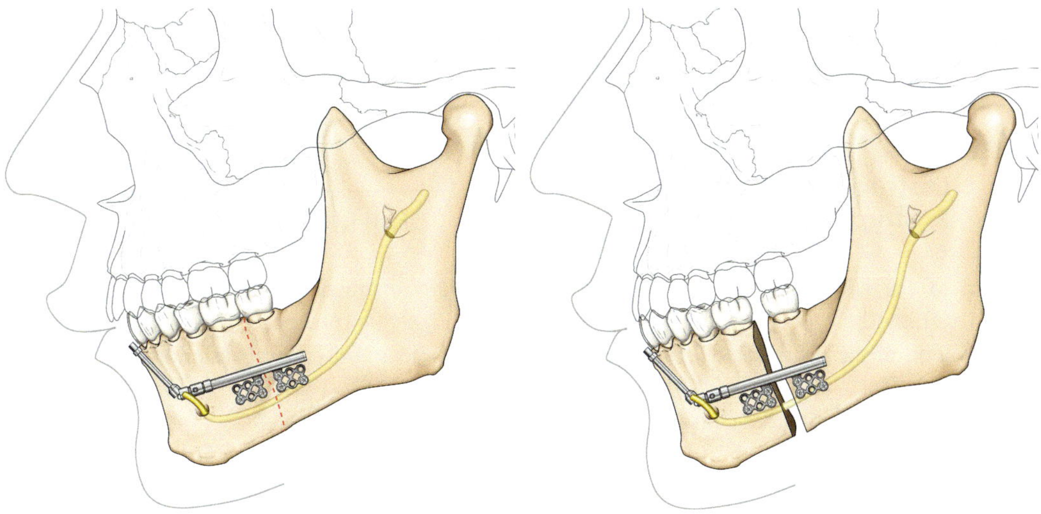

Fig. 24.2 Distractor placement in the molar region of the lower jaw. Osteotomy between first and second molar.

2 Surgical Procedure

The young patients are carefully prepared for the operation, and it is emphasized that after the operation the active distraction phase requires the intensive cooperation of the patient. If possible, a small gap should be created orthodontically between the distal radix of the first mandibular molar and the mesial radix of the second molar. This is where the transverse interradicular osteotomy is performed (Fig. 24.2) [2].

The patients must be aware that two operations are necessary: Insertion and removal of the distractor, usually under general anesthesia.

Different distractors can be selected depending on the size of the mandible. The distraction is unidirectional; care must be taken to ensure that the distraction vector is aligned as parallel as possible to the occlusal plane. If there is a deep bite with a traumatic palatal bite, a slightly divergent direction of the distractor is preferred. The distractor must be able to provide sufficient distraction length.

3 Surgical Steps:

General anesthesia with nasal intubation.

- Weight-adapted local anesthesia with vasoconstriction in oral mucosa in the molar region of the mandible.
- Incision 5-8 mm buccal of the mucogingival border from the premolar region to the base of the masseteric muscle.
- Subperiosteal preparation with preparation of the inferior mandibula rim.
- Identification of the mental foramen.
- Mark the vertical osteotomy line between the first and second molar with a fine fissure drill.
- Fitting of the distractor and temporary fixation with at least 2 screws ventral and dorsal to the osteotomy line.
- Buccal cortical osteotomy with the fine Lindemann drill or with the piezo technique.
- Deepening the osteotomy in between the radices with the 5 mm chisel.
- Cranial, lateral, and caudal osteotomy of the mandibular canal.
- Cautious osteotomy of the lingual cortex with a chisel or piezo. The lingual mucosa must not be harmed.
- Mobilizing the osteotomized jaw segments with the osteotome while protecting the structures in the mandibular canal.
- Identical procedure on the opposite side.
- Positioning of the distractor under vector control.
- Definitive fixation of the distractors.
- Activation of the distractors to check function.
- Hemostasis, wound irrigation with saline, and wound closure with Vicryl 4x0.

- Ensure a convenient port for the distraction arms of the distractors, which are usually located in the cover fold.

4 Distraction/Treatment Protocol:

- Start of the active treatment phase 1 week postoperatively.
- Activation of the distractor once a day by 0.5 mm.
- If there is no midline deviation, symmetrical activation on both sides.
- Duration of the active treatment phase depends on the growth deficit of the mandible.
- Stop activation when cusps and molars are in class I relation.
- Consolidation period after active distraction approximately 8–12 weeks, then distractor removal.
- Continuing orthodontic treatment.

5 The Clinical Treatment Phase

Like any distraction treatment, intermolar DOG is a dynamic procedure that requires regular radiological and clinical monitoring, mainly by the orthodontist (Figs. 24.3, 24.4 and 24.5) [4, 5].

6 Radiological Follow-Up:

See Figs. 24.3, 24.4.

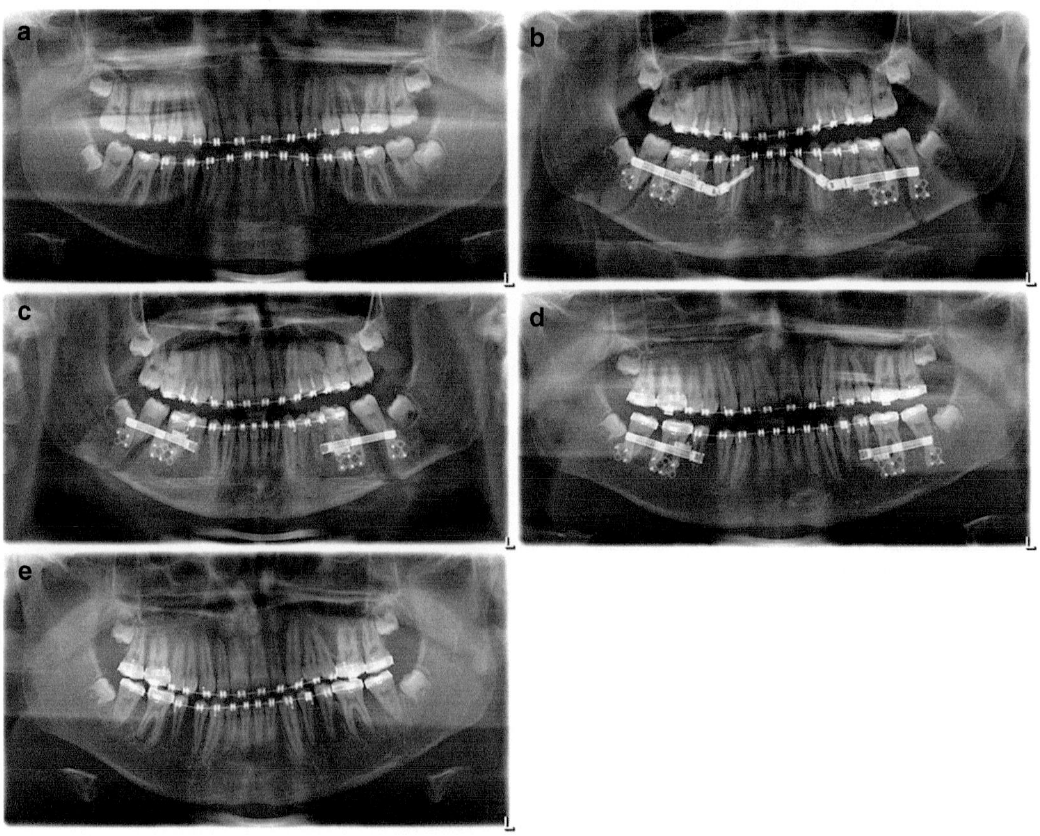

Fig. 24.3 Panoramic X-rays: (**a**) Before intermolar osteotomy and application of distractors. Note the small diastema between the first and second molars of the mandible (**b**) Control after distractor placement. Note the symmetrical axis tilt of the distractors (**c**) End of active distraction treatment and removal of activation rods for more patient comfort (**d**) Bone consolidation 10 weeks after end of distractor activation (**e**) After removal of the distractors

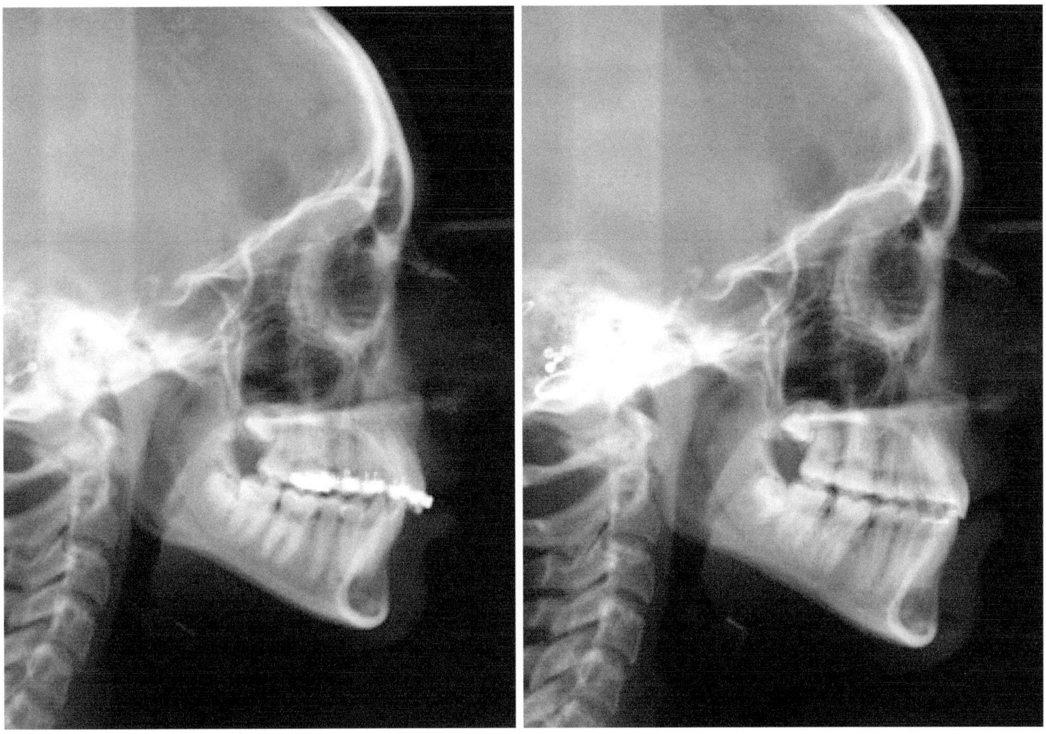

Fig. 24.4 Lateral skull X-ray before and after treatment with intermolar osteotomy and DOG

7 Clinical Follow-Up

See Fig. 24.5.

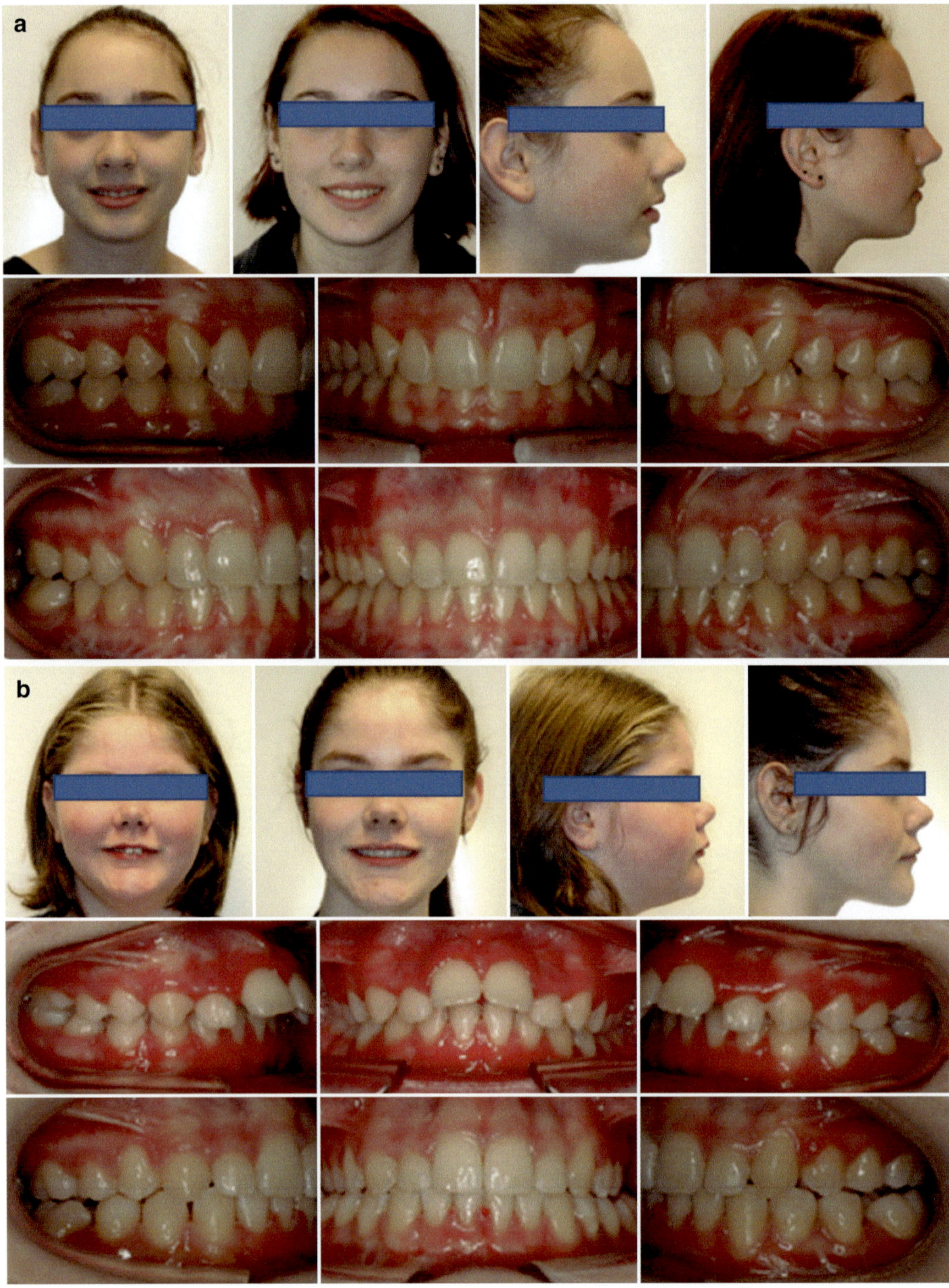

Fig. 24.5 Photographic documentation of two patients: (**a**) 12-year-old patient with class II/2 occlusion before and after end of combined orthodontic and DOG treatment (**b**)12-year-old patient with class II/1 occlusion and traumatic deep bite before and after end of combined orthodontic and distraction treatment. Notice the treatment-related development of the lower third of the face in both cases

7.1 Advantages and Disadvantages of IMDO Treatment

Advantages:

- Treatment at early age.
- Stimulation of self-healing potential by applying DOG on all tissues.
- Dynamic treatment process can be beneficial for TMJ adaptation.
- Positive effects on the posterior airway space.
- Improvement on the position of the cervical spine.
- Increasing width of the mandible and creating space.

Disadvantages:

- Second intervention for distractor removal is needed.
- Risk of wound infection through distractor port.
- Root damage of neighboring teeth during osteotomy (Fig. 24.6).

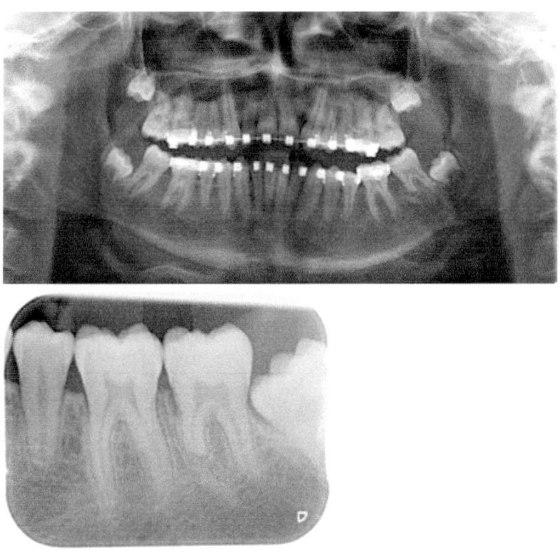

Fig. 24.6 Postoperative X-ray documentation of an unintentional root tip amputation in the second molar in the left mandible after intermolar osteotomy and distraction treatment. Consolidation of the root stump with resorption of the root fragment

8 Conclusion

Satisfactory results can be achieved with intermolar osteotomy and DOG. Despite the risk of tooth damaging during the intermolar osteotomy, a major advantage in terms of patient satisfaction is due to the fact that the entire orthodontic and orthognathic treatment can be completed in a manageable period of time during the pubertal growth spurt. The esthetic benefit of harmonizing the facial features at this sensitive age should not be underestimated in the positive assessment.

References

1. Breik O, Tivey D, Umpathysivam K, Anderson P. Mandibular distraction osteogenesis for the management of upper airway obstruction in children with micrognathia: a systematic review. Int J Oral Maxillofac Surg. 2016;45(6):769–82.
2. Garcia-Piña J, Coceancig P. Inter-molar mandibular distraction osteogenesis (IMDO), why and when to do it. Int J Oral Maxillofac Surg. 2019;48(Suppl 1):118.
3. Kessler P, Wiltfang J, Merten HA, Neukam FW. Distraktionsostogenese der Mandibula bei kraniofazialen Fehlbildungen. Mund Kiefer Gesichtschir. 2000a;4(3):178–82.
4. Kessler P, Wiltfang J, Teschner M, Girod B, Neukam FW. Computergestützte Simulationsmöglichkeiten in der orthopädischen Chirurgie. Mund Kiefer Gesichtschir. 2000b;4(6):373–6.
5. Wiltfang J, Hirschfelder U, Neukam FW, Kessler P. Long-term results of distraction osteogenesis of the maxilla and midface. Br J Oral Maxillofac Surg. 2002;40(6):473–9.

25 Retromolar Mandibular Distraction Osteogenesis RMDO

Suen An Nynke Lie and Peter Kessler

Contents

Abstract

Lengthening the human mandible by distraction osteogenesis (DOG) has become an accepted treatment alternative in selected cases to correct mandibular hypoplasia (Kessler Mund Kiefer Gesichtschir 4(3):178–182, 2000a).

Mandibular DOG is especially used for neonates and infants with upper airway obstruction secondary to micrognathia. In infants extraoral appliances and in young adults intraoral distraction devices are preferred

Keywords

Class II relation · Mandibular retrognathism · Indications for mandibular advancement · Sagittal splitting · BSSO · Mandibular advancement · Special surgical aspects · Modifications and surgical alternatives · Distraction osteogenesis—DOG · Retromolar osteotomy · Soft tissue deficit

As described in this chapter, there are genetically determined differences in the regional occurrence of growth patterns in the viscerocranium. In some regions, class II jaw relations predominate up to 60% of all treatment cases, while in Asian countries class III or relative class III jaw relations are more common. The success of distraction treatments, especially in newborns and

S. A. N. Lie · P. Kessler (✉)
Department of Cranio-Maxillofacial Surgery, Maastricht University Medical Center, Maastricht, The Netherlands
e-mail: suen.lie@mumc.nl; peter.kessler@mumc.nl

P. Kessler et al. (eds.), *Illustrated Manual of Orthognathic Surgery*,
https://doi.org/10.1007/978-3-031-06978-9_25

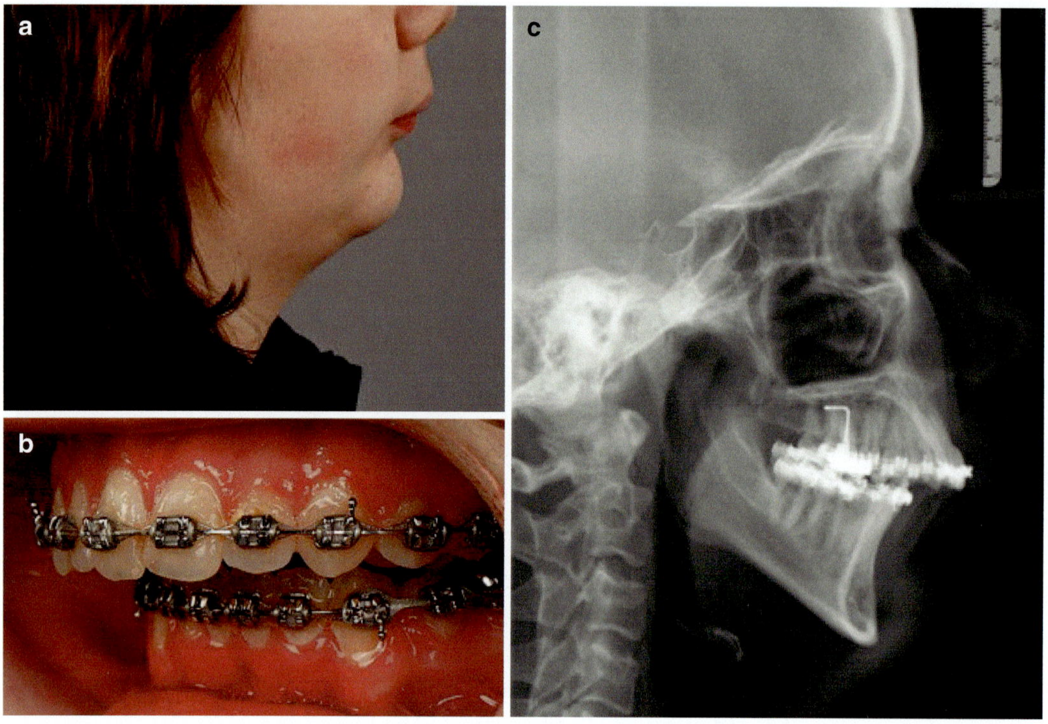

Fig. 25.1 Clinical and radiological situation before treatment: (**a**) Clinical picture of a patient with mandibular deficiency and unfavorable submandibular/submental soft tissue conditions (**b**) Class II/1 malocclusion (**c**) Lateral cephalogram displaying a hypoplastic mandible

patients with syndromal growth disorders affecting the jaws, has led to DOG also being used in classic orthognathic surgery [1, 4, 5, 7].

The structure that stays behind in growth in the mandible is usually the lower jaw body. For special indications or treatment courses, retromolar mandibular distraction osteogenesis treatment—RMDO—represents an additional surgical treatment option (Fig. 25.1).

1 Indication

- Class II/1 or class II/2 malocclusion (Fig. 25.1).
- Short mandible.
- Insufficient length of the suprahyoid soft tissues (geniohyoid muscle).
- Increased risk of relapse with the use of a BSSO.

It is not recommended to perform a RMDO, if the maxillary/midface complex is also retrusive. In this case a bimaxillary advancement is indicated.

2 Surgical Procedure

The patients are carefully prepared for the operation and it is emphasized that after the operation the active distraction phase requires the intensive cooperation of the patient. RMDO like any distraction procedure is a dynamic treatment versus the static treatment in BSSO by osteosynthesis [2].

The patients must be aware that two operations are necessary: Insertion and removal of the distractor, usually under general anesthesia.

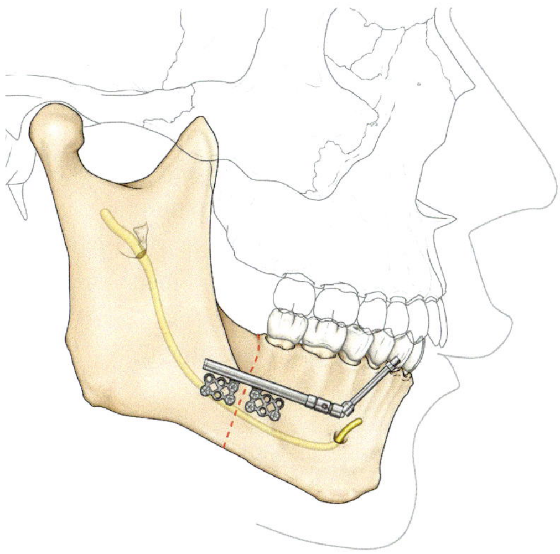

Fig. 25.2 Distractor placement in the retromolar region of the lower jaw. Osteotomy distal of the second molar

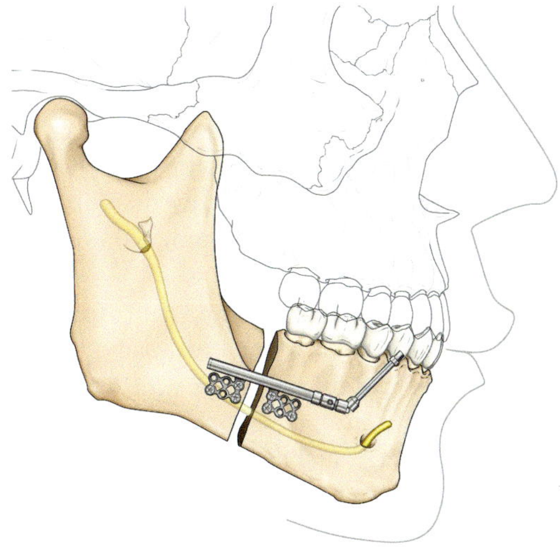

Fig. 25.3 Distractor activated. Distraction gap opens distal of the second molar.

In adults stable distractors must be selected adapted to the size of the mandible. The distraction is unidirectional; care must be taken to ensure that the distraction vector is aligned as parallel as possible to the occlusal plane and in parallel to each other (Figs. 25.2 and 25.3).

If there is a deep bite with a traumatic palatal bite, a slightly divergent direction of the distractor is preferred. The distractor must be able to provide sufficient distraction length.

3 Surgical Steps:

General anesthesia with nasal intubation

- Local infiltration anesthesia with vasoconstriction in oral mucosa in the lateral molar region of the mandible.
- Incision 5–8 mm buccal of the mucogingival border from the premolar region to the retromolar region, comparable to the BSSO approach.

- Subperiosteal preparation with preparation of the inferior mandibula rim.
- Identification of the mental foramen.
- Mark the vertical osteotomy line distal of the second molar with a fine fissure drill.
- Fitting of the distractor and temporary fixation with at least two screws ventral and dorsal to the osteotomy line.
- Buccal cortical osteotomy with the fine Lindemann drill or with piezosurgery.
- Deepening the osteotomy in with the 5 mm chisel.
- Cranial, lateral, and caudal osteotomy of the mandibular canal.
- Cautious osteotomy of the lingual cortex with a chisel or piezo. The lingual mucosa must not be harmed.
- Mobilizing the osteotomized jaw segments with the osteotome while protecting the structures in the mandibular canal.
- Identical procedure on the opposite side.
- Positioning of the distractor under vector control.
- Definitive fixation of the distractors.
- Activation of the distractors to check function.
- Hemostasis, wound irrigation with saline, and wound closure with Vicryl 4x0.
- Ensure a convenient port for the activation rods of the distractors, which are usually located in the vestibular fold.

4 Distraction Protocol:

- Start of the active treatment phase 1 week postoperatively.
- Activation of the distractor twice a day by 0.5 mm (2 x 0.5 mm).
- If there is no midline deviation, symmetrical activation on both sides.
- Duration of the active treatment phase depends on the growth deficit of the mandible.
- Stop activation when cusps and molars are in class I relation with overcorrection.
- Consolidation period after active distraction approximately 12 weeks, then distractor removal.
- Continuing orthodontic treatment.

5 The Clinical Treatment Phase

Like any distraction treatment, RMDO is a dynamic procedure that requires regular radiological and clinical monitoring, mainly by the surgeon (Fig. 25.5).

Distraction treatment not only rebuilds bone but also stimulates redevelopment of soft tissue (Fig. 25.4). The gradual lengthening of muscles, tendons, and connective tissue in general reduces the risk of recurrence.

An advantage of mandibular distraction is that even after the active distraction phase is completed, treatment can be restarted after a break. This time window is about 6 weeks. This may be necessary if one notices a relapse/settling of the mandibular position during follow-up. This concept is called floating bone concept [3, 6].

The clinical case illustrated here is intended to demonstrate that RMDO should only be used in selected cases (Figs. 25.1, 25.4, 25.5). The standard class II treatment is the BSSO with mandibular advancement (Fig. 25.6).

Fig. 25.4 Result after finishing treatment. Note the redevelopment of the submandibular soft tissues

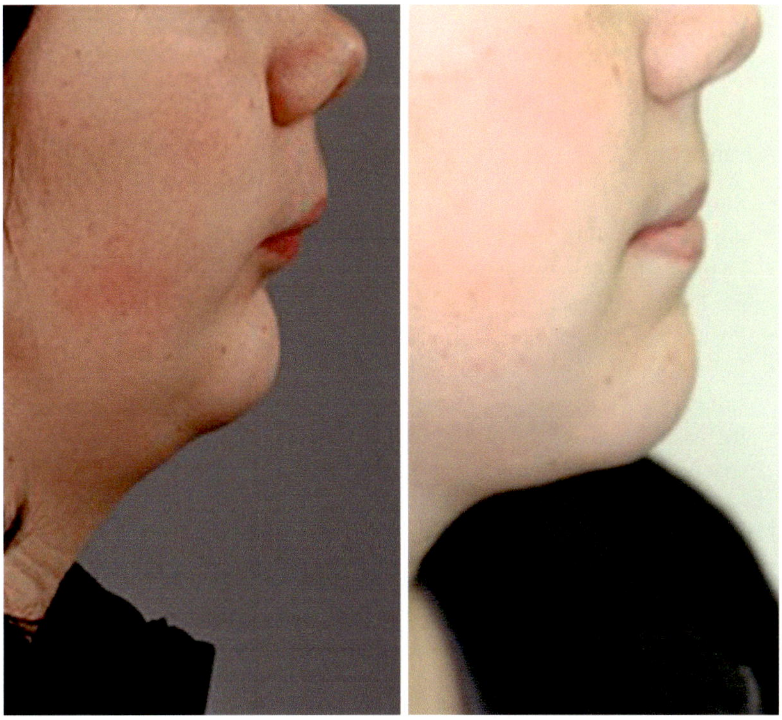

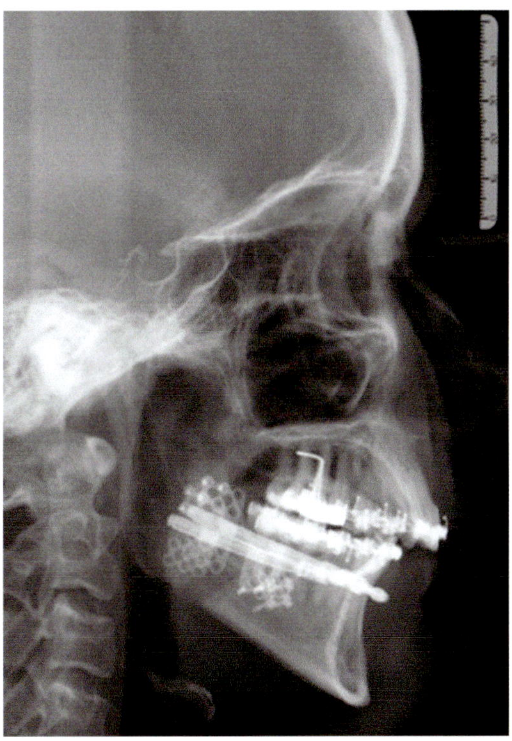

Fig. 25.5 Assessment of mandibular advancement by lateral cephalogram during active distraction treatment. Note the parallel position of the distractors

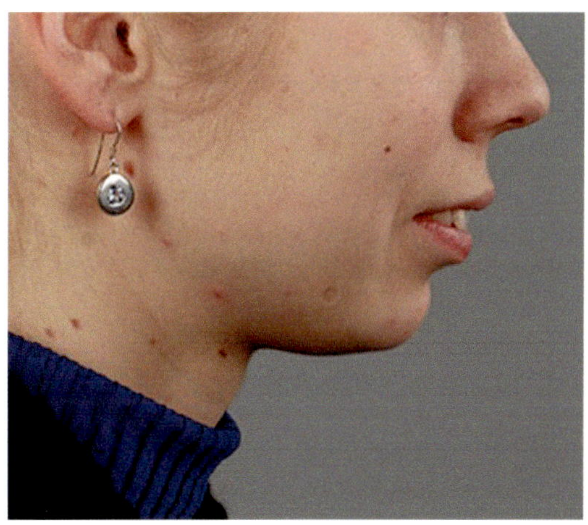

Fig. 25.6 Clinical picture of a patient with II jaw position with standard proportions not requiring RMDO/DOG

5.1 Advantages and Disadvantages of RMDO Treatment

Advantages:

- Stimulation of self-healing potential by applying DOG on all tissues.
- Dynamic treatment process can be beneficial for TMJ adaptation.
- Positive effects on the posterior airway space.
- Improvement on the position of the cervical spine.
- Increasing width of the mandible and creating space.

Disadvantages:

- Second intervention for distractor removal is needed.
- Risk of wound infection through distractor port/activation rod.
- Root damage of neighboring teeth during osteotomy.
- Limited indication.

6 Conclusion

In the surgical treatment of the retrognathic mandible, DOG—RMDO—represents an alternative treatment method that can be used specifically where significant post-development of the mandible and its surrounding soft tissues are a priority.

References

1. Breik O, Tivey D, Umpathysivam K, Anderson P. Mandibular distraction osteogenesis for the management of upper airway obstruction in children with micrognathia: a systematic review. Int J Oral Maxillofac Surg. 2016;45(6):769–82.
2. Baas EM, Pijpe J, De Lange J. Long term stability of mandibula advancement procedures: bilateral sagittal split osteotomy versus distraction osteogenesis. Int J Oral Maxillofac Surg. 2012;41(2):137–41.
3. Hoffmeister B, Marks C, Wolff K. Floating bone concept in mandibular distraction. Int J Oral Maxillofac Surg. 1999;28(1):90.
4. Kessler P, Wiltfang J, Merten HA, Neukam FW. Distraktionsostogenese der Mandibula bei kraniofazialen Fehlbildungen. Mund Kiefer Gesichtschir. 2000a;4(3):178–82.
5. Kessler P, Wiltfang J, Teschner M, Girod B, Neukam FW. Computergestützte simulationsmöglichkeiten in der orthopädischen chirurgie. Mund Kiefer Gesichtschir. 2000b;4(6):373–6.
6. Politi M, Sembronio S, Robiony M, Costa F. The floating bone technique of the vertical ramus in hemifacial microsomia: case report. Int J Adult Orthodon Orthgnath Surg. 2002;17(3):223–9.
7. Wiltfang J, Hirschfelder U, Neukam FW, Kessler P. Long-term results of distraction osteogenesis of the maxilla and midface. Br J Oral Maxillofac Surg. 2002;40(6):473–9.

Part V

Mandibular Excess - Surgical Technique - BSSO

Indications for Mandibular Setback

26

Peter Kessler, Nicolas Hardt, and Suen An Nynke Lie

Contents

Abstract

The word prognathism—class III dysgnathia, mandibular prognathism, class III malocclusion—is derived from Greek πρό (pro, "forward") and γνάθος (gnáthos, "jaw"). Clinical symptoms can be very diverse. They include anterior cross- and headbites, unilateral or bilateral crossbites of various degrees, upper jaw crowding, but also incomplete upper jaw dentitions, compensatory extraverted upper jaw fronts, as well as compensated inverted lower incisors. Furthermore, it must be differentiated whether the respective class III is a forward displacement of the mandible or a backward displacement of the maxilla or a combination of both symptoms. Prognathism can be treated at different ages and stages of development. Depending on this, different therapeutic means can be used, often only with the support of orthognathic surgery. Common to all these means of treatment is that they are visible to the patient's social environment. Non-treatment may remain a limitation in daily life (Severt and Proffit Int J Adult Orthodon Orthoganthic Surg 12:171–176, 1997).

P. Kessler (✉) · S. A. N. Lie
Department of Cranio-Maxillofacial Surgery, Maastricht University Medical Center, Maastricht, The Netherlands
e-mail: peter.kessler@mumc.nl; suen.lie@mumc.nl

N. Hardt (✉)
Kantonsspital Lucerne, Clinic and Policlinic of Cranio-Maxillofacial Surgery, Lucerne, Switzerland

Skeletal class III malocclusion is a widespread, mostly genetically determined malocclusion that can be explained by a growth excess in the mandible and/or growth deficit in the maxilla/midface. A concave facial profile with protruding chin is the result. The prevalence of class III malocclusion varies greatly both among and within populations, and the highest prevalence has been observed in Southeast Asian populations. In pronounced form, biting off food is impossible and the functional range of the temporomandibular joints is limited. This is the functional indication for therapy. The only true option for correction in skeletal class III is surgical. In addition to the BSSO, the inverted L osteot-

P. Kessler et al. (eds.), *Illustrated Manual of Orthognathic Surgery*,
https://doi.org/10.1007/978-3-031-06978-9_26

omy and the intraoral vertical ramus osteotomy (IVRO) can also be used (Bell et al. Surgical correction of dentofacial deformities 2:890–895, 1980).

Keywords

Class III relation · Class III malocclusion · Mandibular prognathism · Maxillary/midface retrusion · Indications for mandibular setback · Sagittal splitting · BSSO · Mandibular setback · Special surgical aspects in mandibular setback · Mandibular segment osteotomy · Modifications and surgical alternatives · Inverted Vertical Ramus Osteotomy - IVRO · Inverted L osteotomy

The morphological characteristics of a mandibular prognathism are responsible for a typical patient appearance, which is judged objectively and subjectively very differently. Patients with class III position of the lower jaw are often dissatisfied with their appearance. At the same time, if the lower face height is enlarged, a prominent chin position can be disturbing (Fig. 26.1).

The clinical image of mandibular prognathism can be assigned to a dentoalveolar or skeletal class III with cause in the mandible or maxilla or a combination of both. Clinical, radiological, and technical analyses (cephalometry), especially in the sagittal plane, are used to determine which diagnosis is applicable [1, 2].

These analyses must provide information about the position and size of the mandibular skeletal structures with respect to the degree of mandibular prognathism within the respective facial growth pattern and clarify the extent of dentoalveolar and/or skeletal involvement in class III malocclusion (Fig. 26.2).

In cephalometric analysis the simple class III cases show a jaw base harmony except for the mandibular prognathism (SNB-angle). The sagittal interbasal relation (ANB-angle) is found to be reduced (negative ANB-angle). If the pogonion prominence is in harmony with the face, it indicates an alveolar mandibular overdevelopment. If the position of the pogonion is also in disharmony—sagittal forward displacement of the pogonion—the situation fulfills the criteria of a skeletal mandibular prognathism (Fig. 26.3) [1, 2].

Vertical and transversal disharmonies or discrepancies may be present in the planning of the procedure, which complicate planning and lead to horizontal and vertical rotational moments in the correction of the malocclusion, which must be observed without fail while avoiding relapse. The more subjective aesthetic distinction between an orthognathic, retrognathic, and prognathic facial type helps to avoid errors in planning and can occasionally lead to the decision to recommend bimaxillary correction in the case of a prognathic facial type even without skeletal disharmony in the maxilla and midface [1, 2].

Special attention must be paid to the relationship of the mandibular base to the skull base plane (ML-NSL) to avoid errors that may lead to an acceptable functional but unsatisfactory aesthetic result. The position of the chin (pogonion-gnathion) requires special attention in order to achieve a satisfactory aesthetic result.

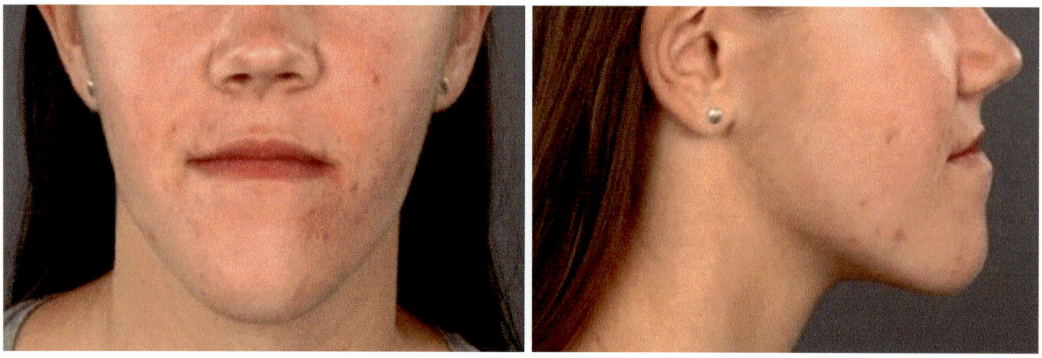

Fig. 26.1 Typical facial appearance in class III malocclusion with mandibular overgrowth

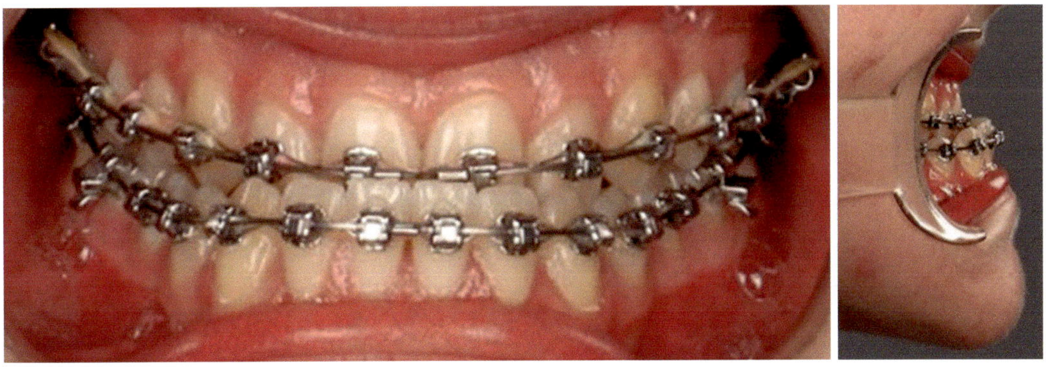

Fig. 26.2 Malocclusion of the patient in Fig. 26.1 with negative dental overjet, anterior and lateral right crossbite

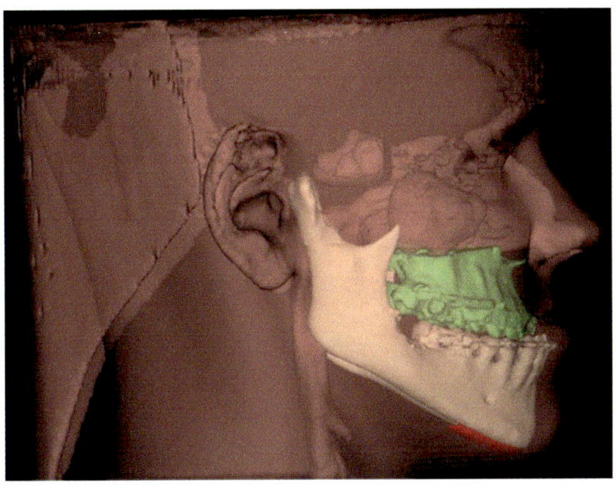

Fig. 26.3 3D imaging of the skeletal class III relation of the patient in Fig. 26.1

Note
- Class III patients often desire correction for aesthetic reasons.
- The indication for correction can be functional or aesthetic or both.
- In planning, special attention must be paid to the vertical sagittal position of the mandibular base—ML-NSL—and the position of the pogonion - SNB, ANB.

1 Conclusion

The diagnosis of mandibular prognathism is usually clear. The assessment of whether it is a pure mandibular prognathism or a combination with maxillary or midface hypoplasia results from the analysis of cephalometry. The resulting correction must take into account aesthetic aspects and desires.

References

1. Bell WH, Hall HD, White RP. Surgical ramus osteotomy. In: Surgical correction of dentofacial deformities. 2. Saunders, Philadelphia, 1980; 890–895.
2. Severt TR, Proffit WF. The prevalence of facial asymmetry in the dentofacial deformities population at the University of North Carolina. Int J Adult Orthodon Orthoganthic Surg. 1997;12:171–6.

Sagittal Split and Mandibular Setback

27

Peter Kessler, Nicolas Hardt, and Suen An Nynke Lie

Contents

Abstract

Surgical treatment of class III malocclusion in most cases involves mandibular setback. After bilateral sagittal split osteotomy (BSSO), mandibular setback, vertical and horizontal rotation is possible. In addition to the standard method of BSSO, segmental osteotomies, intraoral vertical ramus osteotomy (IVRO), and inverted L osteotomy can be used.

Keywords

Class III relation · Class III malocclusion · Mandibular prognathism · Indications for mandibular setback · Sagittal splitting · BSSO - SSRO - IVRO - Inverted L osteotomy · Mandibular setback · Special surgical aspects in mandibular setback · Mandibular segment osteotomies · Modifications and surgical alternatives

The importance of alveolar segmental osteotomies has greatly decreased due to the differentiated orthodontic treatment options. The known risks of alveolar segmental osteotomies—loss of bone, teeth, fractures, and long-term damage to adjacent teeth—are not prevalent with today's surgical correction of the jaw bases.

However there will always be patients in whom orthodontic therapy cannot be performed for various reasons (number of teeth, age of the patient, costs, and patient compliance). For these

P. Kessler (✉) · S. A. N. Lie
Department of Cranio-Maxillofacial Surgery, Maastricht University Medical Center, Maastricht, The Netherlands
e-mail: peter.kessler@mumc.nl; suen.lie@mumc.nl

N. Hardt (✉)
Kantonsspital Lucerne, Clinic and Policlinic of Cranio-Maxillofacial Surgery, Lucerne, Switzerland

P. Kessler et al. (eds.), *Illustrated Manual of Orthognathic Surgery*,
https://doi.org/10.1007/978-3-031-06978-9_27

patients, the segmental osteotomy of alveolar ridge sections may be an alternative therapy. This also applies to those findings in which the extent of correction cannot be resolved by standard combined orthodontic-surgical treatment alone.

1 Mandibular Setback: BSSO

As described in Part I, there are numerous methods of mandibular setback. Of the techniques described there, two are still used regularly today: The osteotomy in the area of the jaw angle and in the area of the ascending mandibular ramus.

The main method, which is used in many places in the mandibular angle area, is the sagittal splitting in the ascending ramus clearly above the jaw angle.

In 1958, Dal Pont then placed the buccal cut in the horizontal mandible at the level of the second molar, resulting in extremely wide bone contact surfaces after sagittal splitting. The masseteric muscle remains on the proximal segment, which is important for its blood supply.

Sagittal split ramus osteotomy (SSRO) and/or bilateral sagittal split osteotomy (BSSO), especially in the Dal Pont modification, are the standard procedures today. Many suggestions for modifying this successful method have been published. These modifications deal with the creation of osteotomy lines, the instruments for tissue retraction, splitting, and especially the fixation of the fragments. Only the most important ones are mentioned here [1–4]. Figs. 27.1 and 27.2 describe the access to the mandibular angle.

In the case of a class III mandibular prognathism, the lower jaw must be shifted backward—mandibular setback—in order to achieve a regular dental occlusion in class I. Regardless of the splitting technique, there will be an overlap of bone segments or bone has to be removed. The two most common osteotomy techniques used are SSRO/BSSO and IVRO. Even with a short lingual osteotomy (SLO) according to

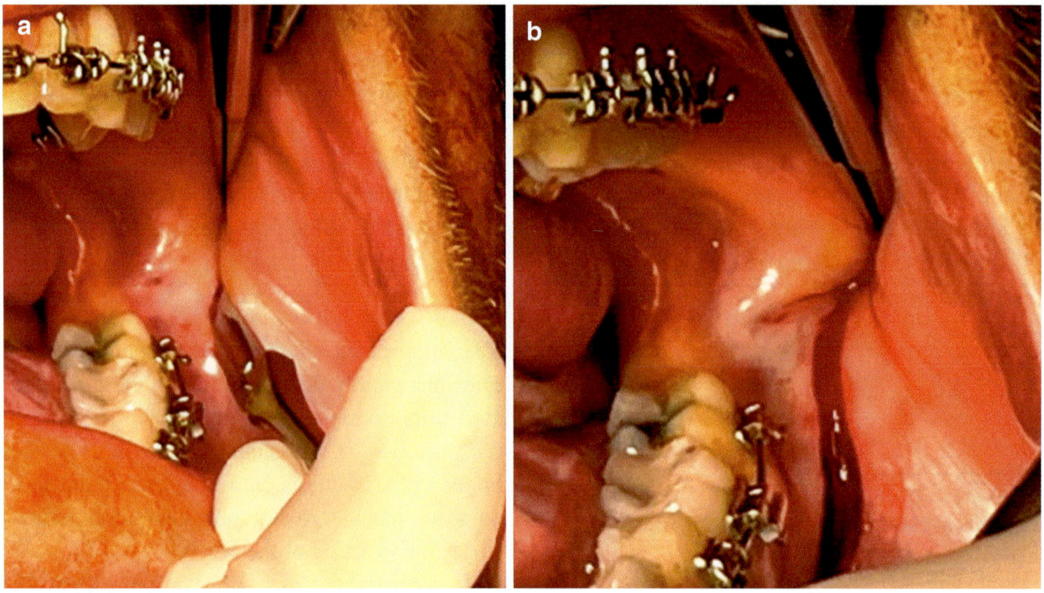

Fig. 27.1 Incision (**a**) The scalpel is inclined at 45° towards the external oblique line (**b**) S-shaped incision in the retro−/para mandibular region

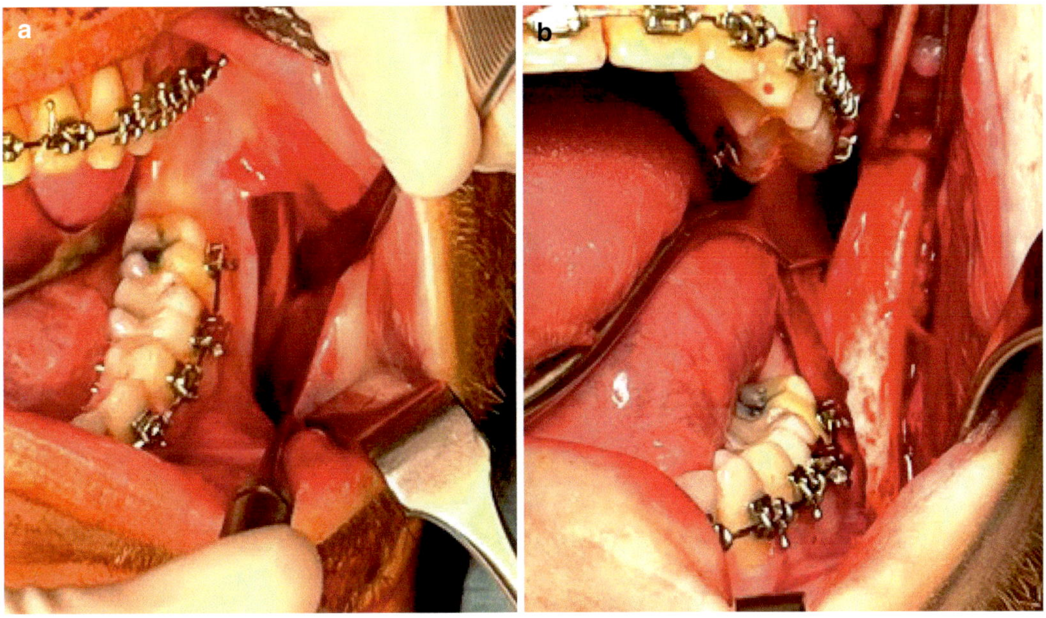

Fig. 27.2 (**a**) Blunt dissection of the buccal pocket without bleeding (**b**) Surgical site prepared for sagittal splitting. All protecting instruments in place

Epker, bony interference/overlap cannot be ruled out [3, 5].

In principle, however, it is irrelevant whether the buccal osteotomy is required at the height of the second molar region or further back. Impacted third molars should have been removed at least 6 months before surgery.

In detail: Under nasal intubation anesthesia and after infiltration of the lingual and buccal jaw angle region with local anesthetics containing vasoconstrictors, the mucosal incision is made slightly lateral to the external oblique line from the distal aspect of the second premolar to the ascending mandibular ramus, but without cutting through the bucco-temporal fascia. This avoids prolapse of the cheek fat body. The periosteum can now be easily pushed away from the mandibular body to the jaw angle by blunt dissection.

A useful instrument for this preparation is the Minnesota retractor. The periosteum should be injured as little as possible. The attachment of the coronoid process is dissected, whereby the connective tissue attachment of the temporal muscle should be detached meticulously. Care is taken not to completely detach the periosteum on the lateral side, so as not to endanger the blood supply to the fragment carrying the joint (proximal segment).

A notched ramus hook is used to retain the soft tissues from the muscular/coronoid process.

The periosteum is now carefully detached lingually at the level of the base of the muscular/coronoid process and a tunnel is made to the posterior edge of the ascending ramus. The lingula with the nerve and vessel exit remains caudally of the periosteal tunnel.

The incisura semilunaris is now identified with a blunt curved elevator, raspatory, or dissector according to Freer. Now a specially formed ramus clamp is inserted, e.g., Satinsky vascular clamp or DeBakey aortic clamp, which retains and protects the soft tissues cranially and lingually (Figs. 27.3 and 27.4).

Next, the more or less prominent edge above the lingula, which represents an offshoot of the mylohyoid line/internal oblique line, can be ablated with a round burr. In class III cases this line can be very prominent. This allows a good view to the dorsal edge of the ascending ramus.

Before the lingual osteotomy is performed, a channel retractor, which surrounds the posterior edge, is inserted to prevent injury to the lingually

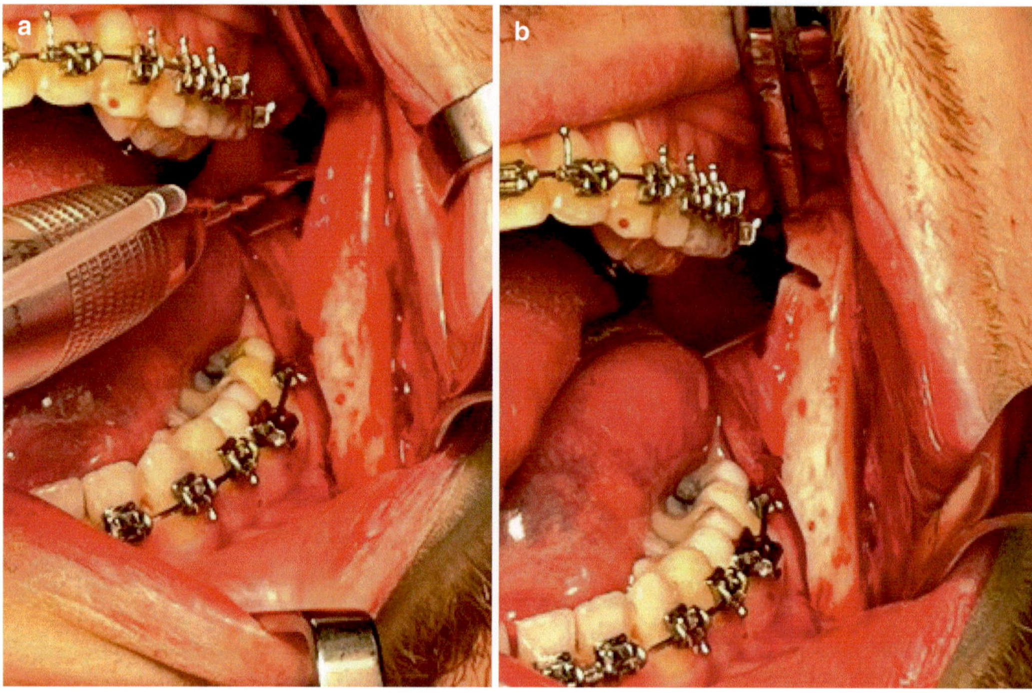

Fig. 27.3 (**a**) Lindemann-burr in correct position on the lingual side. (**b**) Lingual osteotomy

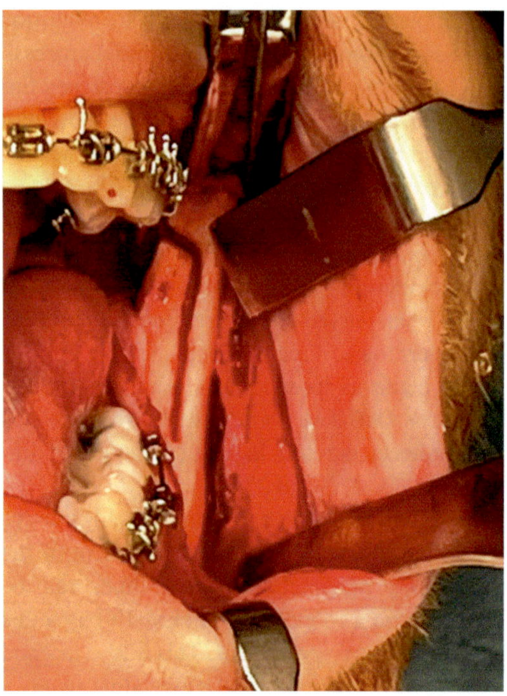

Fig. 27.4 Satinsky-DeBakey clamp in correct position. Connecting osteotomy can be performed before the vertical buccal osteotomy acc. to Dal Pont

located nerves and vessels (Figs. 27.3, 27.4 and 27.5).

A blunt, 90° curved nerve hook can be used for reliable identification of the lingula before the channel retractor is inserted. The channel retractor should lie in contact with the lingual side of the ascending mandibular ramus in such a way that it is turned 45° caudally. In this position, the lingula is protected and at the same time the lingual soft tissues are kept out (Fig. 27.5). The inclination of the Lindemann is decisive. It is recommended to align the drilling plane parallel to the occlusal plane of the mandible (Fig. 27.3).

The short lingual osteotomy is made with the long Lindemann burr at a depth of 1.5–2 mm as described by Epker (SLO) [1, 3]. Caution is required in the middle part of the ascending mandibular ramus, where the bone can be very thin; it is essential to avoid separating the condylar process from the proximal segment.

Now the buccal cortical bone cut is made, which is usually placed in the region of the second molar or distally (short osteotomy). Here, the cortical bone should be completely cut through to

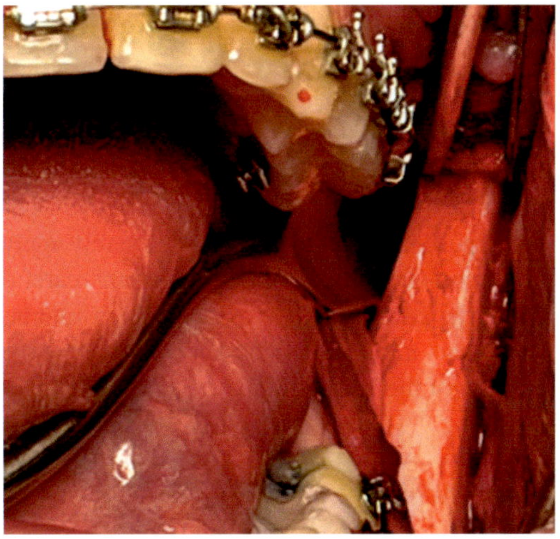

Fig. 27.5 Channel retractor (Dumbach retractor) placed on the lingual side to open the lingual tunnel

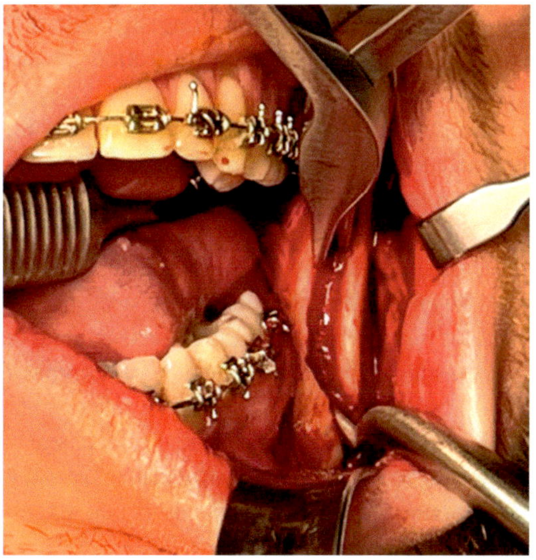

Fig. 27.6 Mandibular split with spreader and Smith separator

ensure easy splitting. A connection between the two cortical incisions is now marked with an excavator drill, which is then completed with a short Lindemann or fissure burr. This bone cut can also be made without predrilling in soft bone types and should safely cut through the cortex along the internal aspect of the buccal cortex. The two cortical cuts can also be connected directly with the saw.

Special attention must be paid to the complete osteotomy with the drill at the transition of the horizontal and buccal osteotomy to the connecting line. No cortical bridges must remain here. It is also recommended to carefully weaken the very solid mandibular base at the lower edge of the buccal osteotomy.

After the buccal edge of the lower jaw is also protected buccally by a channel retractor we then split the mandible with thin, slightly laterally bent chisels to about the middle. Then wide osteotomes can be used with the help of the spreader to widen the gap and finally break the remaining bony connection (Fig. 27.6).

While the osteotomy gap is widened, it is usually possible to identify the course of the mandibular canal. This lies mostly in the distal tooth-bearing segment. If this is successful, the osteotome can also be inserted deeper under the protection of the IAN in order to split bony connections below the course of the canal. Depending on the form of the mandible also straight chisels and osteotomes can be used.

After bilateral osteotomy the tooth-bearing distal segment is now gently mobilized and freely movable. The osteotomized jaw can be relocated dorsally against little resistance. Detaching the masseterico-pterygoidal muscle loop is not recommended. Excess bone on the bucco-lateral side of the proximal segment should be removed if necessary.

The instruments used to split the jaw angle, or the ascending branch of the lower jaw, are chosen differently by each surgeon. After making the connecting osteotomy between the lingual and buccal osteotomy, chisels and osteotomes are preferred. The order of the instruments mentioned seems to be more in keeping with habit.

Freihofer [6] recommended laterally curved chisels that can slide along the buccal cortex to deepen the connecting osteotomy. In many operation theaters this instrument is called Epker osteotome. The splitting itself can be performed with straight osteotomes or a bone spreader or a combination of both. Which instrument is used also has to do with the length of the connecting osteotomy line.

In the classic situation of sagittal splitting according to Dal Pont, the spreader can be inserted close to the buccal osteotomy from above and anteriorly, and then the osteotomes can be used to complete the splitting first buccally and then lingually after identification of the course of the IAN.

If a short connecting osteotomy between the lingual and buccal osteotomy is required, chisels and osteotomes are more likely to be used, as the spreader is less able to expand compact bone. In this case, more energy is required for splitting.

Wire loops of 0.4 or 0.5 mm thick steel wire are used for intermaxillary fixation. These are looped over existing Kobayashi ligature hooks, crimpable hooks, or IMF screws. In any case, a safe and stable IMF must be ensured to avoid displacement of the occlusion during osteosynthesis. Laterally, overlapping of cortical bone may occur. Excess bone should be removed.

With symmetrical initial conditions, less disturbing influences on the proximal segment can be expected than with asymmetrical ones with horizontal deviation of the mandible. If rotational and translational movements are added to the sagittal movement of the mandible, this can lead to an in- and/or outward displacement of the temporomandibular condyle (proximal segment).

This can lead to temporomandibular joint dysfunction and functional restrictions of the lower jaw movements. Part VI describes the procedure for asymmetrically shaped mandibles.

Note

The three moments of BSSO where nerve damage can occur are:

- Preparation of the lingual tunnel.
- Splitting the lower jaw.
- Crushing or direct nerve injury during osteosynthesis, especially when compression or positional screws are used.

2 Conclusions

The correction of mandibular prognathism is the domain of the bilateral sagittal split osteotomy—BSSO. No surgical technique can be applied more universally. The characteristics of this technique must be understood in order to safely apply the technique. Even with the most careful approach, the mandibular split remains a spontaneous fracture that can permanently damage the function of the IAN.

References

1. Epker BN. Vascular considerations in orthognathic surgery. I. Mandibular osteotomies. Oral Surg Oral Med Oral Pathol. 1984;57(5):467–72.
2. Böckmann R, Schön P, Neuking K, Meyns J, Kessler P, Eggeler G. In vitro comparison of the sagittal split osteotomy with and without inferior border osteotomy. J Oral Maxillofac Surg. 2015;73(2):316–23.
3. Epker BN. Modification in the sagittal osteotomy of the mandible. J Oral Surg. 1977;35:157–9.
4. Wolford LM, Davis WM. The mandibular inferior border split: a modification in the sagittal split ramus osteotomy associated with the presence or absence of third molars. J Oral Maxillofac Surg. 2001;59(8):92–4.
5. Hunsuck EE. A modified intraoral sagittal splitting technic for correction of mandibular prognathism. J Oral Surg. 1968;26(4):250–3.
6. Freihofer HP. Probleme der Behandlung der Progenie durch sagittale Spaltung der aufsteigenden Unterkieferäste. Schweiz Mschr Zahnheilk. 1976;86:679.

Special Surgical Aspects in Mandibular Setback

28

Peter Kessler, Nicolas Hardt, and Suen An Nynke Lie

Contents

Abstract

Mandibular repositioning can lead to interference between the proximal and distal mandibular segments depending on the displacement distance and the shape of the mandible. These interferences must be recognized and corrected to avoid temporomandibular joint displacements.

Keywords

Class III relation · Class III malocclusion · Mandibular prognathism · Maxillary retrusion · Indications for mandibular setback · Sagittal splitting · BSSO · Mandibular setback · Special surgical aspects in mandibular setback · Mandibular segment osteotomy · Modifications and surgical alternatives · Intraoral vertical ramus osteotomy—IVRO · Inverted L osteotomy · Temporomandibular joint—TMJ

After repositioning the mandible and adjusting the occlusion, the mandible is usually stabilized with functionally stable 2.0 mm osteosynthesis plates. The bone overlap laterally caused by the repositioning should but does not always have to be removed. This decision depends, among other things, on the posterior dislocation distance of the mandible. If the bone overlap leads to a dislocation of the proximal segment supporting the temporomandibular joint (TMJ), a correction must be performed to relieve the TMJ. In most situations, a moderate correction of the excess bone is sufficient to adapt the two segments in such a way that the bone gap is not too large when the mandible is repositioned (Fig. 28.1).

Gaps of up to 5 mm can be accepted. If the distance in the area of the mandibular split is too large, slight internal rotation of both proximal segments can lead to a satisfactory relation of the split segments, so that a safe osseous regeneration can be guaranteed without damaging the TMJ.

P. Kessler (✉) · S. A. N. Lie
Department of Cranio-Maxillofacial Surgery, Maastricht University Medical Center, Maastricht, The Netherlands
e-mail: peter.kessler@mumc.nl; suen.lie@mumc.nl

N. Hardt (✉)
Kantonsspital Lucerne, Clinic and Policlinic of Cranio-Maxillofacial Surgery, Lucerne, Switzerland

P. Kessler et al. (eds.), *Illustrated Manual of Orthognathic Surgery*,
https://doi.org/10.1007/978-3-031-06978-9_28

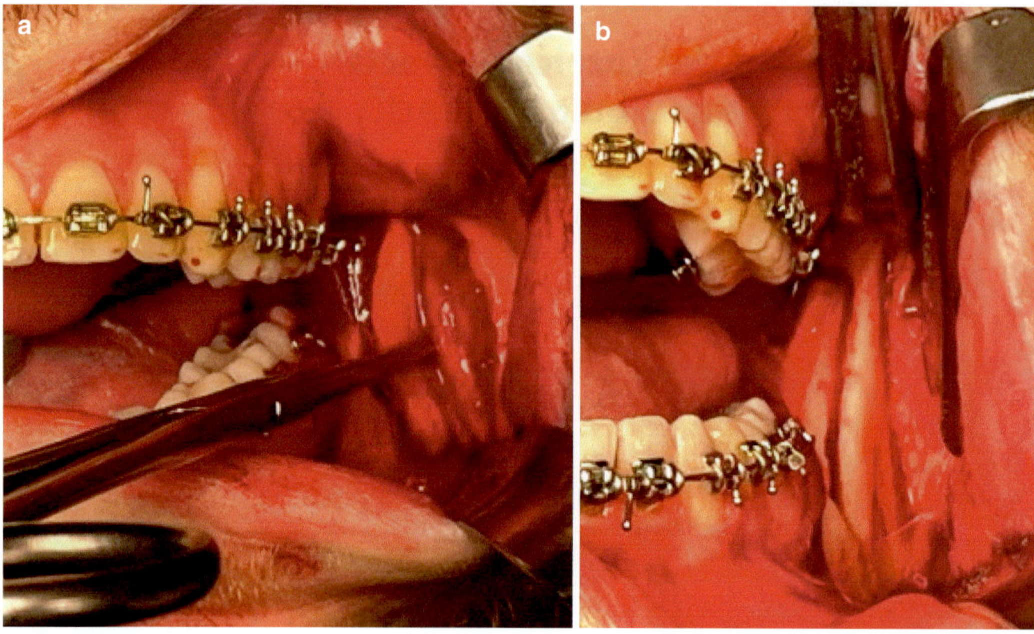

Fig. 28.1 (**a**) Grasping the proximal segment for reduction of bone overlap (**b**) Perfect adaptation of both segments before osteosynthesis

If possible, transfacial access to the surgical site in orthognathic surgery should be avoided. The use of angulated drill hand pieces allows osteosynthesis of the proximal segment while bypassing a transbuccal approach. The angulated hand pieces can also be used for manual screw fixation.

The TMJ should not be pushed deeply into the articular fossa when the lower jaw is repositioned. After the split and sufficient mobilization of the segments, the proximal segments can be grasped transorally with the Kocher clamp and carefully mobilized under manual-digital control preauricularly to prevent unintentional dislocation of the TMJ during the surgery or while positioning the mandible in intermaxillary fixation.

In class III cases the TMJ should be set in the position that corresponds to the habitual occlusion. This means that no forces should act on the TMJ during osteosynthesis when correcting class III mandibles.

A pre-fixation of the lateral segment with the help of an osteosynthesis plate, which must be guided from the lateral mandibular segment to a suitable fixation point on the upper jaw, has become superfluous in the age of digital planning and the possibility of using individualized implants.

1 Conclusions

Three-dimensional planning of orthognathic procedures facilitates the choice of surgical technique and a realistic approach. This helps to avoid intra- and postoperative problems.

29 Mandibular Excess – Modifications and Surgical Alternatives

Peter Kessler, Nicolas Hardt, and Suen An Nynke Lie

Contents

Abstract

Alternatives to BSSO are osteotomies in the region of the ascending mandibular branch. The intraoral vertical ramus osteotomy (IVRO) and the inverted L osteotomy are alternative procedures for mandibular setback (Yamauchi et al. Oral Surg Oral Med Oral Pathol Oral Radiol Endod 104:747–751, 2007; Jung et al, Br J Oral Maxillofac Surg 52:866–867, 2014).

Keywords

Class III relation · Class III malocclusion · Mandibular prognathism · Maxillary retrusion · Indications for mandibular setback · Sagittal splitting · BSSO - SSRO · Mandibular setback · Special surgical aspects in mandibular setback · Mandibular segment osteotomy · Modifications and surgical alternatives · Intraoral vertical ramus osteotomy—IVRO · Inverted L-osteotomy

Computer-based planning is of great help when planning symmetrical or asymmetrical setback operations in mandibular prognathism, as it clearly shows the sagittal and rotational movements of the distal tooth-bearing mandibular segment in relation to the proximal mandibular segment (TMJ) and provides very useful information when selecting the appropriate splitting technique.

In addition, individually manufactured osteosynthesis plates can transmit the preoperatively determined optimal surgical solution to the operating room.

P. Kessler (✉) · S. A. N. Lie
Department of Cranio-Maxillofacial Surgery, Maastricht University Medical Center, Maastricht, The Netherlands
e-mail: peter.kessler@mumc.nl; suen.lie@mumc.nl

N. Hardt (✉)
Kantonsspital Lucerne, Clinic and Policlinic of Cranio-Maxillofacial Surgery, Lucerne, Switzerland

P. Kessler et al. (eds.), *Illustrated Manual of Orthognathic Surgery*,
https://doi.org/10.1007/978-3-031-06978-9_29

Alternatively, a functionally stable osteosynthesis can be deliberately avoided in order to give the proximal segment (TMJ) more freedom to rotate back into a functionally physiological position when the intraoral vertical ramus osteotomy (IVRO) is applied (see: Part VII) [1, 2].

However, this requires a long-lasting intermaxillary fixation (IMF), which in turn requires intensive cooperation from the patient [3]. This, however, means that the decisive advantage of rigid internal fixation avoid is abandoned.

Note

- SSRO/BSSO with short lingual osteotomy—SLO—acc. to Epker is the standard technique in correction of symmetric/asymmetric mandibular prognathism.
- Use 3D planning to avoid negative effects on the TMJ structures due to excessive TMJ rotation/dislocation.
- Asymmetric mandibular prognathism is challenging and needs more attention during planning and surgery.

1 Conclusion

The establishment of alternative splitting procedures resulted from the development in orthognathic surgery per se. The procedures of vertical mandibular splitting are older than the BSSO and are the result of the BSSO, which sometimes cannot be applied perfectly. Nevertheless, the BSSO remains the procedure of first choice in mandibular orthognathic surgery.

References

1. Yamauchi K, Takenobu T, Takahashi T. Condylar luxation following bilateral intraoral vertical ramus osteotomy. Oral Surg Oral Med Oral Pathol Oral Radiol Endod. 2007;104:747–51.
2. Jung HD, Kim SY, Park HS, Jung YS. Modification of intraoral vertical ramus osteotomy. Br J Oral Maxillofac Surg. 2014;52:866–7.
3. Ohba S, Nakao N, Kawasaki T, Miura K, Minamizato T, Koga T, Yoshida N, Asahina I. Skeletal stability after sagittal spit ramus osteotomy with physiological positioning in patients with skeletal mandibula prognathism and facial asymmetry. Br J Oral Maxillofac Surg. 2016;54:920–6.

Part VI

Asymmetries, Vertical and Horizontal Rotation, Mandibular Flaring - Surgical Techniques

Introduction - Asymmetries, Vertical and Horizontal Rotation, Mandibular Flaring - Surgical Techniques

30

Peter Kessler and Kensuke Yamauchi

Contents

Abstract

No face is absolutely symmetrical. Therefore, because of the dentition conditions in the upper jaw and the result of the orthodontic pretreatment, the sagittal forward or backward displacement of the lower jaw always includes a rotational component. Vertical growth differences in the area of the mandibular corpus must be taken into account. Rotation of the distal mandibular segment can lead to unfavorable positional changes of the proximal segment. Three-dimensional complexities can be predicted well using three-dimensional planning tools. If necessary, the surgical technique must be adapted and supplemented by additional procedures to obtain a functionally and esthetically satisfactory result.

P. Kessler (✉)
Department of Cranio-Maxillofacial Surgery, Maastricht University Medical Center, Maastricht, The Netherlands
e-mail: peter.kessler@mumc.nl

K. Yamauchi
Department of Oral & Maxillofacial Surgery, Tohoku University Sendai, Sendai, Miyagi, Japan

The frequency of facial asymmetries is high because a complete symmetry of the right and left half of the face can rarely be found. A distinction is made between structural and physiological asymmetries and genetically determined or acquired asymmetries (trauma). The cause of an asymmetry of the jaws can be in the upper or lower jaw, in both jaws, or also in the area of the skull base. In addition to a bony cause, changes in the number of teeth, tooth loss, and other dental causes could also be possible. In addition to asymmetries that are skeletal or dental in origin, there are a variety of asymmetries that can be caused by volume differences in the surrounding soft tissues or even by space-consuming processes.

Keywords

Vertical and horizontal mandibular rotation · Sagittal split · Mandibular rotation · Special surgical aspects · Hazards and support measures · Surgical modifications · Alternatives · Inverted vertical ramus osteotomy—IVRO · Temporo-mandibular joint—TMJ · Flaring

P. Kessler et al. (eds.), *Illustrated Manual of Orthognathic Surgery*,
https://doi.org/10.1007/978-3-031-06978-9_30

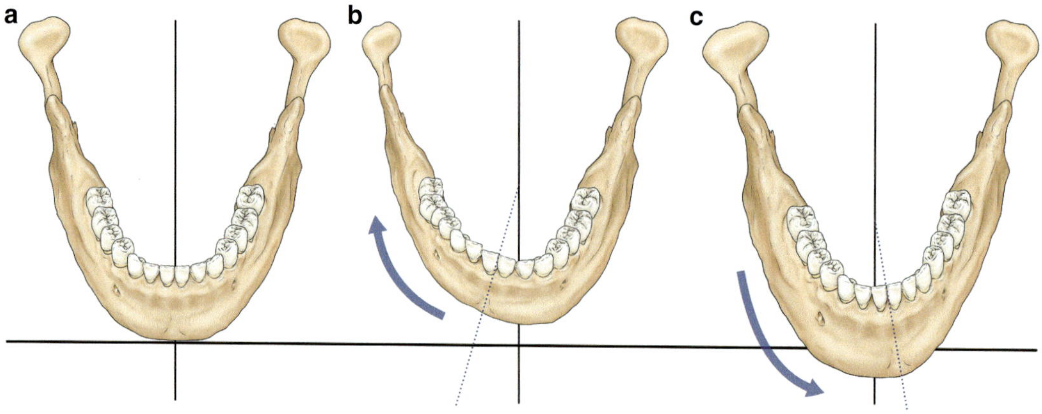

Fig. 30.1 **a–c** adapted from Reichenbach 1952 (**a**)symmetrical form of the mandible, (**b**) mandibular asymmetry due to hypoplasia on the right, (**c**) mandibular asymmetry due to hyperplasia/hypertrophy on the right side. Arrows are indicating the vector of deficiency or overgrowth leading to a rotational component.

In the case of asymmetries that only affect the mandible or are only determined by asymmetric mandibular growth or form, unilateral condylar hyper- or hypoplasia must be mentioned as a special case, as these disorders can be related to autonomous growth disorders.

A clinically relevant classification of condylar hyperplasia or mandibular asymmetry with unilateral involvement was published by [1]. Three categories are distinguished:

The hemimandibular hyperplasia, the hemimandibular elongation, and a mixed form of both first mentioned deviations. Hemimandibular hyperplasia is described as a vertical growth excess in the ascending branch of the jaw or condyle, with the lower jaw showing downward tilting with an ipsilateral open bite, since the growth rate does not allow for dental compensation. A cross bite on the opposite side or chin deviation is not observed.This is also seen with hemimandibular elongation: Cross bite on the opposite, unaffected side of the jaw, midline shift dental and skeletal. The third form is a hybrid of excessive unilateral vertical and horizontal growth (Fig. 30.1).

Since no diagnostic or therapeutic standard has yet been defined for these growth-related mandibular asymmetries, all mandibular asymmetries must be analyzed with extreme caution in order to find the right therapeutic timing and approach.

From what has been said it can be deduced that there can be corresponding deviations that have their cause in unilateral growth deficits up to structural growth deficits, as for example presented in the Pruzansky classification. Hypodontia and ankylosis of teeth or groups of teeth may be present [2].

Genetically caused syndromic changes affecting the development and growth of the mandible and/or the TMJ (first pharyngeal arch) are not explicitly discussed here. Nevertheless, diagnostics, analysis, planning, and therapeutic options can be applied to these patients in most cases.

1 Conclusion

The evaluation of facial asymmetry requires clinical and radiological findings. Different types of excess or deficient growth can lead to three-dimensional asymmetries.

References

1. Obwegeser HL, Makek MS. Hemimandibular hyperplasia—hemimandibular elongation. J Maxillofac Surg. 1986;14(4):183–208.
2. Pruzansky S. Not all dwarfed mandibles are alike. Birth Defects. 1969;1:120–9.

Diagnosis in Mandibular Asymmetries, Vertical and Horizontal Rotation

31

Peter Kessler and Kensuke Yamauchi

Contents

Abstract

The following elements must be considered when assessing hemi- or bilateral mandibular asymmetry morphologically:

- Mandible length.
- Lower jaw shape and size.
- Volume of the mandible/hemimandibles.

Keywords

Facial asymmetry · Vertical and horizontal mandibular rotation · Sagittal split—BSSO · Mandibular rotation · Surgical alternatives · Inverted vertical ramus osteotomy—IVRO · Temporomandibular joint—TMJ · Flaring

1 Photographic and Clinical Analysis

The bipupillary, bizygomatic, bigonial, and mental planes and the stomion must be marked. These planes are placed in relation to a center line through the median of the face—facial midline—and to each other to detect deviations from parallelism and transverse deviations from the midline (Fig. 31.1).

P. Kessler (✉)
Department of Cranio-Maxillofacial Surgery, Maastricht University Medical Center, Maastricht, The Netherlands
e-mail: peter.kessler@mumc.nl

K. Yamauchi
Department of Oral & Maxillofacial Surgery, Tohoku University Sendai, Sendai, Miyagi, Japan

P. Kessler et al. (eds.), *Illustrated Manual of Orthognathic Surgery*,
https://doi.org/10.1007/978-3-031-06978-9_31

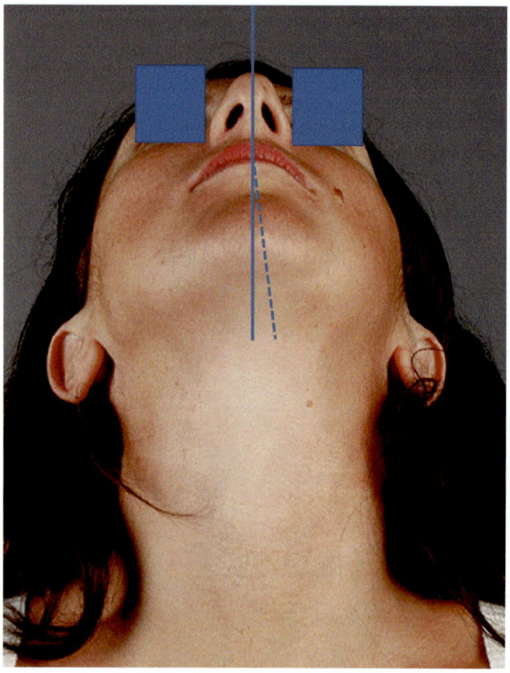

Fig. 31.1 Patient with mild mandibular hyperplasia on the right and deviation of the chin point

2 The Further Clinical Analysis Must Comprise

- Bite position: Class I, II, or III in combination with transverse/transverse-vertical deviation.
- Cross bite ipsi- or contralaterally.
- Lingual/buccal tilting of teeth (premolars, molars).
- Frontal and/or lateral open bite.
- Dental midline deviation.
- Skeletal midline deviation.
- Midline deviation of the chin.
- Participation/involvement of the maxilla: size, form, skull-related position.
- Involvement of the midface (hemifacial asymmetry possible).
- Participation of the orbit/−s (hemifacial growth disturbance).
- Deviation of the nose.

3 Radiological Diagnosis

Panoramic and anterior-posterior two-dimensional radiographs are only useful for screening, but not for the quantitative evaluation, classification, and diagnosis of patients with hemimandibular asymmetry affecting the face [1].

- Quantification of asymmetry is essential for the evaluation of the degree of deformity.
- Quantification is essential for objectification of the deviation and planning.
- Quantification enables a classification of severity.
- Quantification is essential for objective monitoring and follow-up.

The only objective data collection option for planning a correction of facial asymmetries is provided by radiological procedures that generate three-dimensional data sets and images: CBCT, MSCT, and MRI. For the purposes of orthognathic surgery, DICOM (Digital Imaging and Communications in Medicine) data sets of the -CBCT are perfectly sufficient. They are required for the computer-based planning of surgical correction.

In almost all forms of mandibular hyper- or hypoplasia, changes in volume or size in the area of the condylar heads are noticeable. Particularly in the case of enlarged condyles, any doubt about the presence of autonomic growth disturbances in the collum-condylar region should be excluded before surgical correction [1].

This means that further radiological procedures such as SPECT (Single-Photon Emission Tomography) may be required to rule out active growth in the condylar region.

If this is not possible, serial dental casts and photographic documentation of the face as non-invasive procedures are the only way to document changes in facial asymmetry over time [1, 2].

4 The Further Radiological Analysis Must Comprise

- Panoramic X-ray: Evaluation only.
  (a) Shape and size of the condyles.
  (b) Length of the condylar process.
  (c) Dental and/or skeletal midline deviation.
- CBCT: Measurement [3].
  (a) Mark the SN-plane and C-point: deepest point of the semilunar/sigmoid notch.
  (b) Mark Superior Condyle: most cranial point of the condyle.
  (c) Draw parallels between SN-plane and Superior Condyle and C-point: height of the condyle measured between parallels through Superior Condyle and C-point.
  (d) C-Gonion axis: height of the ascending ramus (estimation).
  (e) Gonion-Menton/Gnathion axis: length of the mandibular body (estimation).
  (f) Midline axis through N (Nasion)–ANS (anterior nasal spine)–Sym (mandibular symphysis above the mental tubercle): frontal facial asymmetry.
  (g) Mandibular angle defined by Ar (Articulare) -Gonion axis and Gonion-Menton/Gnathion axis.

Based on 3D analysis, further planes and volumes can be calculated [3]. The volume of the condylar process, the ascending ramus, and the mandibular body can be assessed per side and compared.

Three-dimensional planning with the help of suitable computer programs is the prerequisite for correct planning in general. In the time before the introduction of these techniques, planning based on 2D X-ray images in two or more planes, patient photographs, and plaster models was the standard. These methods never allowed for exact planning. Therefore, documentation, analysis, and planning with 3D techniques are an indispensable prerequisite for surgical therapy today [1, 3].

5 Conclusion

Even comprehensive diagnostics cannot always assign the cause of facial asymmetry, or asymmetry in the mandibular region, to a growth excess or growth deficit. Nevertheless, asymmetries must be carefully considered during planning.

References

1. Nolte JW, Karssemakers LH, Grootendorst DC, Tuinzing DB, Becking AG. Panoramic imaging is not suitable for quantitative evaluation, classification, and follow up in unilateral condylar hyperplasia. Br J Oral Maxillofac Surg. 2015;53(5):446–50.
2. Karssemakers LH, Raijmakers PG, Nolte JW, Tuinzing DB, Becking AG. Interobserver variation of single-photon emission computed tomography bone scans in patients evaluated for unilateral condylar hyperactivity. Oral Surg Oral Med Oral Pathol Oral Radiol. 2013;115(3):399–405.
3. Nolte JW, Verhoeven TJ, Schreurs R, Bergé SJ, Karssemakers LH, Becking AG, Maal TJ. 3-Dimensional CBCT analysis of mandibular asymmetry in unilateral condylar hyperplasia. J Craniomaxillofac Surg. 2016;44(12):1970–6.

Surgical Correction in Mandibular Asymmetry

32

Kensuke Yamauchi and Peter Kessler

Contents

K. Yamauchi
Department of Oral & Maxillofacial Surgery, Tohoku University Sendai, Sendai, Miyagi, Japan

P. Kessler (✉)
Department of Cranio-Maxillofacial Surgery, Maastricht University Medical Center, Maastricht, The Netherlands
e-mail: peter.kessler@mumc.nl

Abstract

A suitable therapy must pursue two goals:

- Correction of asymmetry.
- Elimination of the progressive component of the disease.

Keywords

Vertical and horizontal mandibular rotation · Sagittal split - Unilateral and bilateral sagittal

P. Kessler et al. (eds.), *Illustrated Manual of Orthognathic Surgery*,
https://doi.org/10.1007/978-3-031-06978-9_32

split osteotomy USSO/BSSO - Sagittal split ramus osteotomy SSRO · Mandibular rotation · Special surgical aspects · Surgical modifications · Alternatives · Chin osteotomy · Inverted vertical ramus osteotomy—IVRO · Temporomandibular joint—TMJ · Flaring

It is important to make a distinction between asymmetry and cause of asymmetry or, if necessary, to combine them in the analysis. An expectative behavior can lead to a strong worsening of the asymmetry, which is accordingly more difficult to correct. Since an end to autonomous growth cannot be predicted, interventions on the temporomandibular joint (TMJ) may also be necessary or their combination with classical elements of orthognathic surgery. Interventions on the condyle are not described here [1–6].

Especially in cases of laterognathism, which can be localized in the entire viscerocranium, the choice of the site for the osteotomy is difficult and requires great care and experience. The indication for corrective osteotomy also depends to a great extent on the etiology of the lateral deviation of the corresponding parts of the facial skeleton.

The general rule for the selection of the osteotomy site or the osteotomy sites is that the more asymmetric the face is, i.e., the more pronounced the lateral shift is, the more osteotomies are required to restore facial symmetry and occlusion. For example, a lateral displacement of the chin can be corrected without altering the occlusion by simply shifting the chin margin.

On the other hand, asymmetry caused by malformation of the joint and ascending ramus requires osteotomies on the affected and unaffected side. In most cases, osteotomies must also be performed in the upper jaw to achieve facial symmetry. On this basis, harmonious occlusion is easier to achieve. The same applies to the overdevelopment/excessive growth of a joint or an entire side of the mandible, which can usually also only be corrected by multiple osteotomies [7].

The choice of the osteotomy site will therefore depend essentially on the severity of the facial asymmetry and the corresponding laterognathia, which is usually associated with an occlusion disorder. The main methods affecting the mandible are described here.

1 Chin osteotomies and Corrections of the Mandibular Rim

Mandibular asymmetry without occlusion disorder: correction by genioplasty with lateral displacement and vertical correction (Fig. 32.1). Possible additional corrections at the lower margin of the mandible. Augmentation with tissue transplants—bone, cartilage—is possible, also the implantation of allogenic implants up to patient-specific implants.

Part IX discusses the technique of genioplasty in detail. In addition to the possibilities described there, the lateral chin displacement must be mentioned in laterognathism and mandibular asymmetry.

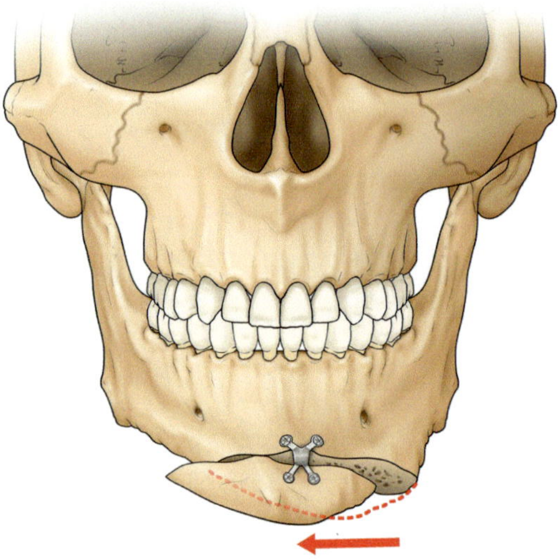

Fig. 32.1 Genioplasty. Shifting the chin point to correct a mandibular midline deviation.

2 Osteotomies in the Mandibular Angle

Mandibular osteotomies to correct laterognathism can be performed unilaterally in the region of the temporomandibular joint, the ascending mandibular ramus or the jaw angle as well as bilaterally, using various surgical techniques. Distraction treatment may also be indicated. Standard procedures are the BSSO/USSO (bilateral/unilateral sagittal split osteotomy) and secondarily IVRO, the inverted ramus osteotomy.

3 Unilateral Sagittal Split Osteotomies—USSO

When planning the operation, the focus must be on the midline of the face, the midline of the rows of teeth, and the chin (Menton = Me). The greater the horizontal deviation of the mandible, the more dislocation/rotation of the proximal segment/TMJ on the side facing away from the asymmetry can be expected, as the dorsal displacement of the distal segment (mandible) is greater (Figs. 32.2 and 32.3).

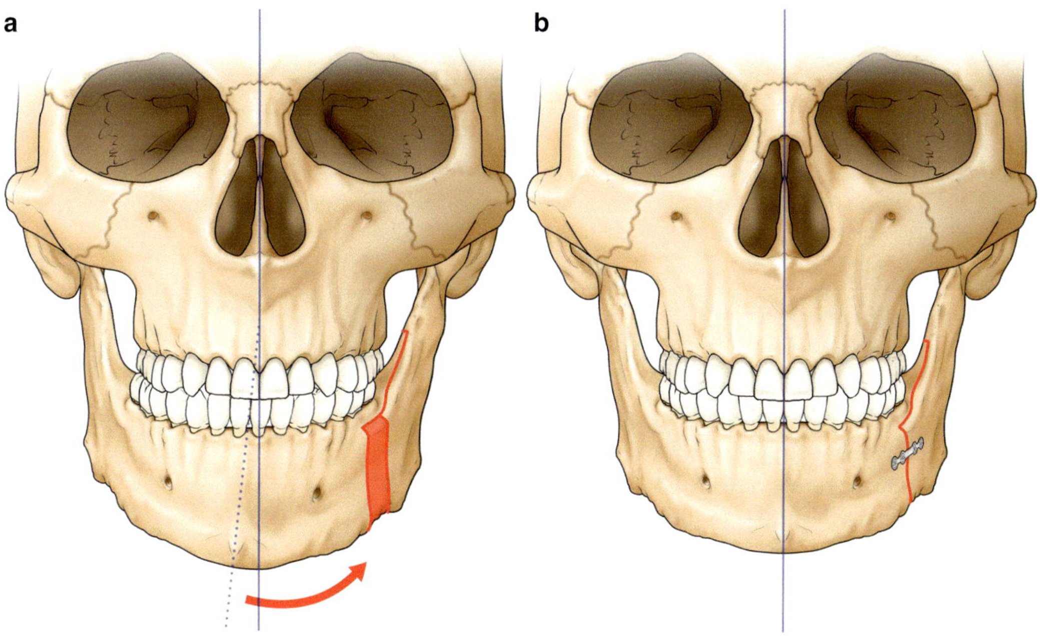

Fig. 32.2 (**a**) SSRO (sagittal split ramus osteotomy) on the left for correction of a mild mandibular asymmetry with (**b**) setback of the mandible on the left side.

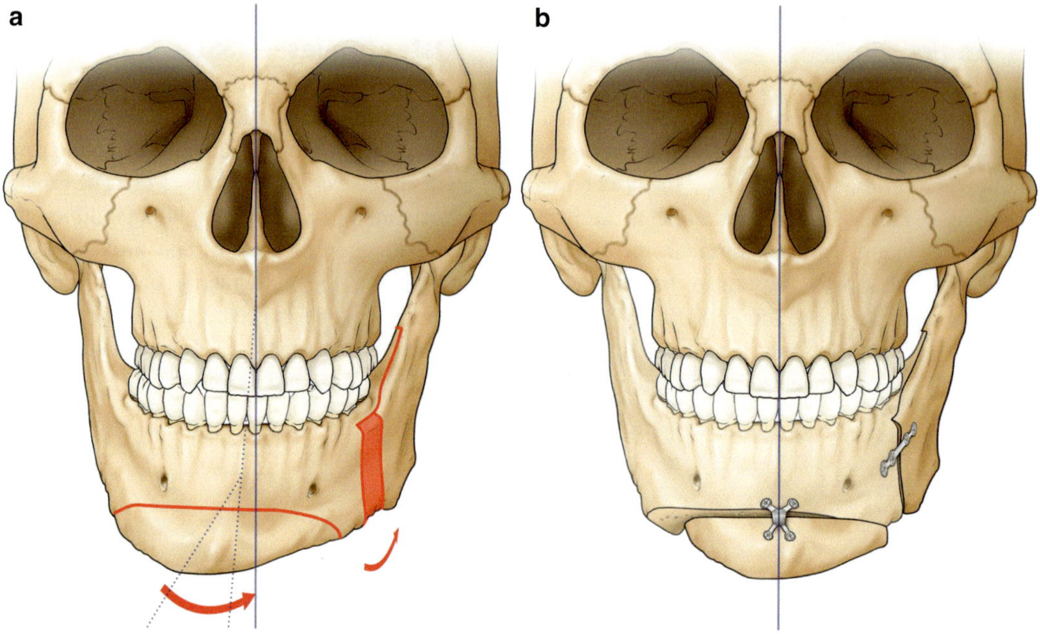

Fig. 32.3 (**a**) SSRO for correction of a mild mandibular asymmetry with (**b**) setback of the mandible on the left side and simultaneous chin correction.

4 Mandibular Asymmetry in Prognathism

The greater the horizontal deviation of the mandible, the more dislocation of the proximal segment on the side facing away from the asymmetry can be expected, as the posterior displacement of the distal mandibular segment is greater and must be included in the correction of the asymmetry (Fig. 32.4).

The rotational adaptability in the TMJ complex consisting of condyle and fossa is limited and amounts to only a few degrees (changes in the Bennett angle). Depending on the selected osteotomy technique, flaring may occur on the affected side.

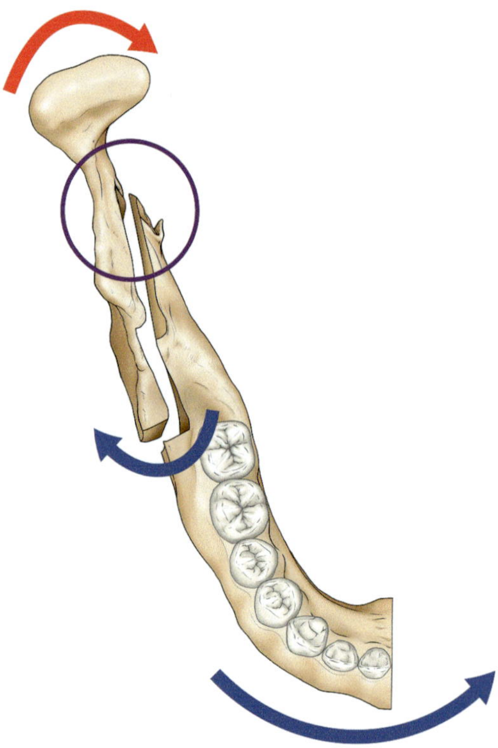

Fig. 32.4 SSRO for correction of mandibular asymmetry with rotation of the mandible on the left side. Risk of joint rotation due to dislocation of the proximal segment. Risk of flaring.

5 Mandibular Asymmetry in orthognathism

Due to the fact that the rotational component is largely eliminated, bilateral osteotomy is usually required in laterognathic cases with transverse displacement of the mandible. In transverse dental orthognathia, a chin correction is often sufficient, possibly in combination with a correction of the mandibular base.

6 Bilateral Sagittal Split Osteotomies—BSSO

A bilateral osteotomy in the area of the ascending ramus or the mandibular angle is not only used to correct mandibular pro- or retrognathism, but may also be indicated in the presence of laterognathism. The surgical technique is the same as described in the Parts III, IV, and V extensively.

If the mandible is displaced laterally at the same time, it is important to note that on the longer side of the mandible the overlapping buccal cortical bone must be shortened (Fig. 32.6). When adjusting the occlusion, it is important to observe the center line of the face and thus also the center line of the chin. This may still be displaced after the occlusion has been set, so that a genioplasty may also be required (Figs. 32.5 and 32.6).

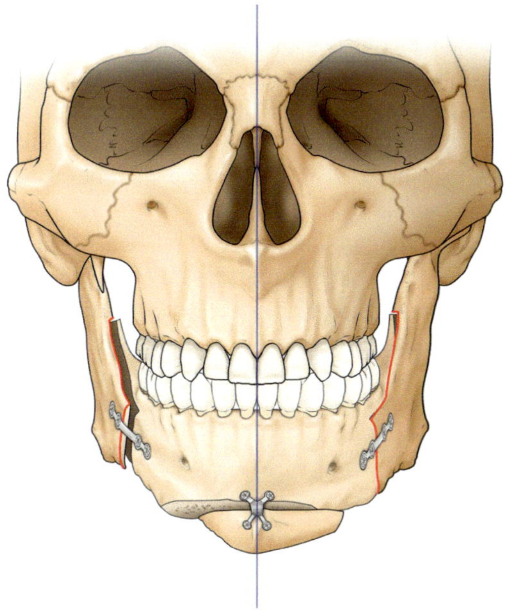

Fig. 32.6 BSSO and correction of mandibular asymmetry including genioplasty.

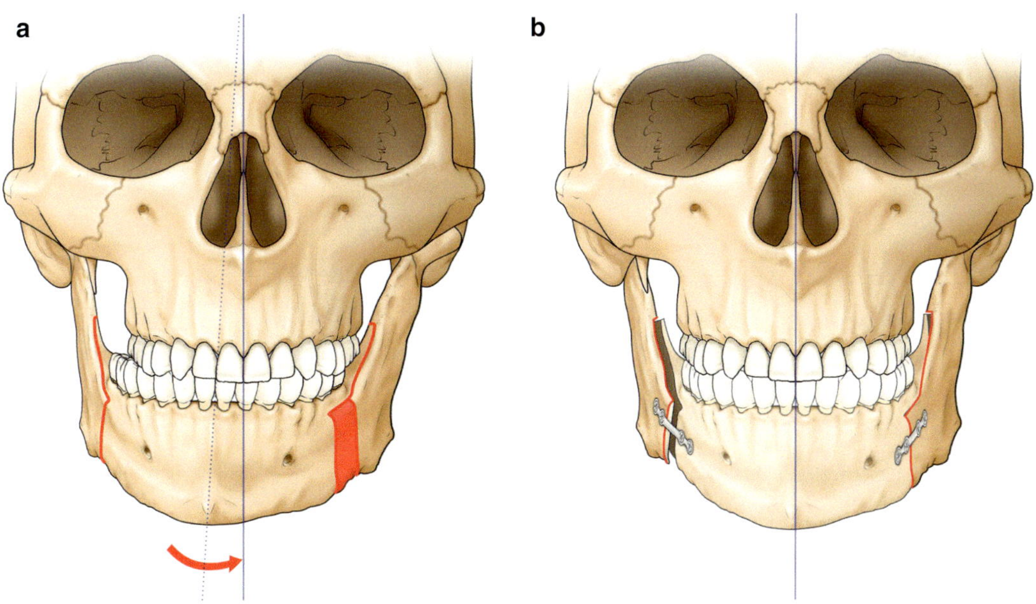

Fig. 32.5 (**a**) BSSO and correction of mandibular asymmetry with (**b**) buccal cortical ostectomy on the hyperplastic left side.

Of course other types of osteotomy in the ascending ramus, such as the intraoral vertical (IVRO) or oblique ramus osteotomy, can also be used. The disadvantage of this method, however, is that the overlapping bone surfaces, especially on the shorter mandibular side, are small, which delays the bony consolidation of the fragments.

In the presence of a laterognathism with mandibular retrognathia, as in condylar hypoplasia e.g., the advancement of the shorter mandibular side can be used to correct the midline at the same time.

Depending on the degree of retrognathism an advancement can be necessary on both sides. On the shorter mandibular side a Dal Pont osteotomy with a long bone overlap is indicated. On the opposite side a short SSO should be preferred to avoid negative rotational effects on the TMJ.

7 Rotation and Side Shift of the TMJ

The rotational movements of the temporomandibular joint head can be anticipated by computerized planning, but not specified exactly in every case. In addition to rotational movements, lateral displacements or canting of the ascending mandibular ramus (proximal segment) can also lead to displacement/tilting of the TMJ (Fig. 32.7).

A further complicating factor is that rigid osteosynthesis may fix the proximal mandibular segment in a functionally unfavorable position. If the condylar head cannot be seated in a physiologically ideal position, abnormal movement of the condyle in the fossa will result. This can lead to temporomandibular joint disorders, TMJ resorption, and relapse.

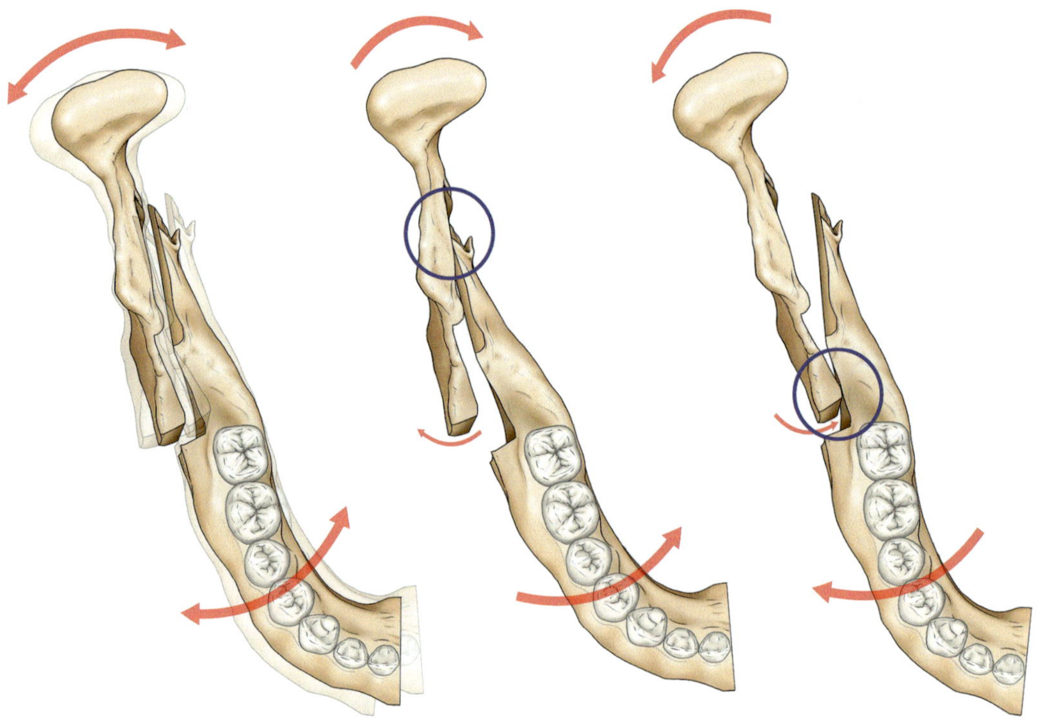

Fig. 32.7 The long overlap in mandibular split according to Dal Pont can lead to a rotational component on the TMJ—proximal segment—depending on the direction of mandibular rotation in the distal segment. Circled in blue undesirable pivot points with dislocation effects on the TMJ.

Rotational influences on the temporomandibular joint can be displayed well with the help of 3D planning. To reduce negative influences on the TMJ, a suitable splitting technique must then be simulated and implemented, if necessary, to protect the joints. With the help of CAD/CAM manufactured splints and possibly patient-specific implants (plates and screws), the planning can be transferred to the OR, even without navigation or intraoperative radiological control.

What cannot be predicted, however, is how the mandible will break in the sagittal splitting procedure. This must be checked and corrected intraoperatively, if splints or osteosynthesis plates do not fit properly. Negative influences on the TMJ by rotation or dislocation increase the risk of a skeletal recurrence [8].

8 Flaring

When IVRO is used in setback surgery, there is a greater overlap of the proximal and distal segments, since this type of osteotomy does not allow for any variation. This means that unfavorable effects can also be exerted on the TMJ in the IVRO. In addition, stripping the pterygomasseteric muscle loop releases the proximal segment from its muscularly determined position and thus exposes the distal segment to movements caused by surgery and displacement, which can lead to serious dislocations in the TMJ (Figs. 32.8 and 32.17).

In the SSRO, the pterygo-masseteric muscle loop, which is not detached, provides additional stability for the TMJ against rotational influences. However, when using the SSRO, a long split similar to the Dal Pont variant can also cause interference between the proximal and distal segments.

If this is recognized intraoperatively, a vertical fracture of the lingually overlapping bone segment on the distal segment—mandibular body—may be necessary after splitting in order to exclude disturbing rotational influences on the position of the proximal segment (Fig. 32.9).

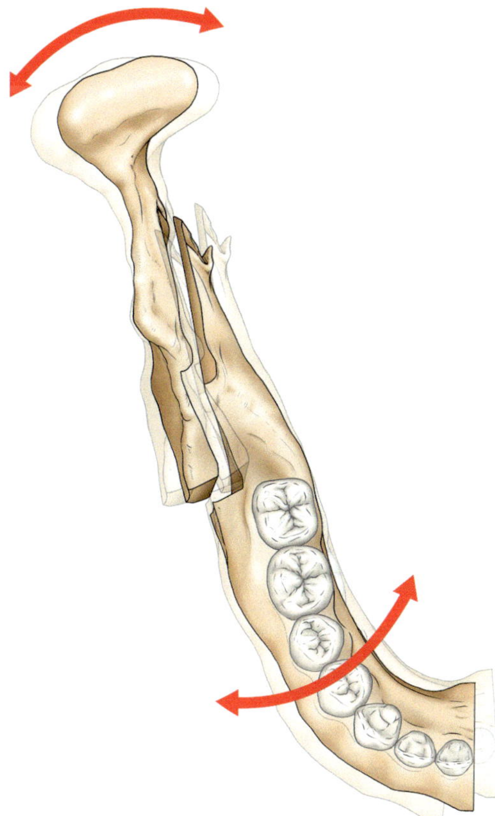

Fig. 32.8 Consequences of mandibular body rotation (distal segment) to both sides with dislocation of the proximal segment and TMJ rotation in SSRO. Compare Fig. 32.8 with Fig. 32.17 IVRO.

This maneuver is delicate and can lead to an increased risk of injury to the surrounding soft tissues, including the lingual and inferior alveolar nerves. Bone healing in the split region may also be at risk if the procedure is too radical and/or the osteosynthetic stabilization is insufficient.

In the case of an asymmetrical mandible shape or asymmetrical horizontal mandibular position, the use of the IVRO can lead to less interference than the SSRO technique.

The SSRO is the standard technique also from the point of view of osteosynthetic stabilization, which is easier to perform with an SSRO than with the IVRO. A short bone overlap should be attempted to avoid the risk of dislocation or even luxation of the TMJ (Fig. 32.10).

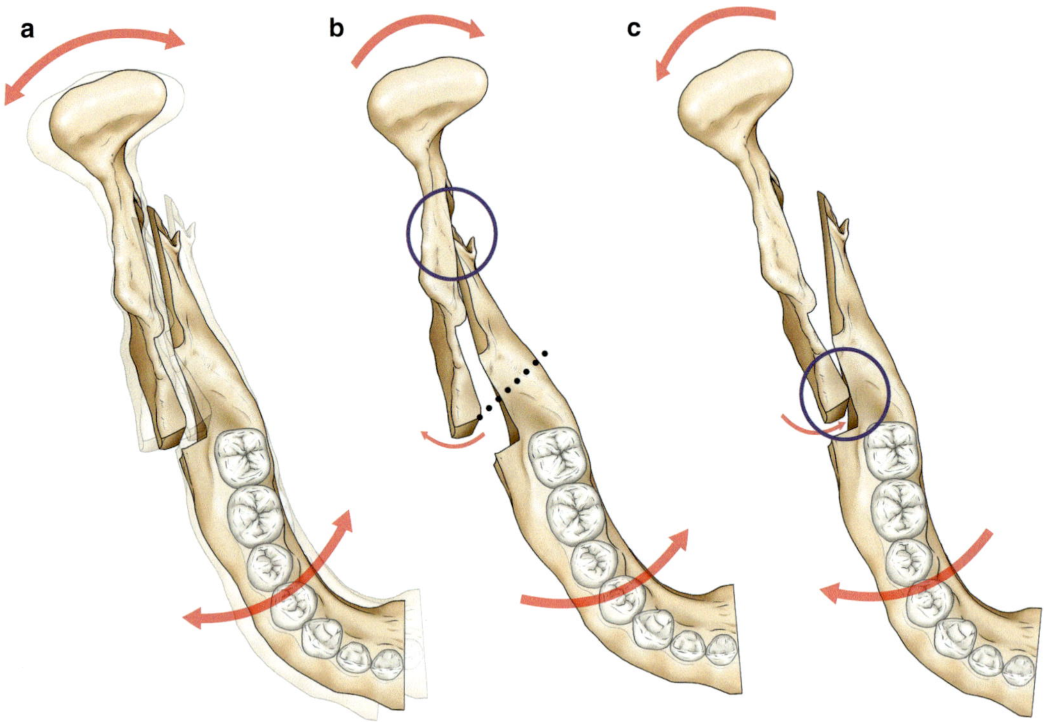

Fig. 32.9 Long bone overlap and possible osteotomy—dotted line—to avoid flaring or rotation/dislocation of the proximal segment (**a**) Illustration rotational effects on the TMJ (**b**) Lateral rotation of the proximal segment will result in an inward rotation of the TMJ. Dotted line indicates osteotomy/fracture for correction of flaring (**c**) Medial rotation of the proximal segment will result in an outward rotation of the TMJ.

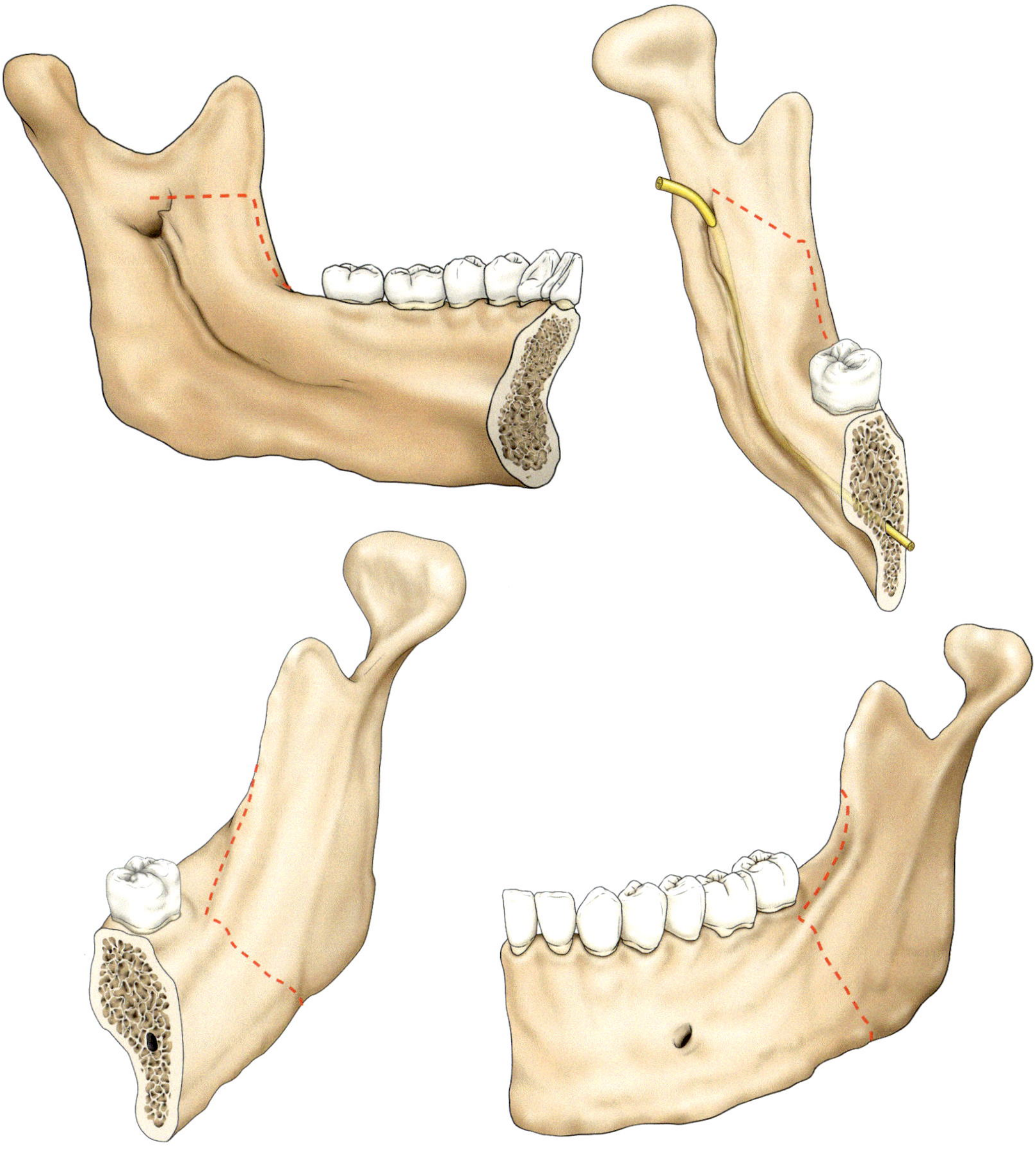

Fig. 32.10 Short bone overlap with oblique buccal osteotomy as alternative to the Dal Pont procedure to avoid or reduce long bone overlap.

9 Osteotomies in the Ascending Ramus—IVRO

9.1 Surgical Technique

As described in Part V the mucosal incision is positioned over the external oblique line and extended from the level of the occlusal plane anteriorly and inferiorly approximately about 3 cm. This incision is positioned to be able to close the wound with intermaxillary fixation at the end of operation. The periosteum is incised and reflected from the lateral surface of the mandible only, extending from sigmoid notch to the antegonial notch [9–11].

At the anterior portion of the ramus and temporalis tendon is stripped off the coronoid process to identify clearly the anterior aspect of the sigmoid notch even at the level of maxillary occlusal plane height. Channel retractors are positioned in the sigmoid notch/posterior rim of the ascending mandibular ramus and the antegonial notch, then almost whole lateral surface of the ramus can be seen by reflecting with the retractors.

The initial point of the osteotomy is located just posterior to the opening of the mandibular foramen and the antilingula prominence is the orientation point at lateral surface of the ramus (Fig. 32.11). See also Part III BSSO Relevant Clinical and Topographic Anatomy.

However, some cases with flat surface do not provide sufficient prominence. The initial point is planned at 7 or 8 mm anteriorly from the posterior border of the ramus (Fig. 32.12).

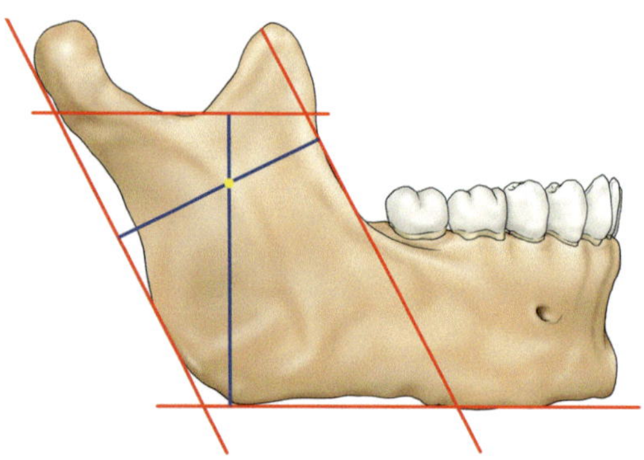

Fig. 32.11 Construction of the antilingula to determine the vertical osteotomy.

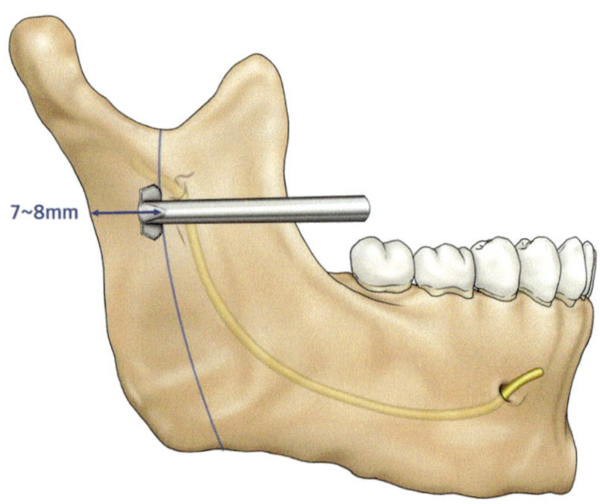

Fig. 32.12 Ideal vertical osteotomy line about 7-8 mm anterior to the posterior border of the ascending ramus, but dorsally from the antilingula.

After confirming the starting point, the osteotomy is completed by using an angulated oscillating saw from the sigmoid to the antegonial notches.

Care has to be taken at the anterior and posterior edge to prevent the injury to the maxillary and facial artery by poor protection with the retractors. So the surgeon has to check the relationship between osteotomy line and the retractors to protect the soft tissue around the notches. Ultrasonic bone cutting device such as Piezo surgery also helps to decrease the risk of damage the soft tissues.

After completing the osteotomy, the proximal segment is mobilized and displaced laterally to check the completeness of the osteotomy. To mobilize the proximal segment, only minimal periosteum is dissected off in the region of the medial pterygoid muscle (Fig. 32.13). Depending on the rotational movement, the proximal and distal segments may overlap or not.

At the contralateral side a short SSRO should be preferred for rigid osteosynthesis. Which side

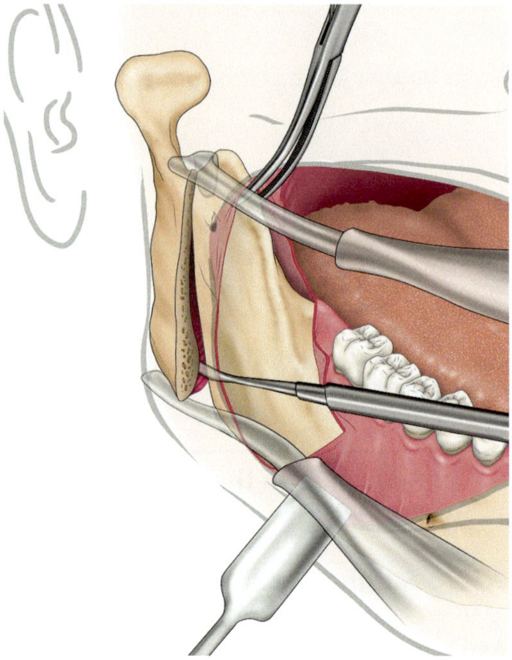

Fig. 32.13 Mobilization of the proximal segment and dissection of the medial pterygoid muscle.

can be treated with IVRO and which side with a conventional SSRO is determined by the preoperative planning. In addition to rotation effects, a lateral displacement of the mandible may also be necessary. This movement and the antero-posterior displacement determine the choice of osteotomy technique in order to avoid larger bone diastases.

In IVRO the condylar proximal segment is usually left floating without being stabilized by osteosynthesis. Nevertheless, rigid fixation with a horizontally oriented osteosynthesis plate is possible, although the spontaneous adjustment of the TMJ is lost (Fig. 32.14).

The mandible is repositioned to the planned occlusion following intermaxillary fixation with wires or elastics. In a case with severe mandibular prognathism with setback, the distal segment in IVRO may block the backward movement to acquire the desired occlusion by interference at the coronoid process. Then a coronoidotomy is needed to acquire adequate space and mobility of the distal segment. In some cases, a lateral flaring of proximal segment is observed, and bone at the inferior rim of the proximal segment has to be removed by reduction with the reciprocating saw [12].

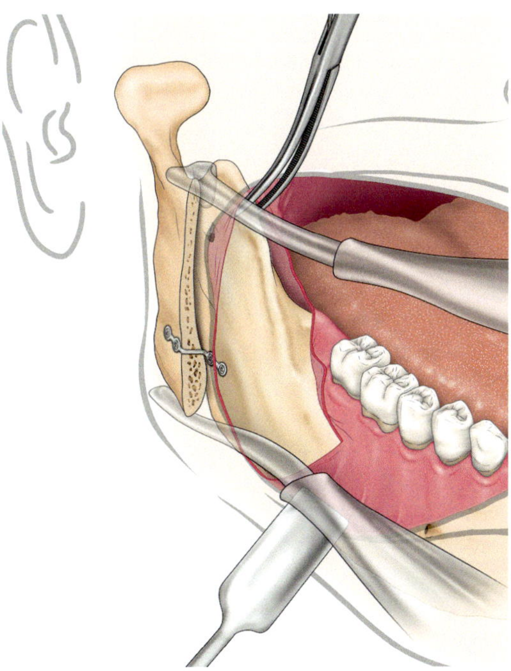

Fig. 32.14 Horizontal osteosynthesis after IVRO with 2.0 mm 4-hole miniplate with bar. ©Copyright Keisuke Koyama 2020. All rights reserved

The medial aspect of the proximal segment must sometimes be trimmed with a burr or saw to facilitate passive adaptation of proximal and distal segment (Fig. 32.15a, b).

Figures 32.16 and 32.17 refer again to the problem of lateral flaring during horizontal mandibular movements to correct midline shifts. The pivot point can be identified during 3D planning so that the appropriate splitting technique can be applied/selected to avoid damaging the TMJ by dislocation or rotation. Several strategies are displayed.

Figure 32.18 depicts BSSO in the correction of mandibular asymmetry. If a classic BSSO is performed and the rotation leads to significant displacements of the proximal segment, the lingually protruding bone of the distal segment should be shortened or fractured to allow passive alignment of the segments. This measure is not necessary in every case and depends on the course of the fracture after splitting.

To prevent the condylar luxation or sagging after surgery, the inferior part of proximal segment is sutured to the periosteum of the surrounding tissues in the retromolar region to tract the proximal segment anteriorly to the inferior part of the distal segment (Fig. 32.19). For this purpose a drill hole has to be made in the base of the proximal segment. After checking the relationship of segments, wound closure is done followed by the insertion of drain tube. For detailed description see Part V.

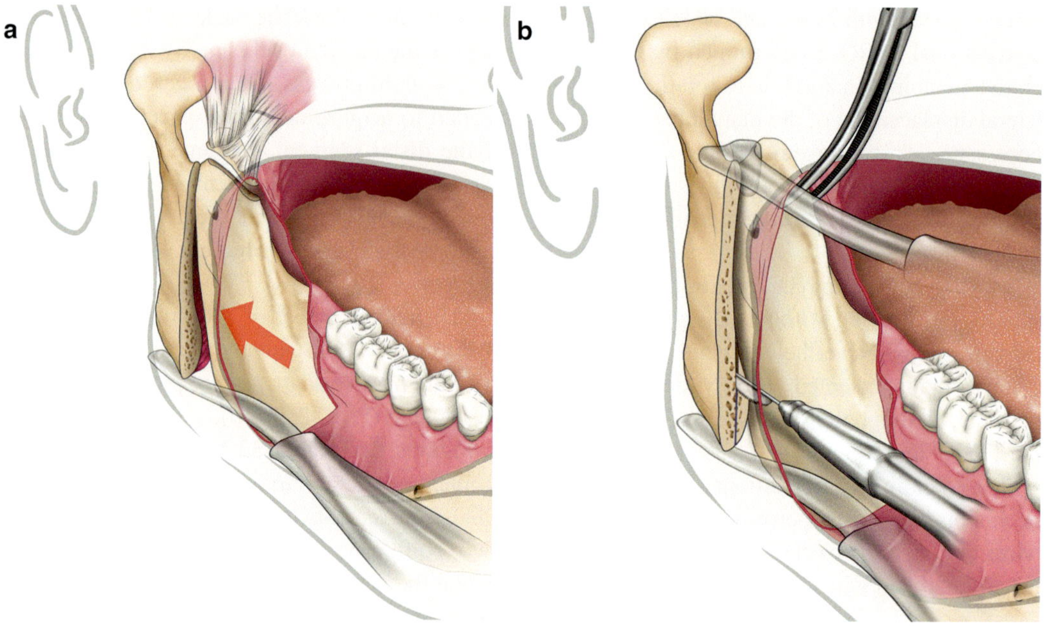

Fig. 32.15 (**a**) Coronoidotomy and backward movement of the distal segment (**b**) Correction of interfering bone edges and lateral superimposition of proximal and distal segment.

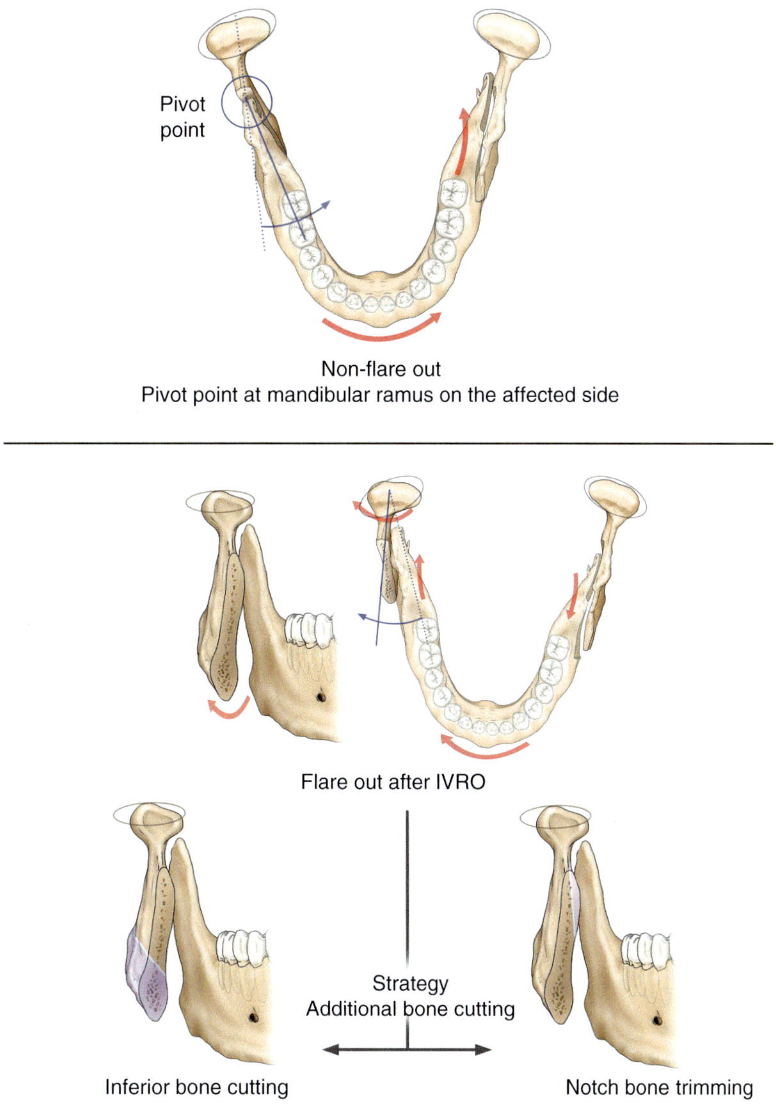

Fig. 32.16 IVRO on the right side with no flare-out and flare-out rotations to the left and right, respectively. No segment interference, if the pivot point lies in the region of the osteotomy and the rotation of the mandible does not lead to segment interference. If pivotal rotation leads to lateral dislocation of the distal segment and inward rotation of the proximal segment, correction may be necessary to avoid TMJ rotation/luxation.

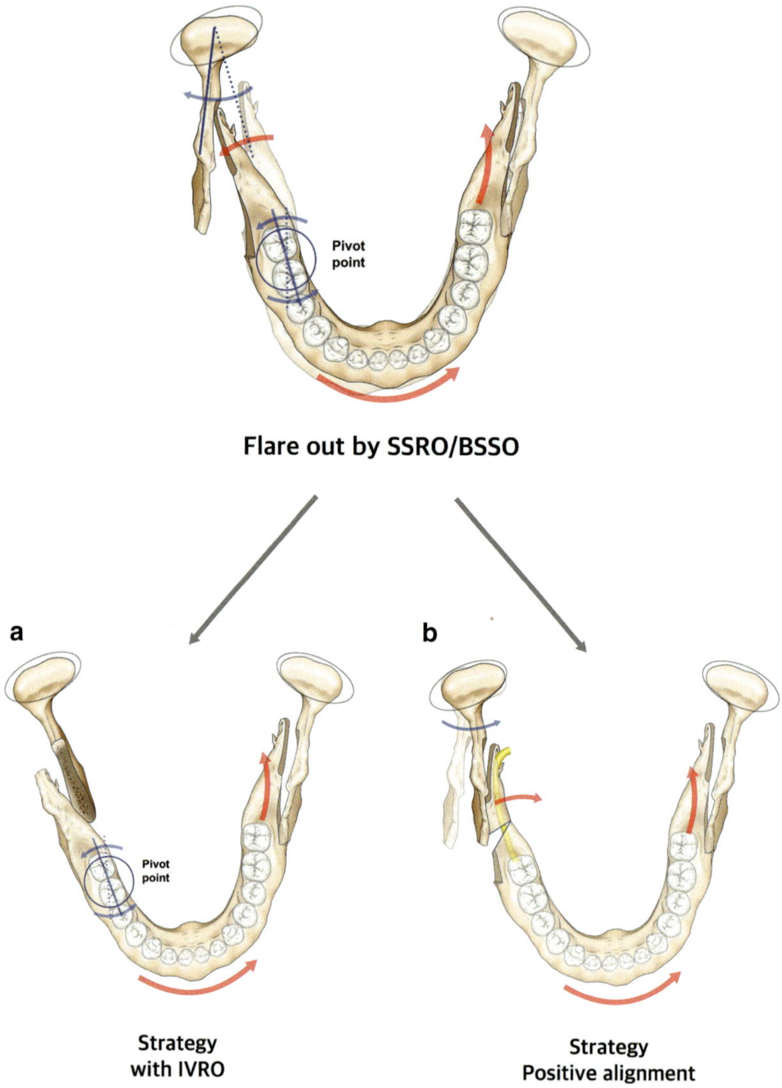

Fig. 32.17 Rotation of the mandible to the left with segment interference in BSSO. Risk of dislocation of the TMJ on the right side. Two strategies are offered: (**a**) IVRO as alternative to BSSO or (**b**) positive alignment with fracture of the overlapping lingual segment. ©Copyright Keisuke Koyama 2020. All rights reserved

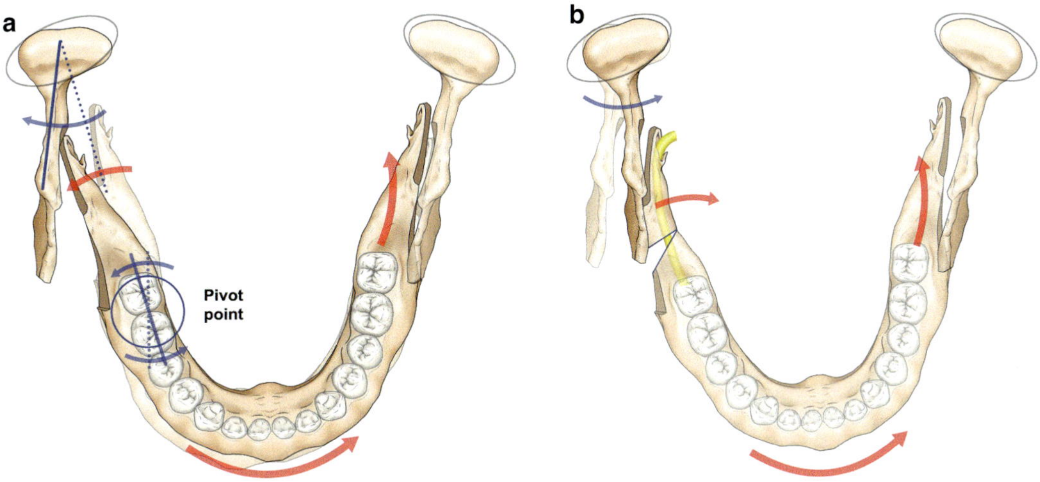

Fig. 32.18 (**a**) Rotation to the left with segment interference is more pronounced when a BSSO is performed (**b**) Passive alignment of the proximal segment with correction of TMJ position is only possible, if the lingually protruding bone of the distal segment is corrected in its axial alignment.

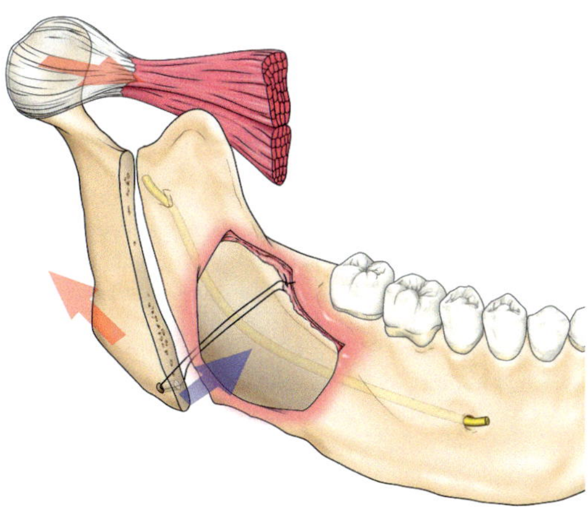

Fig. 32.19 Suturing of the proximal segment.

10 Postoperative Management

If no osteosynthesis is applied on the IVRO side, intermaxillary fixation is maintained for 7 days with/without interocclusal splint. After removing the IMF, light vertical training elastics are placed bilaterally. Without bilateral osteosynthesis the pulling direction must correspond to the midline. You have to keep an eye that no open bite occurs. In such a case, the elastics must be positioned so that the bite is closed again. This is achieved mainly by elastics in the anterior tooth region.

The elastics are changed with the relationship of the occlusion and mandibular movement during the first postoperative month. The exceptions to the use of full-time training elastic therapy are the periods when elastics are removed to facilitate eating, tooth brushing, and exercising mouth opening. After occlusion is stabilized and the elastics are reduced to one per each side, the application of elastics is based on individual needs with postoperative orthodontic treatment.

11 Which Criteria Are Decisive in the Choice of Surgical Technique?

The USSO/BSSO has a wider bony attachment surface than the IVRO:

- Rigid fixation allows mouth opening immediately after the operation.
- Postoperative healing is faster with rigid osteosynthesis.

In IVRO the bony contact is comparatively narrow or missing:

- Rigid osteosynthesis is difficult.
- Long postoperative intermaxillary fixation is required.
- Simple surgical technique.
- Shorter operation time.
- Low risk of damage to the inferior alveolar nerve.

The main advantage of IVRO is that it reduces postoperative temporomandibular joint problems. Instead of intraoperative rigid fixation with rigid condylar positioning, IVRO allows functional and gradual repositioning of the mandibular condyles with postoperative physiotherapy with controlled mouth opening. Stable bony healing depends on patient compliance [12].

12 Conclusion

When correcting vertical and horizontal asymmetries of the mandible, alternative techniques can be used if the distal segment is more displaced in order to avoid functionally harmful influences on the proximal segment and the TMJ. The IVRO is a common technique with different technical challenges than BSSO.

Often patients wish to correct facial asymmetry even before they think about the necessary orthodontic pretreatment. In the case of strong asymmetries, aesthetics is the guiding factor. Often the correction of the lower jaw alone will not be sufficient. Correction of the chin position can be of great advantage and contribute a lot to the elimination of an asymmetry. The upper jaw must not be disregarded in the analyses, since the majority of all corrections to eliminate facial asymmetries must be bimaxillary. Rotational components carry the risk of functional impairment of the TMJ. Computer-aided preoperative planning confidently identifies this and may force adjustment of the surgical approach.

References

1. Delaire J, Gaillard A, Tulasne JF. La place de la condylectomie dans le traitement des hypercondylies. Rev Stomatol Chir Maxillofac. 1983;84(1):11–8.
2. von Eiselsberg F. Über schiefen Biss in Folge Arthritis eines Unterkieferköpfchens. Arch Klin Chir. 1906;79:587–92.
3. Gruca M, Meisels E. Asymmetry of the mandible from unilateral hypertrophy. Ann Surg. 1926;83:755–67.
4. Nolte JW, Karssemakers LH, Grootendorst DC, Tuinzing DB, Becking AG. Panoramic imaging is not suitable for quantitative evaluation, classification, and follow up in unilateral condylar hyperplasia. Br J Oral Maxillofac Surg. 2015;53(5):446–50.
5. Nolte JW, Verhoeven TJ, Schreurs R, Bergé SJ, Karssemakers LH, Becking AG, Maal TJ. 3-Dimensional CBCT analysis of mandibular asymmetry in unilateral condylar hyperplasia. J Craniomaxillofac Surg. 2016;44(12):1970–6.
6. Steinhäuser EW, Rudzki-Janson IM. Kieferorthopädische Chirurgie—Eine interdisziplinäre Aufgabe—Band II. Berlin: Quintessenz; 1994.
7. Bell WH, Hall HD, White RP. Surgical ramus osteotomy. In: Surgical correction of dentofacial deformities. 2. Sanders, Philadelphia, 1980; 890–895.
8. Severt TR, Proffit W. The prevalence of facial asymmetry in the dentofacial deformities population at the University of North Carolina. Int J Adult Orthodon Orthognath Surg. 1997;12:171–6.
9. Jung HD, Kim SY, Park HS, Jung YS. Modification of intraoral vertical ramus osteotomy. Br J Oral Maxillofac Surg. 2014;52:866–7.
10. Yamauchi K, Takenobu T, Takahashi T. Condylar luxation following bilateral intraoral vertical ramus osteotomy. Oral Surg Oral Med Oral Pathol Oral Radiol Endod. 2007;104:747–51.
11. Yamauchi K, Takahashi T, Kaneuji T, Nogami S, Miyamoto I, Lethaus B. Pivot technique combined with mandibular backward distraction osteogenesis for the patient with high risk for relapse. J Craniofac Surg. 2012;23(3):658–60.
12. Ueki K, Marukawa K, Shimada M, Yoshida K, Hashiba Y, Shimizu C, Nakagawa K, Alam S, Yamamoto E. Condylar and disc positions after intraoral vertical ramus osteotomy with and without Le fort I osteotomy. Int J Oral Maxillofac Surg. 2007;36(3):207–13.

Part VII

Mandibular Excess: class III Setback/ Surgical Technique-IVRO

Indications for Mandibular Setback/Advancement Using IVRO or Inverted L Osteotomy

33

Kensuke Yamauchi and Peter Kessler

Contents

Abstract

Vertical splitting of the ascending mandibular branch is an old procedure. This technique is suitable when the mandible is to be repositioned, especially in class III correction, mandibular prognathism. This technique is no longer recommended for mandibular advancement. In regions with predominantly prognathic jaw types, this technique is popular because it can be performed quickly and is gentle on the tissue. Advantages of the BSSO, such as sufficient bone overlay, are eliminated. The stability of osteosynthetic stabilization cannot be compared with the possibilities of the BSSO. Even in the case of strong horizontal rotational movement, a vertical ramus osteotomy can be applied on the side facing the rotation.

Keywords

Class III · Bird-face deformity · Orthognathic · Mandibular setback · Vertical osteotomy and mandibular setback · Mandibular setback–IVRO–BSSO–inverted L osteotomy · Special surgical aspects in mandibular setback · Modifications and surgical alternatives

In the introduction to Parts V and VI, the most important indications for mandibular repositioning or repositioning with correction of asymmetry have already been described in detail. In this chapter, we will discuss alternative methods of mandibular osteotomy, which can be used especially in cases of mandibular setback surgery. The clinical criteria and planning preparation correspond to the procedures described in the above chapters. 3D planning is of even greater importance here, since IVRO and inverted L osteotomy must be seen as alternatives to standard

K. Yamauchi (✉)
Department of Oral & Maxillofacial Surgery, Tohoku University Sendai, Sendai, Miyagi, Japan

P. Kessler (✉)
Department of Cranio-Maxillofacial Surgery, Maastricht University Medical Center, Maastricht, The Netherlands
e-mail: peter.kessler@mumc.nl

P. Kessler et al. (eds.), *Illustrated Manual of Orthognathic Surgery*,
https://doi.org/10.1007/978-3-031-06978-9_33

sagittal splitting surgery and do not have the same status as SSRO or BSSO [1–3].

IVRO and inverted L osteotomy are especially popular in the Asian population, since the mandibular repositioning—often in combination with maxillary advancement—contributes to the idealization of the face with enhancement of the midface prominence and simultaneous reduction of the mandibular or chin prominence. In principle, both techniques are technically simpler than the splitting procedures described in detail in the previous chapters. In addition, the use of osteosynthesis is often unnecessary, which makes the procedure both temporally and logistically attractive.

Patients with class III position of the lower jaw are often dissatisfied with their appearance. At the same time, if the lower face height is enlarged, a prominent chin position can be disturbing.

The clinical image of mandibular prognathism can be assigned to a dento-alveolar or skeletal class III with cause in the mandible or maxilla or a combination of both. Clinical, radiological, and technical analyses (cephalometry), especially in the sagittal plane, are used to determine which diagnosis is applicable.

These analyses must provide information about the position and size of the mandibular skeletal structures with respect to the degree of mandibular prognathism within the respective facial growth pattern and clarify the extent of dento-alveolar and/or skeletal involvement in class III occlusion (Parts V and VI).

However, procedures to idealize facial proportions must be performed in accordance with the patient's wishes and expectations in addition to clinical analysis. After weighing the risks and possibilities, the decision to correct the mandible can be made in favor of IVRO or inverted L osteotomy in the case of a class III mandibular relationship.

Severe class II jaw relations with a bird-face deformity, high Frankfurt-mandibular plane angle, and reduced posterior facial height pose another exceptional indication for vertical ramus osteotomies, if a BSSO cannot be applied. An inverted L osteotomy can facilitate mandibular advancement and ramus lengthening [3].

1 Conclusion

Vertical osteotomies in the ascending mandibular ramus are suitable for repositioning the mandible and correcting the ramus length.

References

1. Caldwell JB, Hayward JR, Lister RL. Correction of mandibular retrognathia by vertical L osteotomy: a new technique. J Oral Surg. 1968;26:259–64.
2. Dattilo DJ, Braun TW, Sotereanos GC. The inverted L osteotomy for treatment of skeletal open-bite deformities. J Oral Maxillofac Surg. 1985;43:440–3.
3. Greaney L, Bhamrah G, Sneddon K, Collyer J. Reinventing the wheel: a modern perspective on the bilateral inverted 'L' osteotomy. Int J Oral Maxillofac Surg. 2015;44:1325–9.

34 Vertical Ramus Osteotomy and Mandibular Setback

Kensuke Yamauchi and Peter Kessler

Contents

Abstract

Vertical splitting of the ascending mandibular branch is an old procedure. This technique is suitable when the mandible is to be repositioned, especially in class III correction, mandibular prognathism. This technique is no longer recommended for mandibular advancement. In regions with predominantly prognathic jaw types, this technique is popular because it can be performed quickly and is gentle on the tissue. Advantages of the BSSO, such as sufficient bone overlay, are eliminated. The stability of osteosynthetic stabilization cannot be compared with the possibilities of the BSSO. Even in the case of strong horizontal rotational movement, a vertical ramus osteotomy can be applied on the side facing the rotation.

Keywords

Class II · Bird-face deformity · Orthognathic surgery · Mandibular setback · Vertical osteotomy and mandibular setback · Mandibular setback–IVRO–BSSO–inverted L osteotomy · Special surgical aspects in mandibular setback · Modifications and surgical alternatives

In the introduction to Parts V and VI, the most important indications for mandibular repositioning or repositioning with correction of asymmetry have already been described in detail. In this chapter, we will discuss alternative methods of mandibular osteotomy, which can be used especially in cases of mandibular setback surgery. The clinical criteria and planning preparation correspond to the procedures described in the above chapters. 3D planning is of even greater importance here, since IVRO and inverted L oste-

K. Yamauchi (✉)
Department of Oral & Maxillofacial Surgery, Tohoku University Sendai, Sendai, Miyagi, Japan

P. Kessler (✉)
Department of Cranio-Maxillofacial Surgery, Maastricht University Medical Center, Maastricht, The Netherlands
e-mail: peter.kessler@mumc.nl

P. Kessler et al. (eds.), *Illustrated Manual of Orthognathic Surgery*,
https://doi.org/10.1007/978-3-031-06978-9_34

otomy must be seen as alternatives to standard sagittal splitting surgery and do not have the same status as SSRO or BSSO [1–3].

IVRO and inverted L osteotomy are especially popular in the Asian population, since the mandibular repositioning—often in combination with maxillary advancement—contributes to the idealization of the face with enhancement of the midface prominence and simultaneous reduction of the mandibular or chin prominence. In principle, both techniques are technically simpler than the splitting procedures described in detail in the previous chapters. In addition, the use of osteosynthesis is often unnecessary, which makes the procedure both temporally and logistically attractive.

Patients with class III position of the lower jaw are often dissatisfied with their appearance. At the same time, if the lower face height is enlarged, a prominent chin position can be disturbing.

The clinical image of mandibular prognathism can be assigned to a dento-alveolar or skeletal class III with cause in the mandible or maxilla or a combination of both. Clinical, radiological, and technical analyses (cephalometry), especially in the sagittal plane, are used to determine which diagnosis is applicable.

These analyses must provide information about the position and size of the mandibular skeletal structures with respect to the degree of mandibular prognathism within the respective facial growth pattern and clarify the extent of dento-alveolar and/or skeletal involvement in class III occlusion (Parts V and VI).

However, procedures to idealize facial proportions must be performed in accordance with the patient's wishes and expectations in addition to clinical analysis. After weighing the risks and possibilities, the decision to correct the mandible can be made in favor of IVRO or inverted L osteotomy in the case of a class III mandibular relationship.

Severe class II jaw relations with a bird-face deformity, high Frankfurt-mandibular plane angle, and reduced posterior facial height pose another exceptional indication for vertical ramus osteotomies, if a BSSO cannot be applied. An inverted L osteotomy can facilitate mandibular advancement and ramus lengthening [3].

1 Conclusion

Vertical osteotomies in the ascending mandibular ramus are suitable for repositioning the mandible and correcting the ramus length.

References

1. Caldwell JB, Hayward JR, Lister RL. Correction of mandibular retrognathia by vertical L osteotomy: a new technique. J Oral Surg. 1968;26:259–64.
2. Dattilo DJ, Braun TW, Sotereanos GC. The inverted L osteotomy for treatment of skeletal open-bite deformities. J Oral Maxillofac Surg. 1985;43:440–3.
3. Greaney L, Bhamrah G, Sneddon K, Collyer J. Reinventing the wheel: a modern perspective on the bilateral inverted 'L' osteotomy. Int J Oral Maxillofac Surg. 2015;44:1325–9.

The Inverted L Osteotomy

35

Kensuke Yamauchi and Peter Kessler

Contents

Abstract

The inverted L-osteotomy represents a variant of vertical osteotomies in the ascending mandibular branch. Attention must be paid to the function of the temporal muscle. Inverted L and vertical ramus osteotomy can also be used when anatomic reasons prohibit BSSO. A longer period of intermaxillary fixation must be accepted.

Keywords

Vertical osteotomy and mandibular setback · IVRO–inverted L osteotomy · Special surgical aspects in mandibular setback · Mandibular advancement · Modifications and surgical alternatives

K. Yamauchi (✉)
Department of Oral & Maxillofacial Surgery, Tohoku University Sendai, Sendai, Miyagi, Japan

P. Kessler (✉)
Department of Cranio-Maxillofacial Surgery, Maastricht University Medical Center, Maastricht, The Netherlands
e-mail: peter.kessler@mumc.nl

The third clinically relevant possibility to fracture the mandible in a controlled manner is the Inverted L Osteotomy (Fig. 35.1).

If the problem of the IVRO in the area of the coronoid process is to be expected, then this procedure offers itself, whereby here elements of the classical BSSO/SSRO and the IVRO merge.

The main indication for the inverted L osteotomy, however, is when the cancellous bone supply between the compact osseous lamellae in the region of the mandibular angle is so low that conventional splitting of the mandible would result in a bad fracture.

The horizontal osteotomy below the coronoid is at the same level as the lingual osteotomy of the Hunsuck-Epker variant of BSSO/SSRO. However, it is an osteotomy and not a split, the bone is completely passed through [1, 2]. The combination of the vertical osteotomy is

P. Kessler et al. (eds.), *Illustrated Manual of Orthognathic Surgery*,
https://doi.org/10.1007/978-3-031-06978-9_35

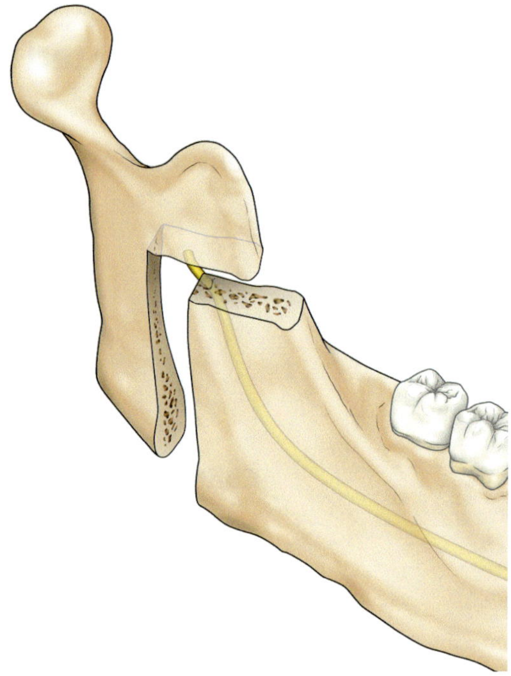

Fig. 35.1 Ideal inverted L osteotomy. ©Copyright Keisuke Koyama 2020. All rights reserved

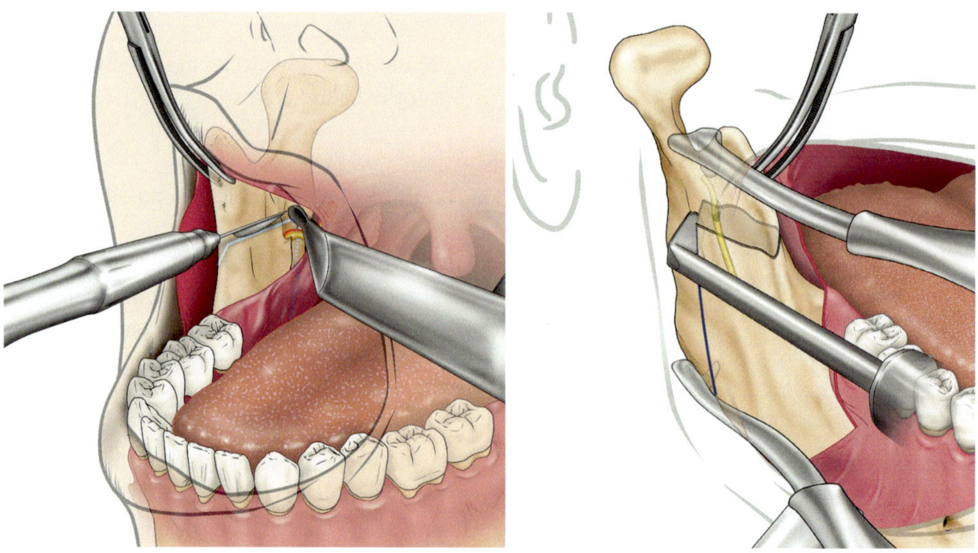

Fig. 35.2 Horizontal and vertical osteotomy with the oscillating saw. Piezosurgery can be applied ©Copyright Keisuke Koyama 2020. All rights reserved

again borrowed from IVRO and, like IVRO, is performed dorsal to the lingula/antilingula of the ascending ramus (Fig. 35.2). The inverted L osteotomy on one side can be combined with an SSRO on the contralateral side [3].

1 Advantages

- Technically simple, quick to perform.
- Ideal in compact bone, where splitting is impossible.

- In mandibular asymmetry with relevant vertical displacement.
- Theoretically more bone overlap than with IVRO, but significantly less than with both BSSO/SSRO.
- Risk of injury to IAN.

2 Disadvantages

- Increased risk of a bad fracture in the area of the semilunar notch.
- Mobilization of the segments more difficult due to more bony interference.
- Osteosynthesis is recommended, especially in cases where inverted L osteotomy replaces the SSRO/BSSO (Fig. 35.3a–c).
- Cranial displacement of distal segment impossible.

Another indication for inverted L osteotomy can be found in mandibular asymmetries where a relevant vertical correction to the caudal is required (Fig. 35.3b).

Pronounced bird-face deformities can be treated by vertical ramus osteotomies with further mandibular advancement and lengthening of the ascending mandibular branch, although prolonged postoperative intermaxillary fixation must be accepted [4].

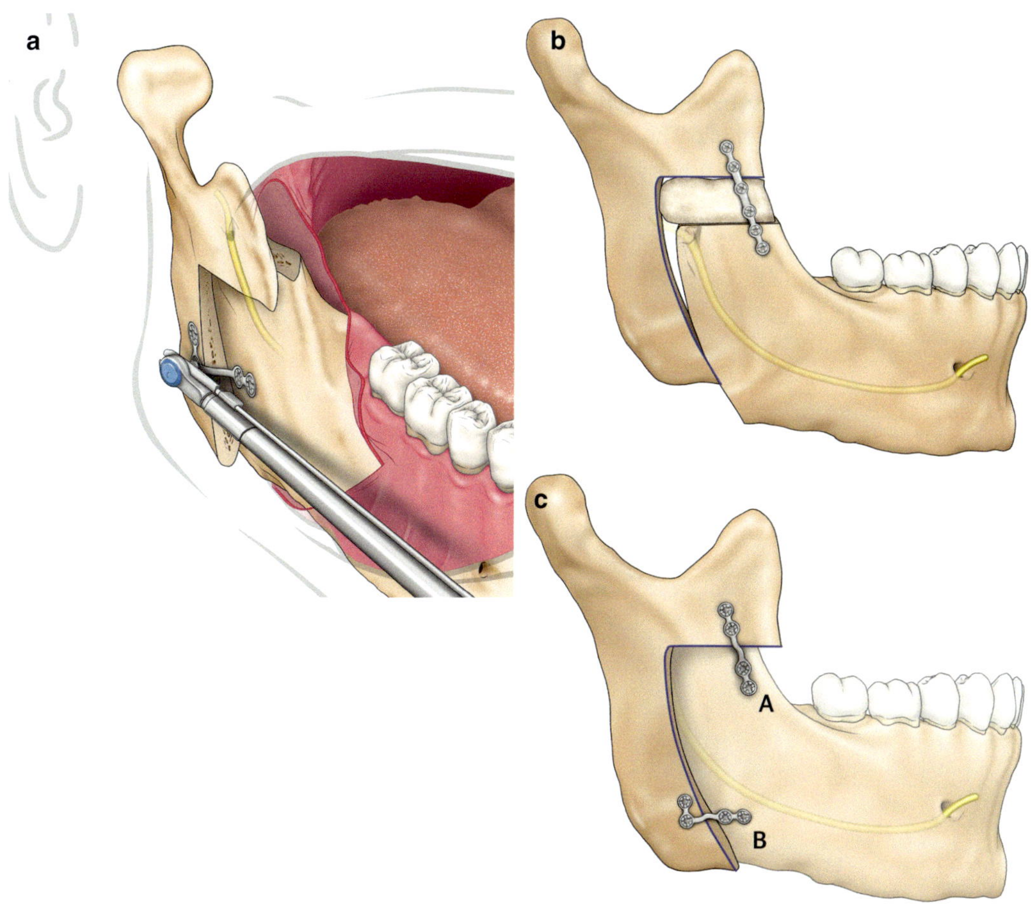

Fig. 35.3 (**a**) Osteosynthesis with the angulated burr/screwdriver (**b**) Vertical osteosynthesis with bone interposition in major vertical correction (**c**) Stable osteosynthesis is recommended for optimal bone healing.

Then the coronoid process with the temporal muscle attached will not block caudal dislocation to the distal segment [5].

The surgical procedure from incision to wound closure corresponds to the procedure in the preceding chapters. In the case of compact bone structure and thin bone layers, stable osteosynthesis is recommended to optimally support bony healing (Fig. 35.3c).

3 Conclusion

Inverted L osteotomy can be considered as an alternative osteotomy technique. It is also suitable for mandibular advancement with limitations.

Inverted L and vertical ramus osteotomy are alternatives when BSSO cannot be performed. Furthermore, the vertical osteotomies are suitable for mandibular repositioning. The procedure is quick to perform and rigid osteosynthesis is often not applied. The functional influxes of the masticatory muscles must be taken into account, and intermaxillary fixation plays an important role in postoperative management.

References

1. Dattilo DJ, Braun TW, Sotereanos GC. The inverted L osteotomy for treatment of skeletal open-bite deformities. J Oral Maxillofac Surg. 1985;43:440–3.
2. DiStefano JF, Spilka C. Inverted L osteotomy for correction of mandibular prognathism after relapse. J Oral Surg. 1978;36:147–9.
3. McMillan B, Jones R, Ward-Booth P, Goss A. Technique for intraoral inverted "L" osteotomy. Br J Oral Maxillofac Surg. 1999;37:324–6.
4. Greaney L, Bhamrah G, Sneddon K, Collyer J. Reinventing the wheel: a modern perspective on the bilateral inverted 'L' osteotomy. Int J Oral Maxillofac Surg. 2015;44:1325–9.
5. Muto T, Akizuki K, Tsuchida N, Sato Y. Modified intraoral inverted-"L" osteotomy: a technique for good visibility, greater bony overlap and rigid fixation. J Oral Maxillofac Surg. 2008;66:1309–15.

Part VIII

Alveolar Segment Osteotomies

Types of Segmental Alveolar Osteotomies in the Mandible

36

Peter Kessler and Nicolas Hardt

Contents

Abstract

Class II division I malocclusions are the most common dentofacial deformities seen in clinical practice. Combined orthodontic and surgical treatment in cases of severe class II dentofacial deformities (*class II division I malocclusion/class II division II malocclusion*) is a routine procedure in these orthodontic patients (Bell et al., American Journal of Orthodontics. 85:1–20, 1984).

Some indications for segment osteotomies in combination with correction of class II deformities are as follows: Excess vertical growth in the anterior dentoalveolar process of the mandible, some types of mandibular vertical alveolar deficiency and anterior open bite, relapse after BSSO, cases of condylar agenesis and hypoplasia, lateral open bite, mandibular dental arch asymmetry, and negative curve of Spee (Köle. Oral Surgery, Oral Medicine, and Oral Pathology 12(3):277–288, 1959; MacIntosh RB Journal of Maxillofacial Surgery. 2:210-218, 1974).

However, the aim will always be to avoid segmental osteotomies by means of suitable orthodontic pretreatment, since the techniques of relocating the entire mandible are safer and involve fewer risks. Nevertheless, there are situations in which the performance of a segmental osteotomy is indicated, either in combination with a BSSO or as a stand-alone procedure. Segmental osteotomies can be performed in the anterior mandibular region, but also laterally.

P. Kessler (✉)
Department of Cranio-Maxillofacial Surgery, Maastricht University Medical Center, Maastricht, The Netherlands
e-mail: peter.kessler@mumc.nl

N. Hardt (✉)
Kantonsspital Lucerne, Clinic and Policlinic of Cranio-Maxillofacial Surgery, Lucerne, Switzerland

P. Kessler et al. (eds.), *Illustrated Manual of Orthognathic Surgery*,
https://doi.org/10.1007/978-3-031-06978-9_36

Keywords

Alveolar osteotomies · Segmental osteotomy · Dentoalveolar retrusion · Anterior deep bite - Class II malocclusion · Dentoalveolar protrusion · Correction of open bite · Posterior subapical osteotomy · Anterior body osteotomy · BSSO

1 Anterior Subapical Segmental Osteotomy

Anterior subapical segmental osteotomies in the mandible involve vertical and horizontal separation and mobilization of the alveolar mandibular segment ideally between the first premolars and canines.

The subapical osteotomized segment is then repositioned:

- Either superiorly to correct an open bite.
- Inferiorly with ostectomy of a horizontal bone segment.
- Posteriorly with ostectomy of a vertical alveolar bone segment or as a combined movement.

Dentoalveolar segment relocation—downwards and backwards—is associated with bone removal; alveolar segment relocation—upwards and forwards—is associated with bone interposition inferiorly or distally.

Segmental anterior mandibular osteotomies may be combined with the anterior maxillary osteotomies in cases with bimaxillary alveolar protrusion [1–3].

2 Posterior Subapical Osteotomy

The posterior subapical osteotomy is performed to correct super-eruption of posterior mandibular teeth or in case of ankylosis of impacted posterior teeth.

3 Variants of an Anterior Segment Osteotomy

- *Lateral mandibular body step osteotomy/ostectomy.*

  The lateral step osteotomy/ostectomy of the mandible is a variant of the anterior segmental block osteotomy to reposition the anterior section of the mandible, e.g., for posterior or superior repositioning [4, 5]
- *Anterior body osteotomy (Straight vertical osteotomy).*

  A vertical osteotomy with ostectomy primarily to reposition the anterior mandibular segment.

4 Conclusion

Segmental osteotomies can be applied in the upper as well as in the lower jaw. Anterior and lateral segmental osteotomies are discerned.

References

1. Bell WH, Jacobs JD, Legan HL. Treatment of class II deep bite by orthodontic and surgical means. Am J Orthod. 1984;85(1):1–20.
2. Köle H. Surgical operations on the alveolar ridge to correct occlusal abnormalities. Oral Surg Oral Med Oral Pathol. 1959;12(3):277–88.
3. MacIntosh RB. Total mandibular alveolar osteotomy: encouraging experiences with an infrequently indicated procedure. J Maxillofac Surg. 1974;2(4):210–8.
4. Fonsecca RJ, Marciani, RD, Turvey TA. Oral and maxillofacial surgery, Bd 1 Saunders/Elesevier, 2009.
5. Harris M, Reynolds IR. Fundamentals of orthognatic surgery. Saunders; 1991.

Indications for Segmental Osteotomies in the Mandible

37

Peter Kessler and Nicolas Hardt

Contents

Abstract

Mandibular subapical segmental osteotomies are not the most common choices to treat patients with dentofacial deformity. However, especially the anterior subapical osteotomy is a very versatile technique that allows the osteotomized segment to be moved in different directions. The surgical technique can also be applied with other dysgnathias and in combination with a BSSO.

P. Kessler (✉)
Department of Cranio-Maxillofacial Surgery, Maastricht University Medical Center, Maastricht, The Netherlands
e-mail: peter.kessler@mumc.nl

N. Hardt (✉)
Kantonsspital Lucerne, Clinic and Policlinic of Cranio-Maxillofacial Surgery, Lucerne, Switzerland

Keywords

Segmental osteotomies · Mandibular osteotomies · Dysgnathia · BSSO · Alveolar protrusion · Open bite

1 Anterior Subapical Osteotomy

It is possible to set the anterior segment backward, forward, upward, and downward, depending on the need. Also, this type of osteotomy may be performed along with a bilateral sagittal split osteotomy (BSSO).

According to *Bell et al.* [1, 2], the mandibular anterior subapical osteotomy may be indicated to level the occlusion, produce anteroposterior changes of the osteotomized segment, correct crowding in the lower anterior arch, correct anterior dentoalveolar asymmetries, alter the axial inclination of the anterior teeth, reduce overall treatment time, and improve treatment stability.

Anterior subapical osteotomy is indicated when there is a skeletal class I relation but a

P. Kessler et al. (eds.), *Illustrated Manual of Orthognathic Surgery*,
https://doi.org/10.1007/978-3-031-06978-9_37

deformity in the frontal mandibular segment cannot be corrected by orthodontic treatment.

1. Alveolar protrusion of the mandibular front segment with possibly negative overjet (*mandibulo-alveolar protrusion*) in contrast to a true mandibular prognathism, the jaw base is normally developed. The maldevelopment is limited to the frontal alveolar process and teeth (dentoalveolar localization). The protrusion of the mandibular front is often associated with a protrusion of the maxillary front (*bimaxillary alveolar protrusion*).
2. Alveolar elevation of the anterior bone segment and teeth as a concomitant symptom of mandibular prognathism. Anterior elevation of the anterior mandibular segment is a fairly regular occurrence in mandibular prognathism and alveolar protrusion in the maxilla (pronounced curve of Spee with elevation of the mandibular front).
3. Marked anteroposterior discrepancy of the anterior bone segment and teeth (*mandibulo-alveolar retrusion*) in class II division II malocclusion .
4. Vertical alveolar bone deficit in the anterior mandibular segment in certain types of anterior open bite (*vertical mandibulo-alveolar deficiency*).
5. Asymmetries of the anterior mandibular dental arch.
6. Vertical height/volume deficits in the anterior mandibular segment may be associated with ankylosing teeth or oligo/hypodontia.

2 Conclusion

There are specific indications in which segmental osteotomy in the anterior mandibular region in particular may be indicated. If orthodontic correction is impossible or unsuccessful, relocation of a defined jaw segment can help. Especially the vertical component may be affected.

References

1. Bell WH, Proffit WR, White RP. Surgical correction of dentofacial deformities. Philadelphia: WB Saunders; 1980.
2. Bell WH, Jacobs JD, Legan HL. Treatment of class II deep bite by orthodontic and surgical means. Am J Orthod. 1984;85(1):1–20.

38 Preoperative Planning and Preparation for Surgery in Segmental Mandibular Osteotomies

Peter Kessler and Nicolas Hardt

Contents

Abstract

The surgical preparations require the same care as for other orthognathic procedures. Particular attention must be paid to the subapical bone supply for creating an osteotomy.

Keywords

Segmental osteotomies · Mandibular osteotomies · Dysgnathia · BSSO · Alveolar protrusion · Open bite · Preoperative planning

P. Kessler (✉)
Department of Cranio-Maxillofacial Surgery, Maastricht University Medical Center, Maastricht, The Netherlands
e-mail: peter.kessler@mumc.nl

N. Hardt (✉)
Kantonsspital Lucerne, Clinic and Policlinic of Cranio-Maxillofacial Surgery, Lucerne, Switzerland

Planning requirements:

- Dental casts and profile photos.
- Dental status.
- Routine radiographs: panoramic radiography, if indicated cone-beam CT (CBCT).

Evaluation of:

- Chin region/bone strength in the region of the mandibular symphysis: mental spine/cortical bone structure in the mental region/position of the mental foramina.
- Assessment of contour of the chin and anterior alveolar process, the root tip region and the interdental septa 35–45.
- Analysis of the lateral projection of the facial skeleton on the lateral cephalogram or CBCT, cephalometry (Fig. 38.1).

P. Kessler et al. (eds.), *Illustrated Manual of Orthognathic Surgery*,
https://doi.org/10.1007/978-3-031-06978-9_38

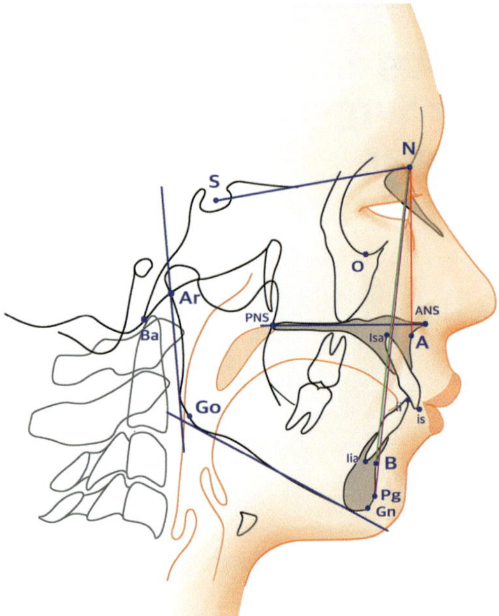

Fig. 38.1 Graphic-cephalometric surgery planning—lateral cephalogram of a case with bi-alveolar protrusion and dental class II relation with large overjet. Lower jaw base and ascending ramus are normally developed.

1 Preparation for Operation

- Planning
- Simulation by means of model operation
- Production of surgical splints

Simple plaster models are sufficient. The correction of the inverted overbite or anterior step, for example, is done by retro positioning the pro- and extruded lower jaw segment by one premolar width. On the plaster model, the corresponding premolar is erased on each side and the segment including the anterior teeth is cut out approximately at right angles.

The three cut surfaces must be such that a harmoniously shaped dental arch with normal anterior overbite is created when the fragment is adjusted. An occlusal splint is made on the corrected model. Preoperatively, individually made dental wire-arches can be prepared.

If posterior teeth are missing, the splint can serve as a prosthesis splint which is temporarily used even after the surgery. The anterior arch of the splint is stiffened with self-curing acrylic at the end of surgery to stabilize the segment on the vestibular and lingual side. With this type of fixation, intermaxillary immobilization is not required.

If the anterior teeth are elongated, only the affected segment from the alveolar process is osteotomized and shortened accordingly.

If preoperative extractions are performed for orthodontic tooth movements, it must be ensured that a 3 mm wide interdental space remains to allow the vertical osteotomy to be performed without damaging the roots. Interdental space can also be created orthodontically without extracting teeth.

If the anterior teeth are positioned too low, the mandibular segment is elevated and supported with a bone graft. Here, too, the segment is adjusted using an occlusal splint and the segment is then fixed using arch-wires supported by self-curing acrylics as described above.

In general, segments are also fixed at their base with mini plates of 1.5 mm and short screws in such a way that the bone segment has maximum stability. Nevertheless, the greatest care must be taken in segmental osteotomies when making and adjusting the occlusal splints [1, 2].

2 Profile Changes

In an anterior subapical segmental osteotomy of the mandible, the lower lip follows a skeletal retro-positioning of approximately 75% at the level of the lip, and a forward movement of the alveolar process segment of 60%.

If the chin position remains unchanged, the labio-mental fold is simultaneously reinforced or flattened. A change in the vertical height of the face is impossible.

3 Conclusion

The planning and preparation of a segmental osteotomy requires thoroughness to be performed successfully at all. This has to do primarily with the limited space available around the segment to be lifted.

References

1. Bell WH, Proffit WR, White RP. Surgical correction of dentofacial deformities. Philadelphia: WB Saunders; 1980.
2. Bell WH, Jacobs JD, Legan HL. Treatment of class II deep bite by orthodontic and surgical means. Am J Orthod. 1984;85(1):1–20.

Anatomical, Surgical, and Technical Aspects

39

Peter Kessler and Nicolas Hardt

Contents

P. Kessler (✉)
Department of Cranio-Maxillofacial Surgery, Maastricht University Medical Center, Maastricht, The Netherlands
e-mail: peter.kessler@mumc.nl

N. Hardt (✉)
Kantonsspital Lucerne, Clinic and Policlinic of Cranio-Maxillofacial Surgery, Lucerne, Switzerland

Abstract

The success of a segmental osteotomy depends on the surgical approach, which must be fully thought out from the initial incision to the suture to be successful. This has to do with segmental perfusion and the limited displace-

P. Kessler et al. (eds.), *Illustrated Manual of Orthognathic Surgery*,
https://doi.org/10.1007/978-3-031-06978-9_39

ment ability of the segment in the mandibular arch. Only well-considered surgical steps guarantee success.

Keywords

Segmental osteotomies · Mandibular osteotomies · Dysgnathia · BSSO · Alveolar protrusion · Open bite · Preoperative planning · Surgical access · Incision · Osteosynthesis

1 Decisive Anatomical Reference Points

1.1 Reference Points

1.1.1 For the Mucosal Incision

Gingival margin.

Labial attachment of the lip ligament.

1.1.2 For Access to the Osteotomy

Aponeurosis of the following muscles and structures:

Mentalis muscle, levator labii muscle and depressor anguli oris muscle as well as:

Mental foramen and lower edge of the mandible in the chin region.

1.1.3 For Vertical or Horizontal Ostectomy

Extraction sockets of premolars; mental foramen; alveolar protuberances; interdental and interalveolar space.

1.2 Surgical Aspects

- Operation simulation as exact and detailed as possible.
- Surgical access as clear as possible.
- Bone cuts/osteotomies as simple as possible.
- Existing tooth gaps in the premolar region can be closed surgically by placing the osteotomy/ostectomy deliberately in the region of the tooth gap.

Note
- Subapical osteotomies need careful planning to ensure a vascular pedicle as large as possible.
- The blood flow through the mandibular periosteum could easily maintain a sufficient blood supply to the teeth of an osteotomized segment, even when the labial periosteum was degloved.
- The greater distance from the apices of the teeth not only minimizes direct pulpal injury but increases the vascular pedicle to the mobile segment.

- If the segmental osteotomy is performed posterior to the mental foramen, the mental nerve may cross the osteotomy field. The vascular nerve bundle must be visualized and released from its bone canal; otherwise there is a risk of permanent damage to the nerve.
- Segment fixation as stable as possible.

1.3 Technical Aspects

1.3.1 Rotating Instruments: Burrs

The degree of mechanical processing of the jawbone when the osteotomies are applied depends on the geometry and shape of the rotating instruments (spherical, conical, cylindrical), the instrument diameter, the roughness of the surface structure of the instruments: diamond-coated, saw-tooth structure (cross-toothed, spiral-toothed) and the speed of rotation.

High rotational speed and strong contact pressure of the rotating instruments lead to more or less pronounced bone necrosis and increase significantly at higher rotational speeds and increasing osteotomy depth.

1.3.2 Piezo-Surgery

Piezo-surgery in segmental osteotomies allows highly precise, uncomplicated interdental vertical separation of alveolar bone without damaging the neighboring teeth and the connecting horizontal incisions with the least possible bone loss and guarantees superior protection of soft tissue (nerves/vessels/mucosa).

This is associated with a significantly reduced bone trauma in the area of the osteotomies and a micromorphologically and histologically verified significant improvement in bone healing and a better hemodynamic microcirculation of the tissues of the surgical site [1, 2]. See Chap. 16.

1.3.3 Segment Fixation

The osteotomized alveolar segment is fixed in position either by an intra-mandibular arch-wire splint with and without prior segmentation, which is reinforced with self-curing plastic during surgery.

or

Fixed by an orthodontically ligated orthodontic arch-wire, which is reinforced with self-curing resins during the operation, supplemented by an intraoperatively integrated lingual-occlusal splint.

in combination with

Mini-plate osteosynthesis bridging the osteotomy gap with 1.5 mm plates and self-tapping cortical screws.

2 Surgical Approach: Detailed Surgical Steps

2.1 Anterior Segment Osteotomy

The anterior segment osteotomy is performed after pre-surgical orthodontic gap formation to safely protect adjacent tooth roots and the mental nerve, preferably between the canine and first premolars.

The osteotomy is placed horizontally subapically about 6–8 mm - minimum 5 mm - below the root apices and ends about 2–3 mm before the mental foramen. Then the horizontal osteotomy is connected to the vertical osteotomies in the area of the extracted first premolars.

If extraction is not planned, the anterior segment can be positioned cranially to close an anterior open bite. A bone graft should be integrated into the horizontal gap.

2.2 Detailed Surgical Steps

2.2.1 Step 1: Intraoral Mucosal Incision

- Expose the surgical area from the first molar on the left to the first molar on the right—from 6–6.
- Mobilization of soft tissues subperiosteal to beyond the lower jaw margin.

Intraoral Muco-Periosteal Incision

The labial mucosa and vestibule are infiltrated with local anesthetics containing vasoconstrictive additives, e.g., a solution of epinephrine 1:100,000. After tensioning the lower lip and exposing the vestibule with Langenbeck retractors and drying the mucosa, the incision is marked with a sterile skin marker.

The mucosa is then incised parabolically from 6–6, distal to the planned vertical bone cuts.

The apex of the incision parabola lies in the median region of the labial mucosa (Fig. 39.1).

This incision design prevents suture dehiscence later on. After cutting through the mucosa and submucosa, the terminal branches of the mental nerve are localized in the submucosal tissues in an atraumatic, blunt manner.

Then, below the mobilized mucosa-submucosa cuff, the chin musculature is severed sharply

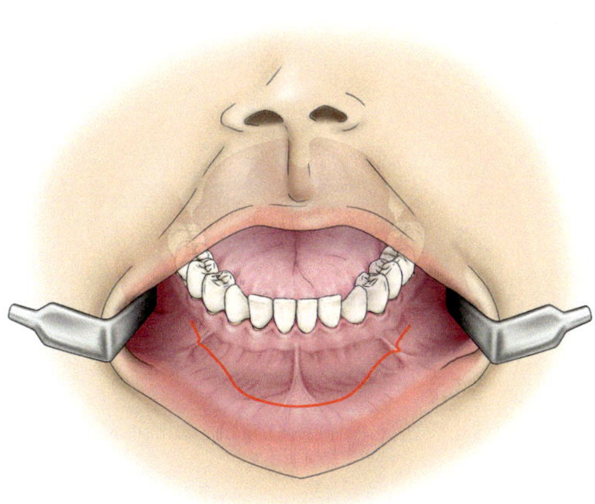

Fig. 39.1 Parabolic incision line from the first molar on the left to the first molar on the right. ©Copyright Keisuke Koyama 2020. All rights reserved

down to the bone—approximately halfway between the gingival margin and the lower limit of the mandible—and the periosteum is incised repeatedly at the same location (Figs. 39.2 and 39.3).

Mucoperiosteal Dissection

The mental nerve is visualized by elevation of the periosteum in distal direction. The periosteum is then elevated below, above, and behind the foramen to form a tunnel, and the periosteal conus is carefully incised and the nerve is prepared freely so that the risk of injury is minimized and the access is considerably widened so that the nerve can be better protected.

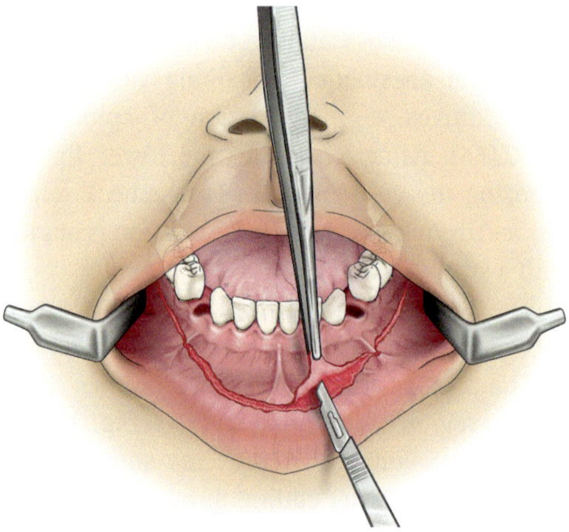

Fig. 39.2 The mucosa incision runs halfway between the inner vermillion border and the mucogingival junction.

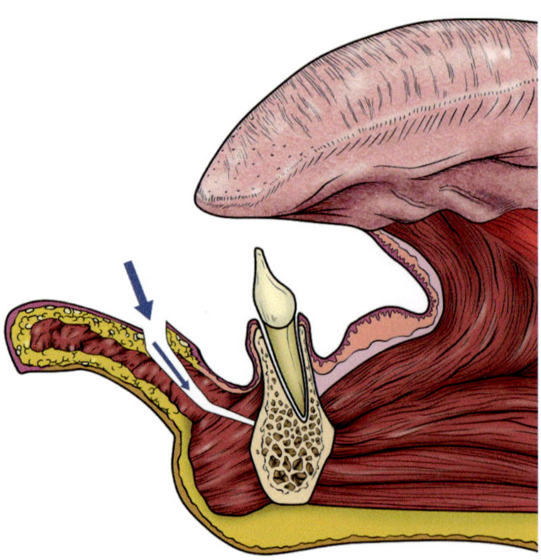

Fig. 39.3 Incision of the muscular tissues of the orbicularis oris and mental muscle.

A smooth, atraumatic detachment of the adhering periosteal-tendinous tissue of the mentalis muscle is best achieved with a sharp-edged, not too wide dissector.

The lateral mimic muscles of the oral fissure can be levered off smoothly, so that it is recommended to start with subperiosteal detachment there first at the height of the mental foramen, and then subperiosteally detach the adherent attachment of the mental muscle (mental tubercula) up to the alveoli of the incisors without tearing.

An elevator is then used to lift the anterior soft tissue package to below the edge of the mandible and a chin retractor is inserted to hold the flap and support the mandible.

If additional reduction of the chin is planned, the soft tissues must be mobilized beyond the edge of the lower jaw.

Clear exposure of the labial bone surface—including the mental foramina—is always necessary. Since the position of the tooth roots are clearly visible, the height of the root tips can be determined easily; transverse osteotomy is performed about 6–8 mm below.

Note

- Deep vestibular mucosal/submucosal incision in the area of the planned segmental osteotomy.
- Sharp cutting of the chin muscles up to the periosteum.
- Periosteal incision and subperiosteal elevation of the vestibular mucosa.
- Elevation of the submucosal periosteum in distal direction with presentation of the mental nerve.
- Tunneling preparation of the gingival mucosa in the area of the vertical interdental osteotomies while preserving the soft tissues for later saliva-tight gingival wound closure in the interdental osteotomy area.

2.2.2 Step 2: Segment Osteotomy

- The interdental bone cuts with burr and micro-saw
- or piezo-surgery and small osteotomes.

It is essential to study the patient's tomograms carefully before performing the osteotomies.

First, usually a premolar is extracted on both sides and the alveolar walls are gently removed. The initial horizontal osteotomy runs about 6–8 mm below the apices of the anterior teeth of the planned alveolar segment. The position of the tooth roots determines the position of the horizontal osteotomy. Danger points of an incorrect subapical osteotomy are injuries to the adjacent roots and root tips and injuries to the mental nerve.

Fine drill holes are made in the cortical bone along the osteotomy line which has been marked with a sterile pencil.

The horizontal and vertical osteotomies are first pre-cut along the cortical perforations with a fissure drill, alternatively with a sagittal oscillating micro-saw.

The completion of the horizontal and vertical osteotomies—including the alveolar bone on the lingual side—is initially performed with fine fissure drills or oscillating saws and, advantageously on the lingual side, atraumatically with piezo-surgery.

If no teeth are to be extracted, the buccal cut can initially only be made through the outer cortex with a fine split drill or oscillating saw.

After very limited loosening the lingual mucoperiosteum vertically from above—using a thin periosteal elevator—the separation of the lingual cortex is performed advantageously by piezo-surgery.

Horizontal and/or vertical alveolar ostectomies/corrections are necessary if the segment is repositioned or lowered (Fig. 39.4).

Note

- Mark vertical osteotomy lines with a fine fissure drill.
- In the case of planned segment repositioning with tooth extraction, the area to be osteotomized is also marked.
- Mark the horizontal connecting osteotomy line with a minimum distance of 6–8 mm to the root tips of the teeth of the segment.
- Completing the osteotomies with fine fissure drills, alternatively fine oscillating saws and chisels or piezo-surgical cutting.

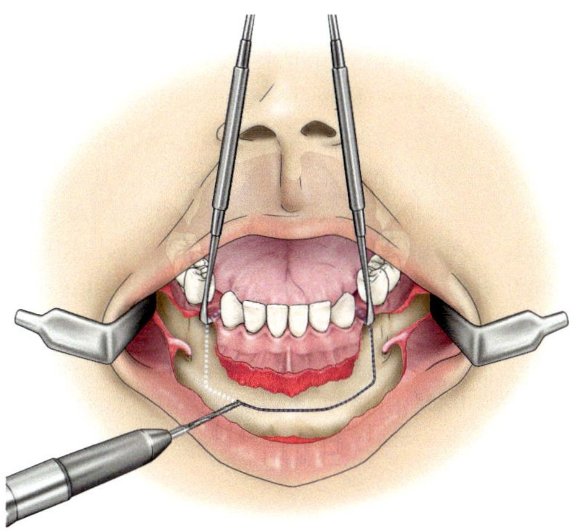

Fig. 39.4 Principle design of vertical and horizontal bone cuts for anterior mandibular segment osteotomy.

2.2.3 Step 3: Segment Mobilization

Mobilization of the Segment with Small Osteotomes

The osteotomized segment is then mobilized with narrow 3–5 mm osteotomes and small lever movements.

The fragment can be lifted by the muscle and mucosa of the lingual side and tilt. A very narrow pear-shaped burr is used for its further processing of the segment. The aim is to shape the cut surfaces according to the model template.

In order to achieve a normal overbite, the segment must either be shifted back, lowered, raised, or rotated. If this results in a horizontal gap open to the front or a continuous vertical gap (Fig. 39.5), this gap is filled with a regional bone graft from the lower edge of the chin.

2.2.4 Step 4: Setting the Segment and Intraoral Fixation

Occlusion-Related Setting of the Osteotomized Segment

After the osteotomized and sufficiently mobilized segment has been precisely adjusted to the occlusion, the preplanned occlusion is secured intraoperatively. This is done either with an applied mono-maxillary dental/occlusal splint which should cover the lingual side of the mandibular teeth and include them for stabilization.

The segment is secured by the mono-maxillary splint which is connected and fixed by wire ligatures and self-curing plastic. The fragment is now firmly locked in its new position (Fig. 39.6). An intermaxillary immobilization is not necessary.

Rigid Segment Fixation

The final fixation of the secured alveolar segment is then performed by rigid osteosynthesis with 1.5 mm miniplates and self-tapping cortical screws.

After 2 weeks, the splint is removed to prevent gingivitis on the lingual side, and since a rigid wire-arch bandage enforced by self-curing plastic is applied labially, the splint can be already dispensed with after this short time.

If the bone segment is still too mobile or the intermaxillary relation can lead to a masticatory overload, the fixation splint must be re-implanted. This should no longer be necessary after a maximum of 6 weeks.

Note

- Setting the front block to the planned position.
- Segment stabilization with preoperatively fabricated occlusal-lingual splint enforced with self-curing plastic.
- Definitive positionally stable fixation using osteosynthesis plates and monocortical screws.

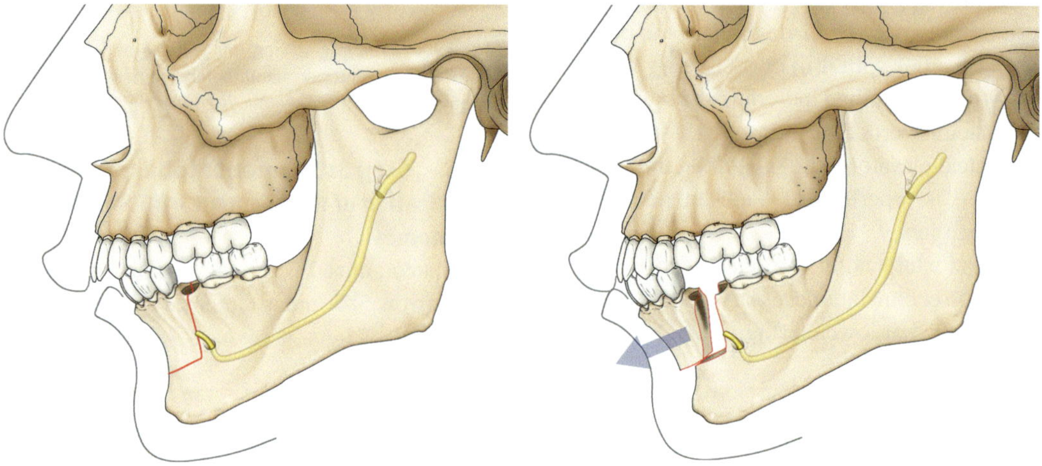

Fig. 39.5 Frontal segment osteotomy: mandible before and after anterior relocation. The resulting bone gaps are in turn filled with bone grafts.

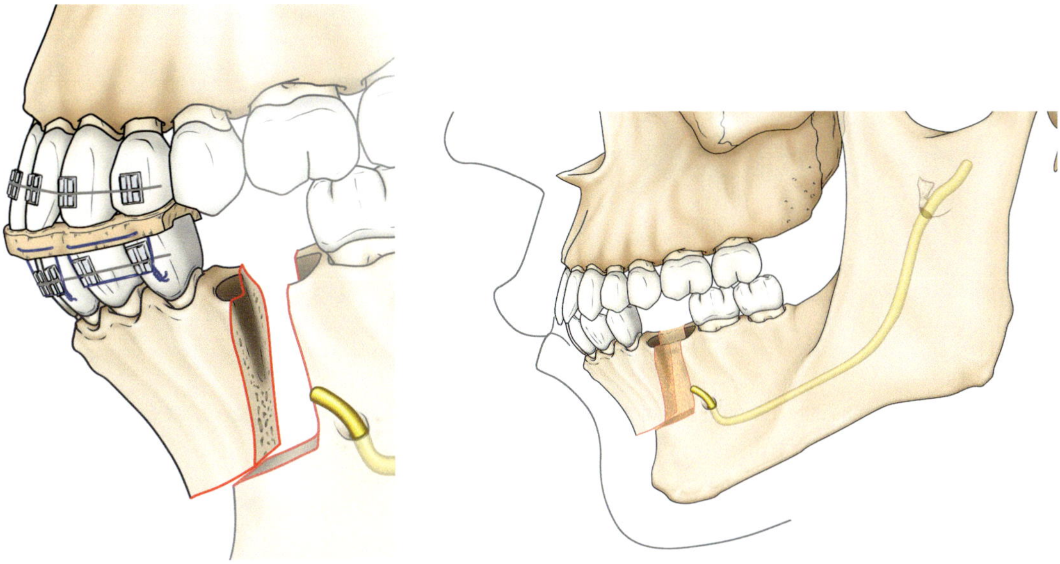

Fig. 39.6 Anterior mandibular segment fixed with an occlusal splint and wires. The osteotomy gap is filled with bone graft.

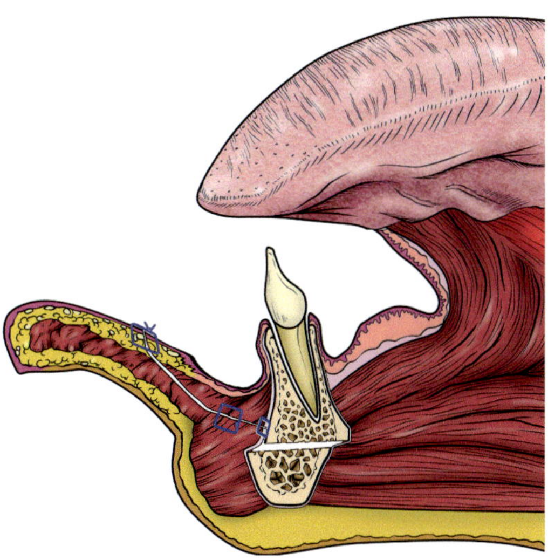

Fig. 39.7 Wound closure in layers.

2.2.5 Step 5: Wound Closure

- Two-layer wound closure.
- Periosteum and musculature with Vicryl 4 × 0 and mattress sutures.
- Mucosa continuous—Vicryl 4 × 0 and 5 × 0.

For practical reasons, the wound is not closed until the segment fixation is complete. Due to the manipulation during splinting, the mucosal suture would be torn open again. Thus, the wound remains covered with a saline compress during splinting. The wound and oral cavity are then thoroughly cleaned with a saline lavage under constant suction.

The wound is closed in two layers: periosteum and muscles are attached to the bone/periosteum with Vicryl mattress sutures 4 × 0. This succeeds well laterally, while possible periosteal incisions are required in the midline area, as the mental aponeurosis is difficult to pull up. The mucosa is sutured with interrupted Vicryl 4 × 0 and 5 × 0 continuously (Fig. 39.7).

2.3 Technical Variants

2.3.1 Downward and Posterior Movement

The two premolars should be carefully extracted and the interdental bone accurately removed/ostectomized to create sufficient space for distal repositioning (Fig. 39.8).

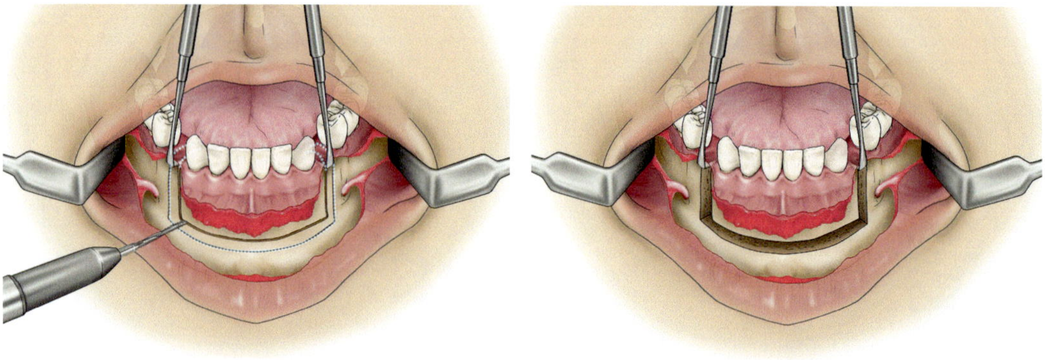

Fig. 39.8 Posterior relocation and lowering of the anterior segment (horizontal/vertical bone cut)

1 and 2 Horizontal and vertical double osteotomies and vertical interseptal and alveolar ostectomy in the residual extraction socket

3. Subapical horizontal ostectomy
4. Bone sculpturing after mobilization of the segment on the lingual side.

2.3.2 Vertical Segment Movement

For exclusively vertical movements—without extractions—it is imperative that there is sufficient space between the roots of the teeth adjacent to the vertical osteotomies. The orthodontist should prepare the patient with a sufficient interdental space for later osteotomy.

Sometimes the mobilized segment cannot be satisfactorily positioned. In this case, all cortical osteotomy margins, especially in the angular region, must be carefully controlled and interfering bone tips must be removed with a well-cooled, narrow drill (bone sculpturing).

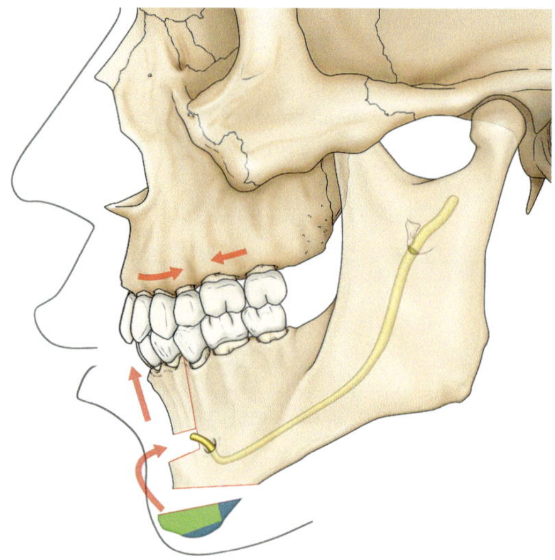

Fig. 39.9 Transplantation of cortical symphyseal bone into the subapical gap [3]. The arrows in the upper jaw indicate orthodontic corrections.

2.3.3 Upward Movement

The segment osteotomy is performed as described and the bone defect in the subapical region resulting from the upward movement is filled with cancellous bone chips. In a simultaneous sagittal split osteotomy, buccal bone can be used to fill the subapical gap.

Alternatively, the subapical bone gap can be closed by grafting the gap with cortical symphyseal bone chips from the chin, especially when the segment is moved vertically to close an anterior open bite (Fig. 39.9). Bone replacement material can be used as well.

2.3.4 Forward Movement

Occasionally, a forward segment movement is necessary to correct a class II division I with a deep bite and large overjet.

The segment may include one or more of the premolars. This requires mobilization of the mental nerve from its canal by removing the lateral cortical bone to the vertical osteotomy with a drill, cutting two parallel grooves starting at the upper and lower end of the mental foramen.

The intervening bone is carefully removed with a trimmer, and the exposed neurovascular bundle is displaced gently from the canal. During this procedure the contents of the nerve canal can be protected with the Ash filling instrument inserted into the canal.

Once the alveolar segment has been mobilized anteriorly and fixed with a splint, the residual vertical gaps are filled with cortico-cancellous bone chips from the iliac crest, e.g., and covered with a buccal mucosa flap.

2.3.5 Optional Variants and Combinations

Correction of bimaxillary protrusion and anterior open bite by anterior maxillary and mandibular subapical ostectomies (Fig. 39.10).

Correction of mandibular deficiency by mandibular subapical osteotomy and sagittal split ramus osteotomies and orthodontic treatment (Fig. 39.11).

Correction of anterior open bite with excessive chin height by subapical osteotomy and transplantation of the symphysis bone in the bone gap (Fig. 39.12).

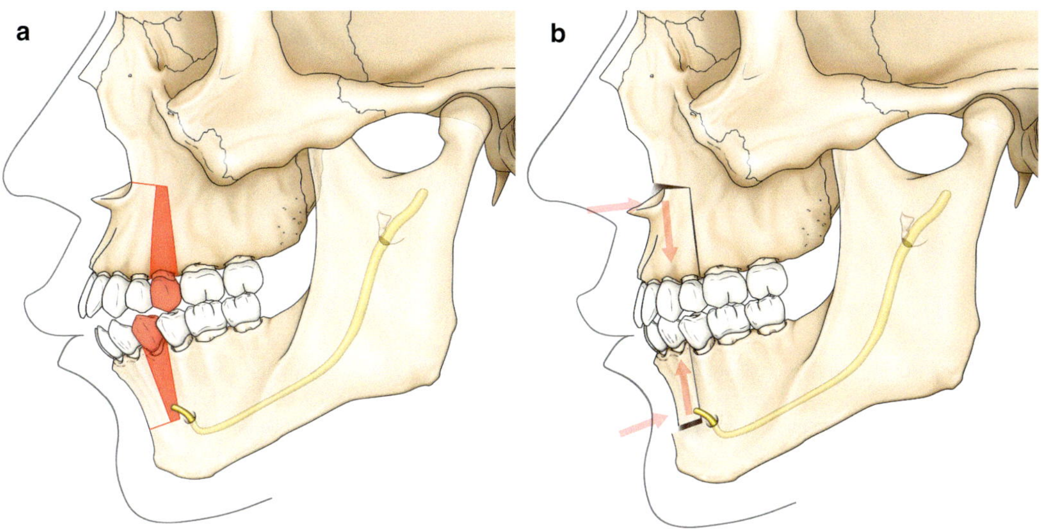

Fig. 39.10 (**a**) Dental, skeletal, and facial features associated with bimaxillary protrusion and anterior open bite (**b**) Maxillary and mandibular subapical dentoalveolar segment osteotomies to close anterior open bite and reduce facial convexity. Arrows indicate planned directional movements. ©Copyright Keisuke Koyama 2020. All rights reserved

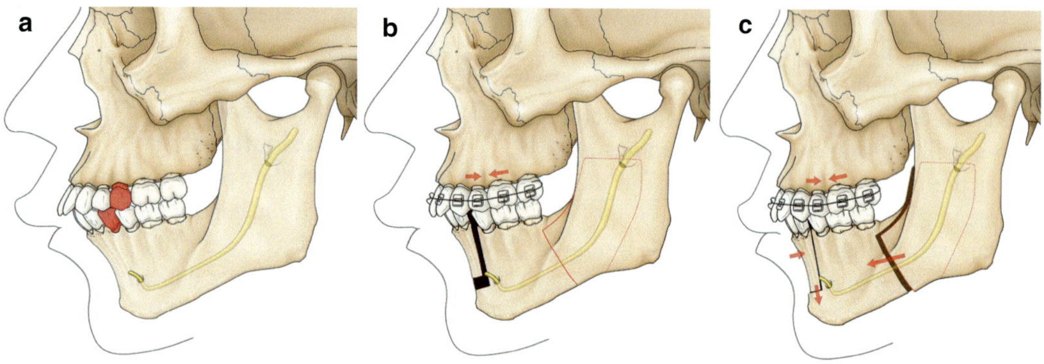

Fig. 39.11 (**a**) Pretreatment: Typical dental, skeletal, and facial features associated with mandibular deficiency—class II division 1 malocclusion—with mandible in centric relation (**b**) Pre-surgery: Maxillary second premolars and mandibular first premolar teeth are extracted to allow correction of misaligned teeth by orthodontic means (**c**) Post-surgery: Mandibular subapical osteotomy to partially level mandibular occlusal plane, mandible surgically advanced into class I occlusion by bilateral sagittal split ramus osteotomy.

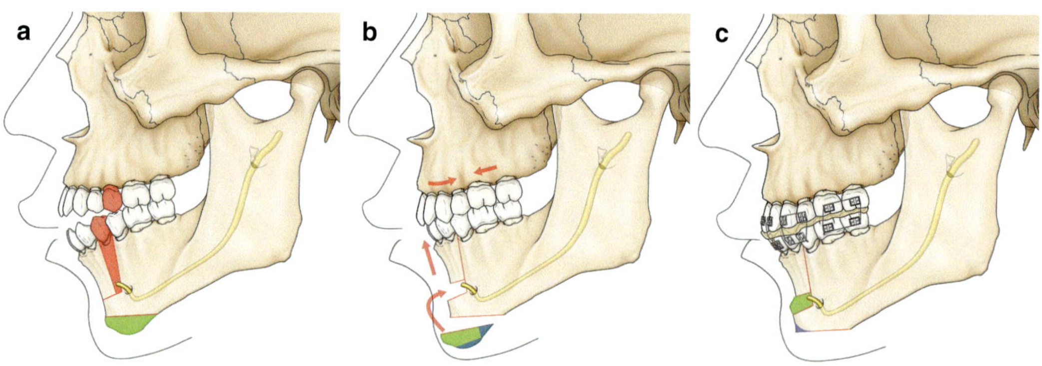

Fig. 39.12 (**a**) Pretreatment: Typical dental, skeletal, and facial features associated with severe anterior open bite—class I occlusion—with mandible in centric relation. (**b**) Presurgery: Maxillary second premolars and mandibular first premolar teeth are extracted to allow correction of malaligned teeth by orthodontic means. Reposition of the osteomized segment in the planned position and resection of the inferior aspect of the chin for bone augmentation. (**c**) Post-surgery: Mandibular subapical osteotomy to partially level mandibular occlusal plane. Resected bone is sculptured to proper dimensions to facilitate its placement into bony gap created by closure of open bite. Anterior mandibular segment fixed by an interocclusal splint and the mandibular arch wire.

3 Conclusion

Segmental osteotomies are complementary procedures in orthognathic surgery. In addition to the limited options for segment shifting, segment stabilization also requires prudence and experience. 3D planning can help with this. Splints and the patient's cooperation are required to achieve primary healing.

References

1. Möhlhenrich SC, Modabber A, Steiner T, Mitchell DA, Hölzle F. Heat generation and drill wear during dental implant site preparation: systematic review. Br J Oral Maxillofac Surg. 2015;53(8):679–89.
2. Siegel SC, Fraunhofer JA. Irrigating solution and pressure effects on tooth sectioning with surgical burs. Oral Surg Oral Med Oral Pathol Oral Radiol Endod. 1999;87(5):552–6.
3. Köle H. Surgical operations on the alveolar ridge to correct occlusal abnormalities. Oral Surg Oral Med Oral Pathol. 1959;12(3):277–88.

Lateral Mandibular Step Osteotomy/Ostectomy, Posterior Subapical Osteotomy and Anterior Body Osteotomy

40

Peter Kessler and Nicolas Hardt

Contents

P. Kessler (✉)
Department of Cranio-Maxillofacial Surgery, Maastricht University Medical Center, Maastricht, The Netherlands
e-mail: peter.kessler@mumc.nl

N. Hardt (✉)
Kantonsspital Lucerne, Clinic and Policlinic of Cranio-Maxillofacial Surgery, Lucerne, Switzerland

Abstract

The principle of the lateral mandibular body step osteotomy/ostectomy and the anterior vertical body osteotomy are variants of anterior segment osteotomy for mandibular prognathism but can also be used to reposition the anterior segment of the mandible backward or

P. Kessler et al. (eds.), *Illustrated Manual of Orthognathic Surgery*,
https://doi.org/10.1007/978-3-031-06978-9_40

vertically. This procedure is reserved for special indications and individual treatment situations and is not one of the first-choice forms of therapy. Posterior subapical osteotomy/ostectomy is also reserved for specific indications.

Keywords

Segment osteotomies · Lateral mandibular step osteotomy · Vertical osteotomy · Ostectomy · Mandibular osteotomies · Dysgnathia · BSSO · Alveolar protrusion - Mandibular prognathism · Open bite · Deep bite · Preoperative planning · Surgical access · Incision · Osteosynthesis

1 Lateral Mandibular Step Osteotomy/Ostectomy

In most cases this is a procedure with osteotomies in the region of the second premolar. The step-shaped bone cut avoids displacement of the mental nerve in the osteotomy area (Fig. 40.1).

The method is indicated in cases of:
1. Mandibular anterior open bite.
2. Excessive mandibular sagittal growth.
3. Asymmetries of the mandibular dental arch.
4. Mandibular retrognathia.

1.1 Detailed Surgical Steps

1.1.1 Step 1: Mucoperiosteal Incision

- After extraction of the first/second premolars, a transoral circum-vestibular incision is made distal to the second molar, and the bone of the mandibular body is then exposed subperiosteally only in the region of the canines/premolars up to the inferior mandibular rim in order to keep the soft tissues attached and not to compromise blood circulation of the mandible.
- The soft tissue flap should be extended to behind the second premolar to provide adequate access to the prospective osteotomy area and thus avoid unnecessary soft tissue trauma.

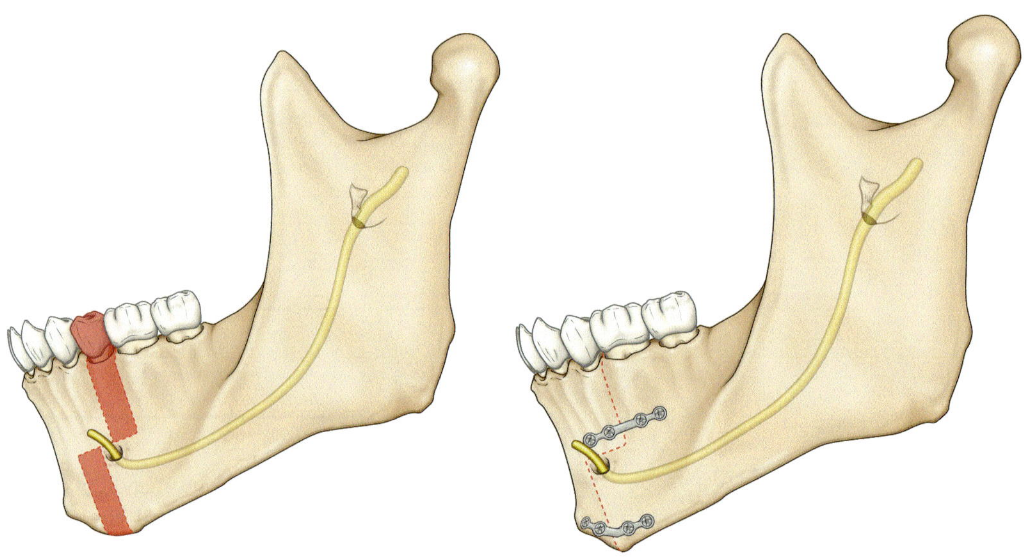

Fig. 40.1 Principle of lateral mandibular body step osteotomy/ostectomy as a variant of an anterior segment osteotomy for correction of mandibular prognathism [1].

1.1.2 Step 2: Osteotomy (Fig. 40.1)

- After adequate exposure of the mental nerve and the subapical premolar region, a horizontal osteotomy is performed 5 mm below the premolar apices and above the foramen.
- Two vertical osteotomies are then made in the extracted first/second premolar region and the interdental bone segment is removed.
- To preserve the inferior alveolar neurovascular bundle, the anterior vertical alveolar osteotomy in front of the foramen is extended caudally to the edge of the mandible—corresponding to a step osteotomy—and a second anterior vertical osteotomy is placed parallel and mesial to it. The width of this bone segment corresponds to the width of the interdental bone segment.

1.1.3 Step 3: Setting the Segment and Fixation (Fig. 40.1)

- After mobilization, the anterior segment is positioned posteriorly, thereby closing the defect of the extraction socket. Care must be taken to ensure sufficient bone contact in order to avoid periodontal problems later on.
- If no extraction is planned, the anterior segment is positioned cranially, closing the open bite.
- After securing the segment position with monomaxillary splinting, rigid segment fixation must be performed with miniplates and self-tapping bone screws where appropriate (1.5/2.0 mm miniplates and self-tapping cortical screws) [2].

2 Posterior Subapical Osteotomy

2.1 Indications

- Correction of super-eruption of teeth in the posterior mandible.
- Ankylosis of premolars and/or molars.
- Abnormal transverse position of the posterior teeth/alveolar process tilting, if orthodontic treatment is not possible or not successful.

2.2 Detailed Surgical Steps

2.2.1 Step 1: Mucoperiosteal Incision

The transoral incision begins at the front edge of the ascending mandibular ramus and extends to the canine region.

In the area of the intended osteotomy, the vestibular incision is made marginally, starting one tooth width behind the intended posterior, respectively anterior osteotomy.

The periosteal attachment is detached, but the inferior border of the mandible is left untouched to preserve soft tissue contour and not to compromise blood supply, the neurovascular bundle is identified, and the horizontal incision is carefully extended into the anterior premolar region.

2.2.2 Step 2: Osteotomy

The horizontal osteotomy is performed subapically, about 5 mm from the root tips. Special attention must be paid to the course and integrity of the mandibular canal and its contents.

The horizontal osteotomy is connected to two vertical osteotomies posterior to the last molar and in front of the first/second premolar. The interdental and horizontal bone incisions should be made carefully with a fine chisel or better with the piezo device to avoid injury to the roots. After mobilization of the segment, the posterior segment can be repositioned.

2.2.3 Step 3: Stabilization

The mobilized and splinted segment is definitely stabilized with mono-cortical 1.5 mm miniplates.

3 Anterior Body Osteotomy (Straight Vertical Osteotomy)

3.1 Detailed Surgical Steps

3.1.1 Step 1

Bilateral circum-vestibular incision with preservation of the attached gingiva in the area of the first or second premolar, depending on the intended extraction (Fig.40.2).

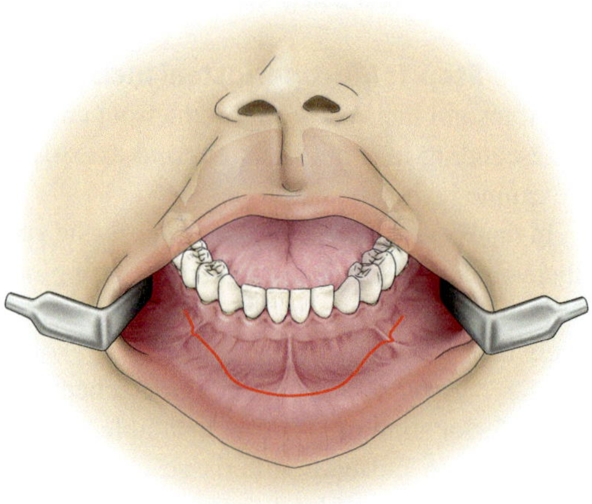

Fig. 40.2 Incision line

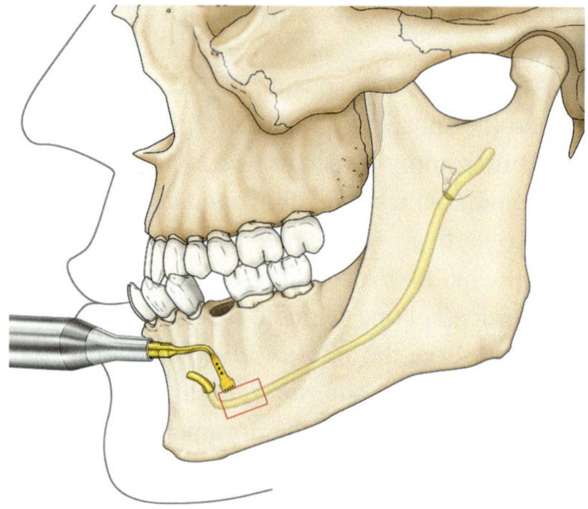

Fig. 40.4 Identification of the mandibular canal

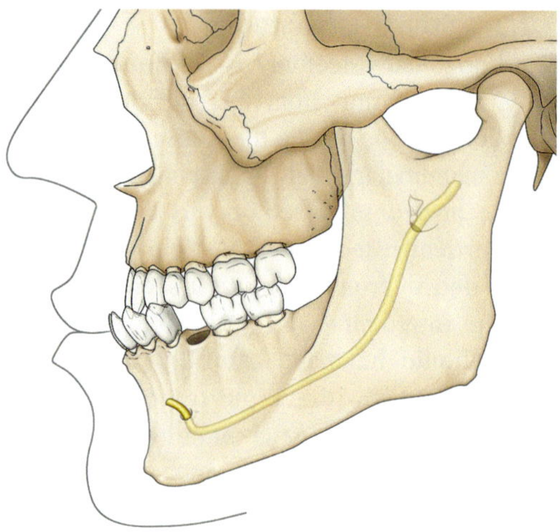

Fig. 40.3 Extraction of premolars

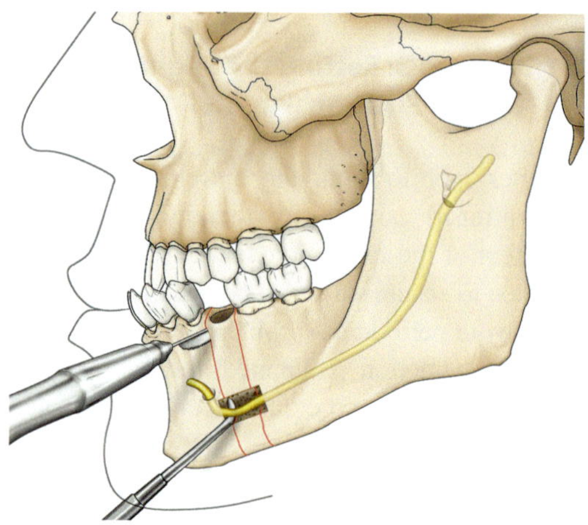

Fig. 40.5 Vertical osteotomy

3.1.2 Step 2

Extraction of premolars before performing osteotomies in the region where the resection is planned (Fig. 40.3).

3.1.3 Step 3

Removal of the lateral cortex above the terminal end of the nerve (piezosurgery) and identification and mobilization of the inferior alveolar nerve (Fig. 40.4).

3.1.4 Step 4

After the inferior alveolar nerve is identified and mobilized, two parallel vertical osteotomy lines are created with a fine drill marked on the cortical bone surface, then the lingual mucoperiosteum is detached from the bone with a fine dissector and the osteotomy is performed with a saw/drill/piezosurgery (Fig. 40.5).

3.1.5 Step 5

After completion of the two osteotomies, the bone segment is removed (Fig. 40.6).

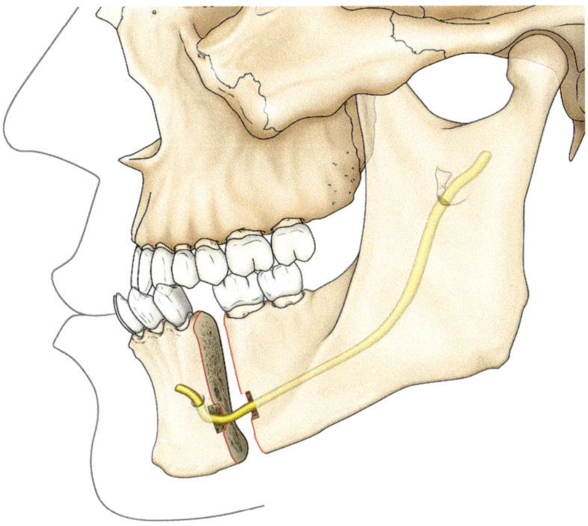

Fig. 40.6 Ostectomy of mandibular segment ©Copyright Keisuke Koyama 2020. All rights reserved

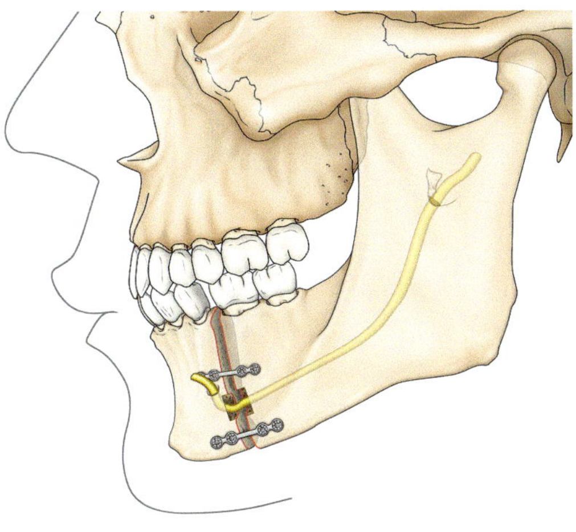

Fig. 40.7 Rigid internal fixation with two 2.0 mm osteosynthesis plates ©Copyright Keisuke Koyama 2020. All rights reserved

3.1.6 Step 6

After bilateral resection, the anterior segment is placed in the pre-planned posterior mandibulo-maxillary position. Mandibulo-maxillary fixation is achieved with a prefabricated surgical splint and using intermaxillary ligatures.

3.1.7 Step 7

Rigid internal fixation is usually achieved with two straight 2.0 mm miniplates above and below the mandibular canal/mental foramen (Fig. 40.7).

4 Conclusion

Excessive mandibular growth in three-dimensional space, but also deficient vertical mandibular growth—open bite, but also especially sagittal mandibular growth deficits can be an indication for supplementary segmental osteotomies of the mandible. Pronounced asymmetries can also be improved in the bite relation by segment osteotomies. Combinations with other osteotomy procedures are possible.

Osteosynthetic stabilization is challenging and may not always meet the definition of rigid osteosynthesis. The dentition plays an important role in segmental osteotomies, as osteotomies have to be placed in interdental spaces.

References

1. Fonsecca RJ, Marciani RD, Turvey TA. Oral and maxillofacial surgery, vol. 1. Saunders/Elsevier; 2009.
2. Shafer DM, Assael LA. Rigid internal fixation of mandibular segmental osteotomies. Atlas Oral Maxillofac Surg Clin North Am. 1993;1:41–51.

Intraoperative Risks in Segment Osteotomies: Danger Points and Errors

41

Peter Kessler and Nicolas Hardt

Contents

Abstract

The risks of surgery are defined by the anatomy, the surgical intervention, and the chance of success, among other factors. Segmental osteotomies present a particular challenge because they must be performed in an anatomically limited space, but at the same time the greatest attention must be paid to perfusion of the osteotomized segment. The segmental stability that can be achieved may not always be satisfactory.

Keywords

Segment osteotomies · Mandibular osteotomies · Preoperative planning · Surgical access · Incision · Osteosynthesis · Mental foramen · Mental nerve · Tooth damage · Infection · Wound dehiscence

P. Kessler (✉)
Department of Cranio-Maxillofacial Surgery, Maastricht University Medical Center, Maastricht, The Netherlands
e-mail: peter.kessler@mumc.nl

N. Hardt (✉)
Kantonsspital Lucerne, Clinic and Policlinic of Cranio-Maxillofacial Surgery, Lucerne, Switzerland

P. Kessler et al. (eds.), *Illustrated Manual of Orthognathic Surgery*,
https://doi.org/10.1007/978-3-031-06978-9_41

1 Vascularization of the Segment

The vascularization of the osteotomized segment/segments is performed exclusively through the lingual soft tissue attachment. This implies that intraoperative injuries to the lingual soft tissue attachment during surgery must be strictly avoided [1].

Soft tissue trauma to the lingual mucosa, as well as injury and denudation of the lingual periosteal stalk, results in delayed revascularization and compromises bone healing.

Note

- Muscle stripping of the adherent muscles should be kept to a minimum, since segmental vascularization occurs by the inserting muscles on the lingual side.
- Excessive soft tissue trauma can lead to devitalization of the segment.
- It is also advisable to segment the alveolar process of a jaw into only a few major segments, as multiple segmentation reduces blood supply.

2 Injury of the Mental Nerve

The mental nerve should be carefully protected during the operation. Injuries to the mental nerve during segmental and chin osteotomies can result in up to 5% in long-term dysfunction and pain.

3 Injuries to Teeth, Periodontium, and Alveolar Ridge

Note

- Loss of teeth in osteotomized segment due to loss of lingual tissue attachment, decrease in blood supply.
- Bone cuts placed close to the teeth—loss of vitality and periodontal defects.
- Tooth root injuries caused by osteosynthesis screws.

4 Injury of Adjacent Tooth Roots

Injuries to adjacent tooth roots can occur due to the bone cut during vertical and horizontal osteotomy as well as due to osteosynthesis screws during segment fixation. If osteotomies are performed in close vicinity to the roots of neighboring teeth or resection of root tips occurs, pulp necrosis with discoloration of the teeth may occur, resulting in endodontic treatment.

Tooth root injuries due to surgery [2].

- Injury rate through segmental osteotomies approx. 4–12%.
- Temporary loss of sensitivity for 6–12 months.
- Direct damage to the roots of teeth heals in about 90% of cases.

Note

The vascular supply of teeth in the segment requires that the horizontal osteotomy be placed ≥5 mm from the root tips of the teeth in the segment.

5 Injuries Due to Osteosynthesis Screws

The contact rate between osteosynthesis screws and tooth roots in segmental osteotomies is 12%. Postoperatively, however, pulp necrosis, devitalization of the teeth, or pain related to the screw injury are rarely observed. If the tooth root is immediately pierced or the root canal is perforated, the tooth may be lost.

6 Injury of Periodontium and Alveolar Crest

The alveolar ridge and the periodontium of teeth neighboring the vertical osteotomy must be protected. If these structures are injured during the operation, deep periodontal pockets may form. Ankylosis or loss of teeth may result.

Intensive irrigation of the drilling and cutting instruments minimizes thermal bone damage.

Whenever an alveolar bone defect develops, a bone graft should be considered for the defect.

6.1 Thermal Damage

High-speed drilling and high contact pressure combined with insufficient water cooling can cause bone necrosis with increasing osteotomy depth.

6.2 Insufficient Wound Closure with Dehiscence

Incorrect wound closure can lead to wound dehiscence, hematoma formation, soft tissue and bone infection, and bone/tooth loss—an undesirable postoperative outcome.

6.3 Insufficient Segment Stabilization

Good segment immobilization and fixation are necessary to prevent segment instability and segment displacement due to fibrous pseudarthrosis (pseudarthrosis formation—malunion) or non-union (delayed bone healing) of the osteotomized segments.

7 Conclusion

The risks of damage to adjacent tooth structures, insufficient segmental blood supply, and insufficient stability are realistic and must be discussed in detail with the patient. Alternative treatments should always be considered.

References

1. Bell WH, Proffit WR, White RP. Surgical correction of dentofacial deformities. Philadelphia: WB Saunders; 1980.
2. Young Kyun K. Complications associated with orthognathic surgery. J Korean Assoc Oral Maxillofac Surg. 2017;43(1):3–15.

42 Tricks and Typical Mistakes

Peter Kessler and Nicolas Hardt

Contents

Abstract

Segment osteotomies can present challenges to even the most experienced surgeon because the surgical margin of maneuver is limited. Tips and tricks help to recognize and treat unexpected problems intraoperatively. The limits of the method must be known and adhered to.

P. Kessler (✉)
Department of Cranio-Maxillofacial Surgery, Maastricht University Medical Center, Maastricht, The Netherlands
e-mail: peter.kessler@mumc.nl

N. Hardt (✉)
Kantonsspital Lucerne, Clinic and Policlinic of Cranio-Maxillofacial Surgery, Lucerne, Switzerland

Keywords

Segment osteotomies · Mandibular osteotomies · Tips and tricks · Incision · Nerve injuries · Tissue traumatization · Segment stability

1 Intraoperative Tricks

- Labial extension of the parabolic vestibular mucosa incision—infra-submucous preparation up to the periosteum—two layers.
- Segment position control with occlusal splint and temporary securing of the segment.
- Two-layer wound closure: first muscle and periosteum then mucosa.

P. Kessler et al. (eds.), *Illustrated Manual of Orthognathic Surgery*,
https://doi.org/10.1007/978-3-031-06978-9_42

- Before wound closure: thorough mechanical cleaning of the wound with saline and constant suction.
- Wound closure only after definitive stabilization of the segment.

2 Intraoperative Errors

- Intraoral access/incision not wide enough.
- Thus missing overlook and unnecessary soft tissue traumatization.
- Crushing of soft tissues, resulting in edema, hematoma, and postoperative pain.
- Tearing/detachment of the periosteum resulting in delayed or compromised wound healing.
- Exaggerated denudation thereby increased risk of devitalization of the fragment ends.
- Too high speed and too little cooling during drilling causing bone necrosis.
- Mental/inferior alveolar nerve injuries—directly related to the size of surgical trauma.

3 Management After Surgery

After segmental mandibular osteotomy, an external tight pressure dressing is applied to prevent the formation of hematomas in the surgical site and to limit the mobility of the lip and chin region in the first days of healing. This allows the soft tissues to be reattached to the bony base.

A 1 in. (2.5 cm) elastic tape is cut and folded butterfly-wise so that there is no adhesive in the center section. Two of these tapes each are placed in front of and under the chin.

If patient hygiene requires the tapes to be changed, the adhesive tapes can be removed without touching the skin over the surgical site, which facilitates their removal or replacement.

4 Limitations and Contraindications

All segmental osteotomies share some potential complications, which may be mild, moderate, or severe [1].

- Mild complications include periodontal defects, pulp necrosis, infection, and delayed union.
- Moderate complications may include infection, delayed union, and malunion.
- Severe complications include nonunion and tooth and/or bone loss.

Because the mandible presents a thick cortical bone, the blood supply may be threatened after soft tissue detachment. Therefore, osteotomies that involve small segments of bone, with one or two teeth mobilized, should be discouraged.

Also, because the soft tissue pedicle attached to the mobilized segment is the exclusive blood supply, the more it is mobilized or manipulated surgically and the further it is repositioned, the greater the potential for detachment of the pedicle and thus compromise of its vasculature.

The anterior subapical osteotomy is mostly contraindicated when the anterior mandible is short in height. In some cases the apices of the anterior teeth, especially the canines, are close to the inferior border of the mandible, impeding performance of the osteotomy. Even if enough space is available to complete the osteotomy, at least 1 cm of basilar bone should remain to ensure the integrity of the mandible.

5 Conclusion

Segment osteotomies represent an addition to the possibilities of performing corrections in the area of the alveolar process that have not been successful orthodontically or cannot be successful because the anatomical conditions do not allow it. In rare cases, segmental osteotomies may be indicated as the sole surgical correction.

The basic methods in orthognathic surgery concern the relocation of the complete jaws [2]. Partial or segmental osteotomies help where, due to unfavorable local anatomical, genetic, or technical possibilities, there is no other option than to improve occlusion by partial osteotomy. From an esthetic point of view, segmental osteotomies often include too small volumes to affect the appearance of the face. Technically, segmental osteotomies are challenging and carry typical risks that are significantly different from those of mandibular relocation in toto.

References

1. Epker BN, Fish LC. Dentofacial deformities: integrated orthodontic and surgical correction. St. Louis: C.V. Mosby; 1986.
2. Kashani H, Rasmusson L. Osteotomies in orthognathic surgery. In: Motamedi M, editor. A textbook of advanced oral and maxillofacial surgery, vol. 3. London: Intech; 2016.

Part IX

Chin Osteotomies

Indications for Chin Osteotomy/ Genioplasty and Standard Procedures

43

Peter Kessler and Nicolas Hardt

Contents

Abstract

The chin is one of the most important units of facial structures responsible for the overall appearance and esthetics of the face. Chin osteotomies are routine esthetic procedures to create a harmonious appearance of the face in terms of shape, position, and size.

Generally, surgeons use the standard sliding osteotomy with anteroposterior displacement, which is used to correct both the retrusive and protrusive chin. There are many modifications, such as curved osteotomy, M-shaped osteotomy, transverse reduction osteotomy, and others. Mandibular anatomy is highly variable, as are the patient's esthetic requirements. Therefore, the solution should be individualized in each clinical case, including the position of the chin.

The 3D technologies with simulation of the covering soft tissue are suitable for simulating the desired result.

P. Kessler (✉)
Department of Cranio-Maxillofacial Surgery, Maastricht University Medical Center, Maastricht, The Netherlands
e-mail: peter.kessler@mumc.nl

N. Hardt (✉)
Kantonsspital Lucerne, Clinic and Policlinic of Cranio-Maxillofacial Surgery, Lucerne, Switzerland

P. Kessler et al. (eds.), *Illustrated Manual of Orthognathic Surgery*,
https://doi.org/10.1007/978-3-031-06978-9_43

Keywords

Chin · Progenia · Retrogenia · Receding chin · Preoperative 3D planning · Standard procedures · Facial profile changes - Transgender surgery · Surgical techniques · Genioplasty · Chin osteotomy · Intraoperative risks and tricks · Postoperative complications

Note

- The facial appearance forms the basis for the typological characteristics and personality of a human being.
- The chin is one of the most prominent elements of the face.
- Chin deformities manifest themselves three-dimensionally, but the majority is related to horizontal deviations.

Chin osteotomy was first described by Hofer in 1942 [1]. Genioplasty also carries risks: esthetic deformation and asymmetry, step-like shape of the mandibular contour depending on the chin dimension and distance of displacement, notching of the mandibular body, and worsening of the labiomental fold after advancement genioplasty. In order to avoid abovementioned disadvantages, numerous modifications have been developed [2].

Facial profiles in the lower facial third can be classified as of normal proportion, or as pro-genic with a horizontal excess in volume and size, or as retro-genic with a sagittal setback and decreased volume. The anterior vertical height if increased is regarded as disturbing.

Surgical correction is indicated, if:

- The chin is receding or even micro-genic as an independent anomaly without malocclusion.
- In mandibular advancement or correction of mandibular asymmetry the basic surgical correction is not esthetically satisfactory.
- In the case of a very pronounced chin-lip furrow, e.g., as a result of a deep bite, where the wrinkle between chin and lip skin is disturbing.
- In extremely protruding and square formed or pointed chins.
- In excessive vertical triangular growth—often related to vertical excess in the lower third of the face.
- In mandibular prognathism, if the mandibular setback does not lead to an esthetically balanced face.
- Exostotic humps.
- Asymmetric chin hyperplasia.

1 Standard Procedures in Genioplasty

Corrections of the form or position of the chin can be achieved by various surgical techniques leading to a three-dimensional positional change of the chin point in the sagittal, vertical, and transverse dimension. Genioplasties can be combined with all kind of orthognathic surgical interventions in the mandible, the maxilla, or both [3, 4].

Most often horizontal chin osteotomies are used for the sagittal correction in anterior or posterior direction (Fig. 43.1).

1.1 Horizontal Osteotomy for Chin Advancement

See Fig. 43.1.

1.2 Horizontal Osteotomy for Chin Repositioning

Surgically same procedure as for chin advancement with reduction of tips or overlapping bone steps of the mobilized chin segment to ensure a smooth transition to the mandibular margin to avoid palpable steps.

Note

Increase of the anterior vertical height of the lower jaw.

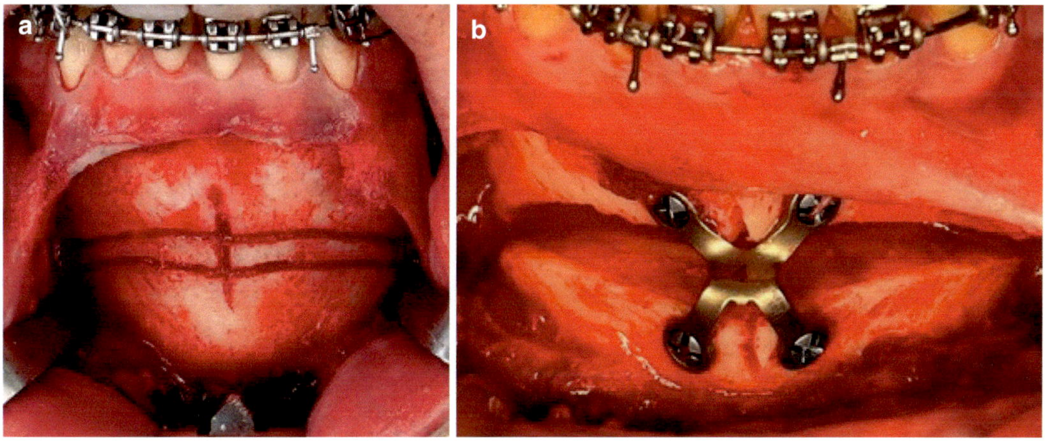

Fig. 43.1 (**a**) Horizontal osteotomy with chin advancement: Double creation of a horizontal osteotomy line for ostectomy of a segment, shortening of the chin height and chin advancement. Vertical line to mark the center line. (**b**) Osteosynthesis

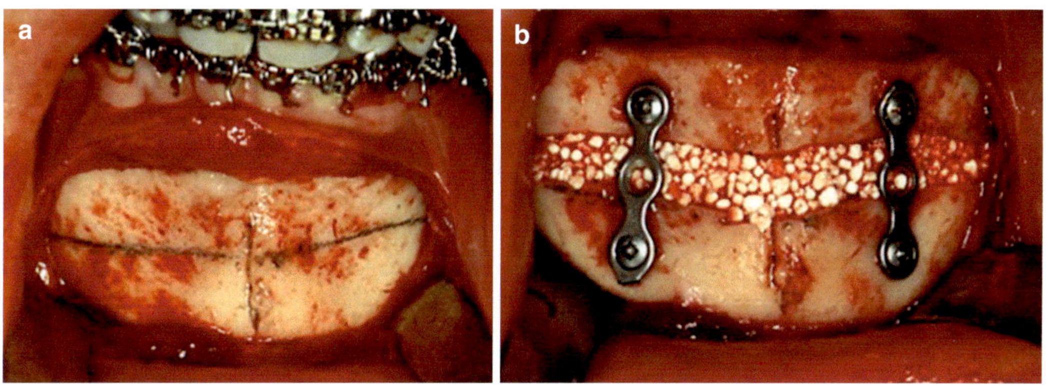

Fig. 43.2 Horizontal sliding osteotomy of the chin with vertical elongation (**a**) Marking the center lines and the horizontal osteotomy (**b**) Intraoperative view with vertical elongation, osteosynthesis, and interposition of bone substitute material

1.3 Horizontal Sliding Osteotomy

The sliding osteotomy is performed either to extend or to reduce the chin height (Figs. 43.2 and 43.3).

In the case of a sliding osteotomy with vertical extension, the chin is moved downwards and possibly forward. The downward movement of the chin segment is associated with the formation of a gap.

If the vertical defect is larger than 5 mm, augmentation of the gap with autogenous bone or bone replacement material must be considered to ensure a perfect contour.

1.4 Double Sliding Chin Osteotomy to Reduce Chin Height

In the double sliding chin osteotomy, a bone strip is removed to vertically reduce the chin height and an anterior or posterior reduction of the segment can be performed in conjunction with the vertical shortening (Fig. 43.3).

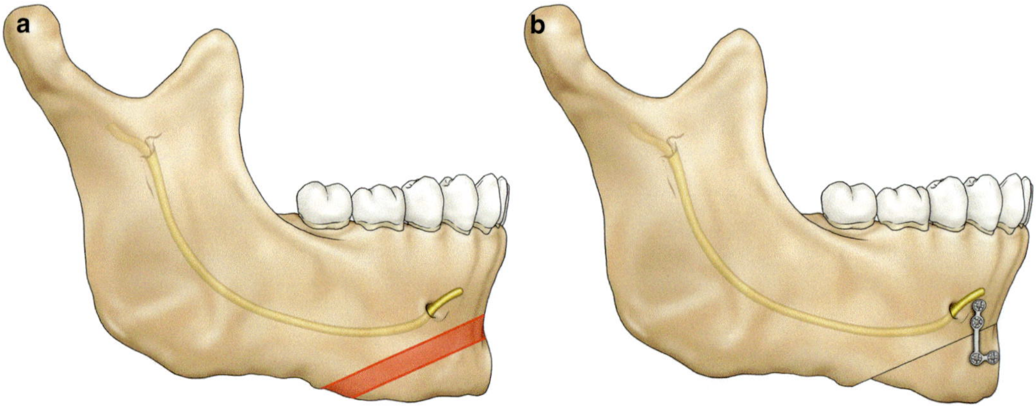

Fig. 43.3 Double Sliding Osteotomy to reduce chin height. (**a**) The bone strip marked red is resected (**b**) Miniplate stabilization ©Copyright Keisuke Koyama 2020. All rights reserved

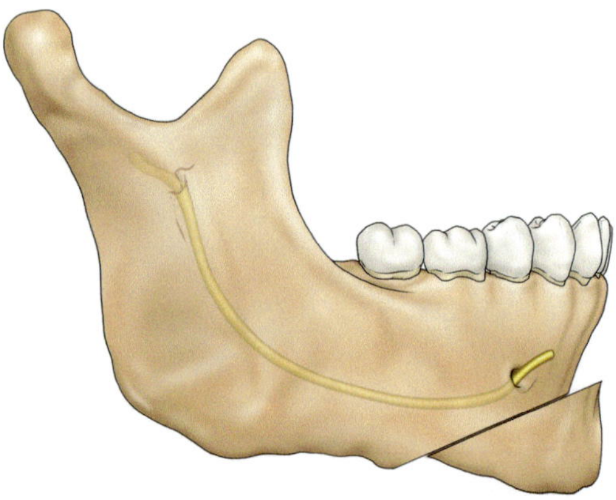

Fig. 43.4 Diagram of the oblique/slanted osteotomy for chin advancement ©Copyright Keisuke Koyama 2020. All rights reserved

1.5 Slanted Osteotomy for Chin Advancement

In an oblique chin osteotomy, a forward displacement is performed with simultaneous rotation of the chin segment upwards (Fig. 43.4) [5].

The advantage is that a maximum forward and upward displacement of the chin apex is possible. An essential element of this technique is that the muscles remain attached to the bony chin. As a result, the muscle attachments are also shifted upwards and forward, thus relaxing the entire perioral region. The contour of the chin determined by the soft tissue is not changed.

1.6 Transverse Narrowing/ Widening Genioplasty

Vertical osteotomies/ostectomies can be added to a horizontal chin osteotomy for transverse, but also sagittal chin deformities. This allows the chin to be widened or narrowed (Fig. 43.5). Reduction or augmentation genioplasty requires combined work in the horizontal, sagittal and transverse planes so as to obtain a harmonious result.

The transversal dimension of the chin can be changed by segmenting the symphyseal region. In case of widening, additional bone grafts or alloplastic materials (resorbable or non-resorbable blocks) are integrated into the median gap.

If reduction of the transverse dimension of the chin is planned, two parallel vertical osteotomies are performed laterally of the midline and a bone segment is removed.

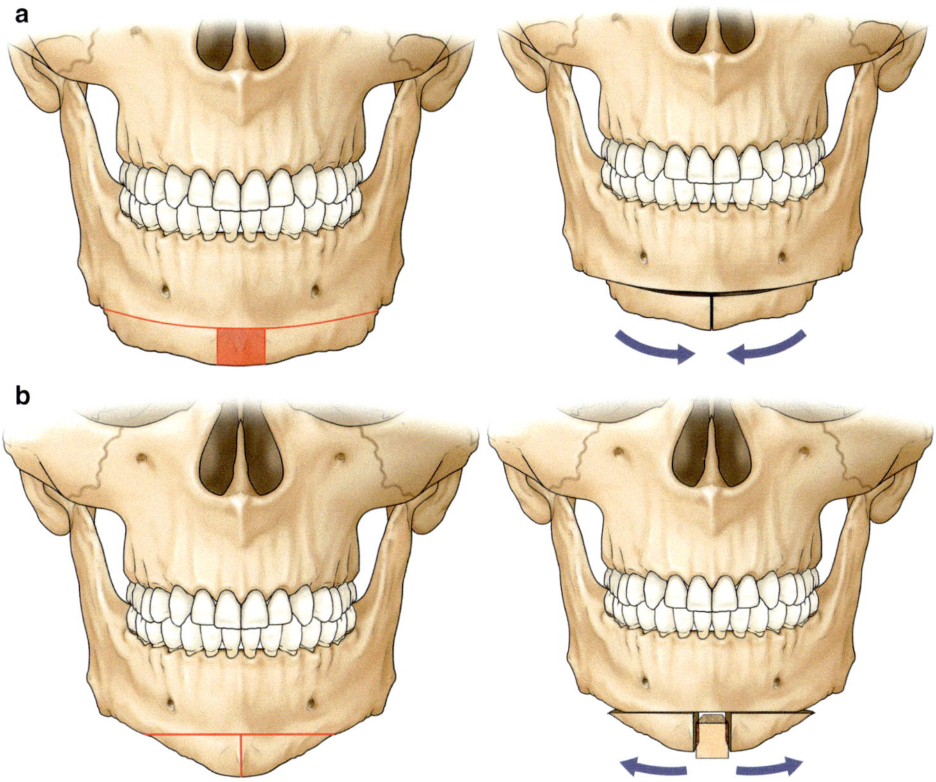

Fig. 43.5 (**a**) Reduction of the transverse width of the chin (**b**) Widening of the transverse dimension of the chin

2 Genioplasty and Facial Profile Changes

Profile changes after chin osteotomies are highly dependent on the surgical method, the bony base, and the soft tissue volume of the chin region. Profile predictions prior to chin plastic surgery should therefore—with appropriate education of the patient—only be understood as guidelines.

Displacements of the bony chin after horizontal osteotomy lead to a 90% reduction of the visible soft tissue pogonion when the segment is repositioned and to an augmentation of the chin soft tissue by approximately 75% of the bony displacement distance after forward displacement.

At the same time, the labiomental fold is flattened or reinforced.

Chin displacements with simultaneous ostectomy or bone interposition (sandwich plastic surgery) are associated with a shortening or lengthening of the soft tissue relief of the lower face of 90% of the skeletal displacements.

3D planning programs with soft tissue simulation are an enormous help in the preoperative assessment of the perceptible changes in the facial profile in the chin region. Thus, changes in the position of the chin are among the most esthetically effective visible changes in the profile of the face.

3 Preoperative Planning

Genioplasty requires careful preoperative planning based primarily on two- and three-dimensional cephalometry and its analysis. Simulation can be performed based on CBCT images and facial photos, 3D reconstruction of bones and soft tissues of the face. The virtual planning based on specialized medical software programs creates the possibility of 3D printing of anatomic models and surgical guides as well as prefabrication of osteosynthesis plates for fixation.

4 Conclusion

Changing the position of the chin is an essential part of corrective orthognathic surgery, but it belongs to facial esthetic surgery. The technique is simple and varied.

References

1. Hofer O. Die operative Behandlung der alveolären Retraktion des Unterkiefers und ihre Anwendungsmöglichkeit für Prognathie und Mikrogenie. Dtsch Zahn Mund Kieferheilk. 1942;9:142–4.
2. Haggerty CJ, Laughlin RM. Operative atlas of oral and maxillofacial surgery. Wiley-Blackwell; 2015.
3. Bell WH, Proffit WR, White RP. Surgical correction of dentofacial deformities, band 1–3. Saunders; 1980.
4. Kelly JP. Mandibular osteotomies. In: Keith DA, editor. Atlas of oral and maxillofacial surgery. Saunders; 1992.
5. Joos U, Delaire J, Scheibe B, Schilli W. Funktionelle Aspekte der Kinnplastik. Fortschr Kiefer Gesichtschir. 1981;26:86.

44 Principle Surgical Technique

Peter Kessler and Nicolas Hardt

Contents

Abstract

Genioplasty can be performed so that the chin can be relocated as a whole or divided. The inclination of the osteotomy line can be adjusted to the chin displacement. The chin wing osteotomy is a lateral extension of the genioplasty.

P. Kessler (✉)
Department of Cranio-Maxillofacial Surgery, Maastricht University Medical Center, Maastricht, The Netherlands
e-mail: peter.kessler@mumc.nl

N. Hardt (✉)
Kantonsspital Lucerne, Clinic and Policlinic of Cranio-Maxillofacial Surgery, Lucerne, Switzerland

Keywords

Genioplasty · Chin osteotomy · Horizontal chin osteotomy · Sliding chin osteotomy · Chin wing osteotomy

1 Anatomical Reference Points

- Labial insertion of the frenulum of the lower lip.
- Mental foramen with mental nerve.
- Alveolar yokes.
- Base of the mandible.
- Digastric fossa.
- Mental protuberance.

P. Kessler et al. (eds.), *Illustrated Manual of Orthognathic Surgery*,
https://doi.org/10.1007/978-3-031-06978-9_44

Note

- Three main neural branches emerge from the mental foramen (Fig. 44.1).
- One branch innervates the mental skin area.
- The two other branches innervate the skin of the lower lip area, the vestibular mucosa and the gingiva to posterior of the second premolar.

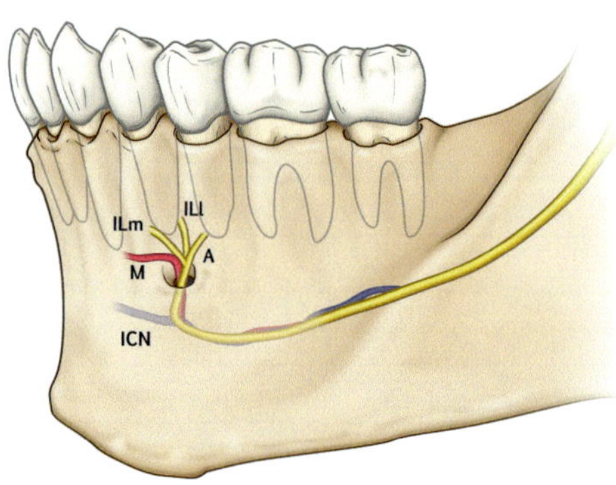

Fig. 44.1 Branching pattern and intrabony and extrabony course of the mental nerve. *A* angular branch, *M* medial branch, *ILm* inferior labial medial, *Ill* inferior labial lateral, *ICN* incisive nerve [1, 2]

2 Technical Notes

Prior to the osteotomy of the chin (genioplasty), the midline of the chin and mandible should be marked after exposure of the chin area. This step is important for controlled midline shifts (Fig. 44.2).

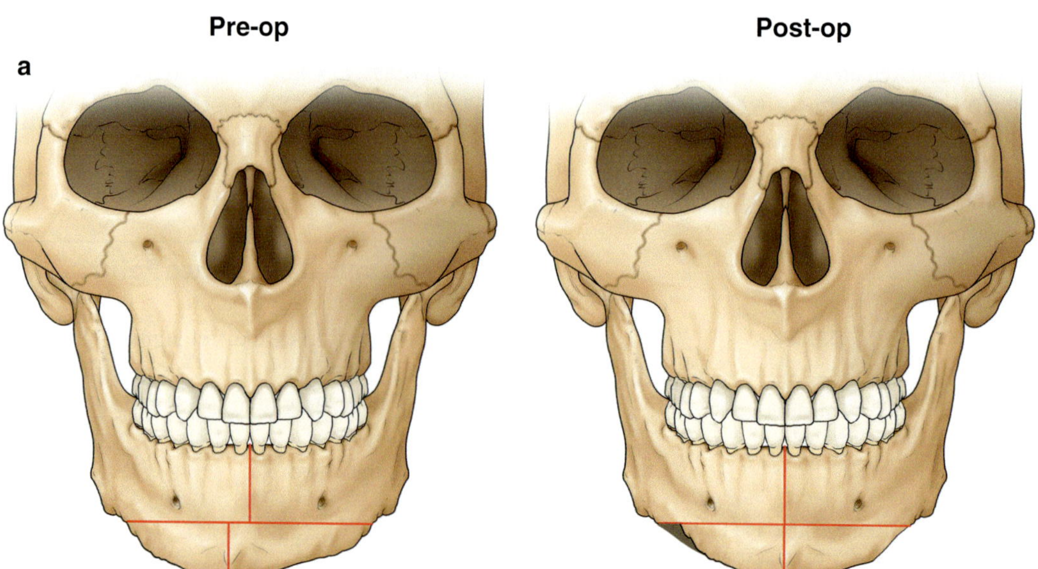

Fig. 44.2 (**a**) The center line of the mandible and the center line of the chin and the horizontal osteotomy line should be marked as reference points/lines using a drill or fine saw. This marking avoids intraoperative misalignment of the osteotomized chin segment. (**b**) Horizontal osteotomy line about 5 mm below the root apices of the front teeth. ©Copyright Keisuke Koyama 2020. All rights reserved

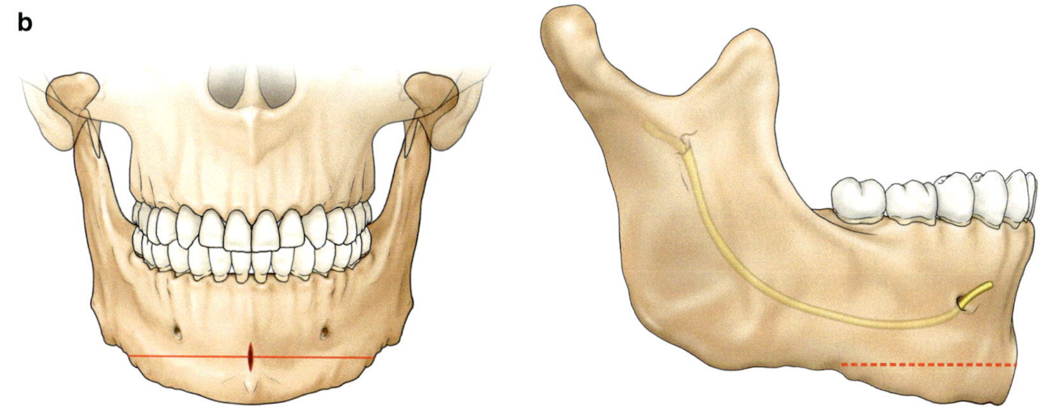

Fig. 44.2 continued

3 Horizontal Chin Osteotomy

3.1 Stepwise Surgical Approach

Step 1: Mucosal Incision and Mucoperiosteal Dissection

The labial mucosa and the vestibule are infiltrated with a local anesthetic containing vasoconstrictive additives before incision. After retraction of the lower lip and exposure of the vestibule with Langenbeck hooks and drying of the mucosa, the incision is color-marked.

Subsequently, the mucosa is cut parabolically from element 35–45. The apex of the incision parabola lies in the median area of the labial mucosa. This incision guide prevents subsequent suture dehiscence. After cutting through the mucosa and submucosa, the mental foramina and the mental nerves are identified and dissected bluntly (Figs. 44.1 and 44.3).

The periosteum is then incised below, above, and behind the foramen and lifted slightly under traction so that the periosteal conus can be carefully incised along the course of the nerve and the mental nerve can be prepared freely in order to minimize the risk of injury on the one hand and to better protect the nerve on the other hand due to the considerably wider access and better overview.

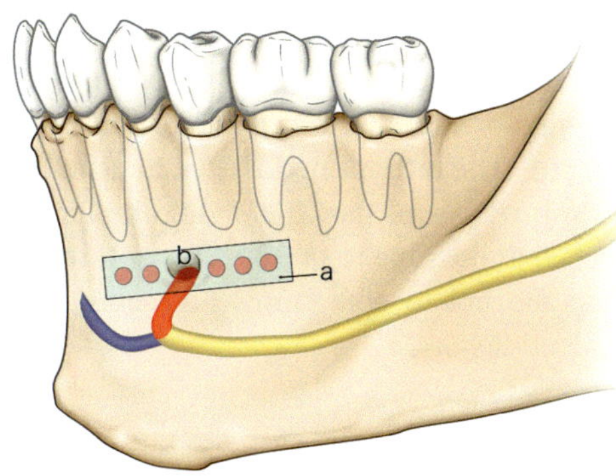

Fig. 44.3 Anatomical variations of the horizontal position of the mental foramen. Blue: mental incisive canal (MIC), red: mental canal, yellow: mandibular canal (*acc* [3, 4]). (**a**) Possible positions of the mental foramen in horizontal plane. (**b**) Average location of the mental foramen in the Caucasian population. ©Copyright Keisuke Koyama 2020. All rights reserved

Note

- Exposition of the surgical field to the first molars on both sides.
- Preparation of the mental foramina on bilaterally.
- Exposition of the mental nerve.

Then, below the mobilized mucosal-submucosal cuff, the chin muscles are cut sharply down to the bone approximately halfway between the marginal gingiva and the inferior rim of the lower jaw. The periosteum is incised in the same place.

A smooth, atraumatic detachment of the adherent tendon tissue of the mental muscle especially at the mental protuberances is best achieved with a sharp-edged, not too wide dissector.

The mimic muscles of the oral fissure insert laterally and can be levered off smoothly, so that it is recommended to start with the subperiosteal dissection here first (height: mental foramen) and then subperiosteally detach the adherent attachment of the mental muscle (mental tubercle/protuberances) up to the alveoli of the central incisors without tearing the periosteum.

An elevator is then used to lift the periosteum to the edge of the inferior border of the mandibular rim. The inferior periosteum attachment of the soft tissues of the chin should be left as untouched as possible to preserve the soft tissue contour and not to compromise the chin segment blood flow.

Note

- Subperiosteal mobilization of the soft tissues in the chin region takes place up to the inferior edge of the lower jaw.
- The inferior periosteal attachment of the soft tissues of the chin should remain unaffected as far as possible.
- Also maintain a 5 × 10 mm field of the periosteal attachment in the center of the chin symphysis to ensure soft tissue attachment and blood supply.

Step 2: Osteotomy

For the subsequent osteotomy, the center line should be marked crosswise as a reference point with a small Lindemann drill (Fig. 44.2).

The position of the root tips determines the position and course of the horizontal osteotomy. The osteotomy runs about 5–10 mm horizontally

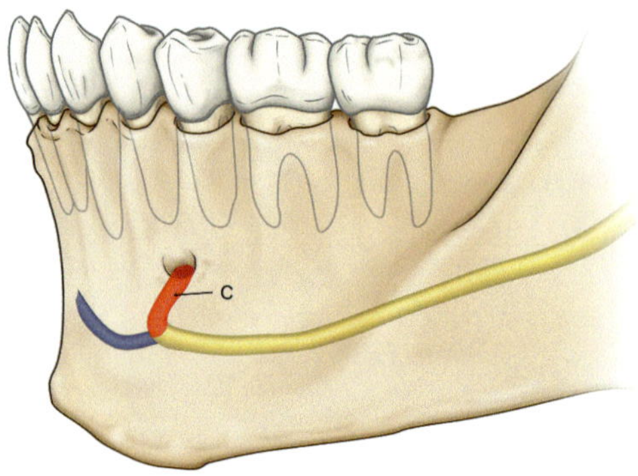

Fig. 44.4 Nerve loop of the mental nerve in the mental canal. The region marked "c" marks the most common position of the mental foramen (*acc* [3, 4]). Blue = incisive canal; red = mental canal (the opening of the mandibular canal); yellow = mandibular canal. ©Copyright Keisuke Koyama 2020. All rights reserved

below the apices and laterally to the edge of the lower jaw (Figs. 44.2 and 44.4).

Laterally of the canines the osteotomy should be 4–5 mm below the mental foramen to avoid injury to the nerve bundle.

The nerve canal itself lies up to 4–5 mm below the mental foramen. The lateral end of the osteotomy is determined by the shape of the chin [1].

Note

- The osteotomy line should be 5–10 mm below the apices of the front teeth.
- 5 mm below the apices of the canines.
- 4–5 mm below the mental foramen.
- 10–15 mm above the lower mandibular edge.

Note

It is important that the osteotomy runs 4–5 mm below the visible mental foramen so that no injury to the anterior loop of the mental nerve occurs while the mental nerve ascends within the canal before leaving the foramen.

Fine cortical drill holes are made along the color-marked osteotomy line. The horizontal line is then pre-cut along the cortical perforations with a hard-metal fissure drill, alternatively an oscillating saw can be used.

The completion of the horizontal osteotomy—including the lingual cortical bone—is initially performed with fine Lindemann burrs or the oscillating saw. Fine osteotomes can be helpful.

Of course, the piezo technique is ideal for a maximally atraumatic procedure, especially on the lingual side of the chin region to avoid bleeding from the floor of the mouth.

> **Note**
> The more parallel the osteotomy line is made to the occlusal and the mandibular plane, the easier it is to relocate the chin segment.

If the vertical dimension of the chin is to be increased, the osteotomy gap can be augmented with bone or bone replacement material.

If a reduction of the vertical height is planned, a parallel osteotomy is performed and the mobilized bone segment is removed.

Step 3: Chin Segment Adjustment
Before the chin segment is adjusted to the exact median, vertical, transverse, and sagittal position, excess bone is removed and the osteotomy margins are smoothed and contoured.

Step 4: Chin Segment Fixation
The chin segment is secured with pre-bent osteosynthesis plates or individually bent mini plates (Fig. 44.5). Especially in the case of vertical chin elongation and laterally displaced segments to compensate for an existing asymmetry, the osteosynthesis should be sufficiently stable.

If necessary, bone chips may also be added to cover the terraced step between the mandible and the advanced chinpoint.

Step 5: Osteosynthesis of the Chin Segment
Prefabricated plates with horizontal steps of 3, 5, 7, and 10 mm are available for chin forward and backward displacements.

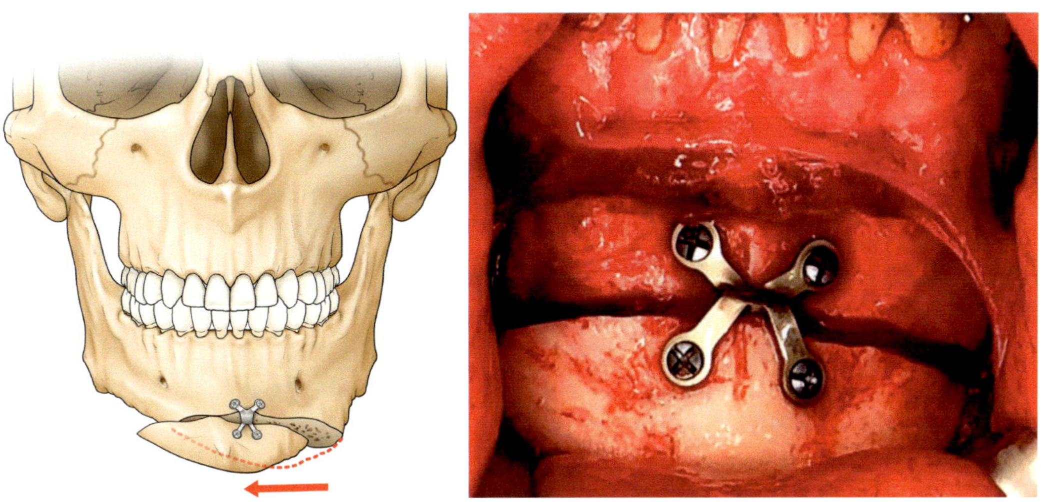

Fig. 44.5 Genioplasty with a preformed and individually adapted osteosynthesis plate.

3.2 Fixation Technique

Positioning of the mobilized chin segment. Adaptation of the plate. Drill the screw holes with the drill bit and insert short screws. To better determine the definitive position of the chin, it is advisable to start at one of the two bone segments, so that the plate can be used to control the chin to the mandible or vice versa to fix the chin segment to the plate pre-fixed to the mandible in a controlled manner.

Step 6: Wound Closure

After fixation is complete, a two-layer wound closure is performed. It is important to ensure the anatomically exact position of the mental muscles. For the readaptation of the mentalis aponeurosis, the periosteum and muscles are sutured to the bone periosteum with Vicryl 4 × 0 mattress sutures. This is successful laterally, while possible periosteal incisions are required in the midline region, since the mentalis aponeurosis is difficult to raise.

Only then is the mucosa readapted with single button sutures (Vicryl 4 × 0) and finally sutured continuously with Vicryl 5 × 0.

Note

- 2-layer wound closure.
- Periosteum and musculature Vicryl 4 × 0 with mattress sutures.
- Mucosa readaptation with single button sutures Vicryl 4 × 0, then continuously with Vicryl 5 × 0.

4 Chin Wing Osteotomy

4.1 Surgical Principle

The chin wing osteotomy is performed transorally as an esthetic correction and contour enhancement of the entire mandibular lower margin and covers the entire mandibular base from jaw angle to jaw angle (Fig. 44.6).

This operation allows a sagittal, vertical, as well as transversal repositioning of the mandibular base in all three planes and has the additional advantage that with the position correction of the entire mandibular base, the jaw angles can also be influenced in their position [5].

Depending on the anatomy, variations have been described. The mini chin wing is a variant of the chin wing osteotomy that ends before the mandibular angle. Its design extends from the chin region to the horizontal branch of the mandible as in a traditional genioplasty. However, the posterior cut ends in the submandibular notch. It corresponds to a posteriorly extended genioplasty. Its advantage is the possibility to be combined with a bilateral sagittal split osteotomy (BSSO).

There are no contraindications to the realization of a mini chin wing. Contrarily to the traditional chin wing, a very low positioned inferior alveolar nerve (IAN) is not a contraindication to the short version of the chin wing osteotomy [6].

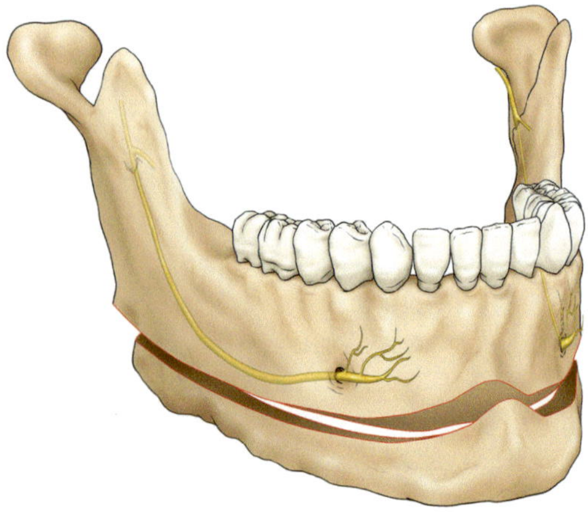

Fig. 44.6 Principle of chin wing osteotomy. ©Copyright Keisuke Koyama 2020. All rights reserved

4.2 Stepwise Surgical Approach

Step 1: Mucoperiosteal Incision

The intraoral incision corresponds to the frontal incision in genioplasty. The mental foramen and nerve is dissected at the foramen so that it can be safely protected.

The mucosal incision is continued approximately 10 mm above the deepest point of the oral vestibule to the jaw angle and directed towards the mandible.

The periosteum is dissected from the cortex to the level where the chin wing osteotomy is planned. It is important that the periosteum is not further detached caudally in order not to compromise the blood perfusion.

The caudal masseter attachments are also bluntly detached from the masseteric tuberosity.

The lingual periosteum and the muscle attachments are left untouched to maintain vascularization of the osteotomized segment.

Step 2: Osteotomy

First, the horizontal chin osteotomy is performed. The horizontal bicortical osteotomy is best performed piezo-surgically.

Approximately 10 mm before the mental foramen, the horizontal bicortical osteotomy is transferred to a more vertically oriented monocortical osteotomy. The further monocortical osteotomy runs latero-caudally from superior to inferior to the jaw angle to avoid any IAN injury.

The monocortical osteotomy can also be performed with a microsaw or a thin burr. Special care must be taken when performing the osteotomy near the mental foramen.

Before performing this osteotomy, it is necessary to carefully identify the location of the mandibular canal by CBCT examination.

After the complete osteotomy of the mandibular base, mobilization should be performed very carefully to avoid fracturing the basal mandibular segment.

The most dangerous place for fracture is in the area around the mental foramen. Osteosynthesis is challenging as the osteotomized bone segment is fragile. Great care must be taken when attaching plates and screws.

> **Note**
> The osteotomy cannot be performed if the mandibular canal runs close to the buccal cortical bone, because the osteotomy will split the buccal cortex in a beveled angulation from above the mandibular canal to inferior and would inevitably cut the nerve.

5 Conclusion

Genioplasty is a simple, varied, and effective technique to redefine the chin position. Changing the chin position changes the esthetics of the face. The combination with all other osteotomy techniques of the facial skeleton makes the chin osteotomy a very versatile technique.

References

1. Hu KS, Yun HS, Hur MS, Kwon HJ, Abe S, Kim HJ. Branching patterns and intraosseous course of the mental nerve. J Oral Maxillofac Surg. 2007;65(11):2288–94.
2. Kieser J, Kieser D, Hauman T. The course and distribution of the inferior alveolar nerve. J Craniofac Surg. 2005;16(1):6–9.
3. Juodzbalys G, Wang HL, Sabalys G. Anatomy of mandibular vital structures. Part II: mandibular incisive canal, mental foramen and associated neurovascular bundles in relation with dental Implantology. J Oral Maxillofac Res. 2010a;1(1):e3.
4. Juodzbalys G, Wang HL, Sabalys G. Anatomy of mandibular vital structures. Part I: mandibular canal and inferior alveolar neurovascular bundle in relation with dental implantology. J Oral Maxillofac Res. 2010b;1(1):e2.
5. Triaca A, Brusco D, Guijarro-Martinez R. Chin wing osteotomy for the correction of hyper-divergent skeletal class III deformity: technical modification. Br J Oral Maxillofac Surg. 2015;53:775–7.
6. Cordier G, Sigaux N, Carlier A, Ibrahim B, Cresseaux P. Mini wing osteotmy: avariant o chin wing osteotomy. J Stomatol Oral and Maxillofac Surg. 2020;121(3):282–5.

Intraoperative Risks: Danger Points—Postoperative Complications

45

Peter Kessler and Nicolas Hardt

Contents

Abstract

During the genioplasty procedure, the mental nerve is at risk of injury. Careful subperiosteal dissection, retraction, and protection of the nerve during the osteotomy helps to prevent injuries to the nerve (Bell et al. Surgical correction of dentofacial deformities, Band 1–3. Saunders, 1980; Joos et al. Fortschr Kiefer Gesichtschir 26:86, 1981; Fonsecca et al. Oral and maxillofacial surgery, Saunders, 2009; Hofer. Dtsch Zahn Mund Kieferheilk 9:142–144, 1942).

Keywords

Genioplasty · Incision and preparation · Nerve injury · Hematoma · Mandibular osteotomy · Esthetics - Transgender surgery · Wound dehiscence

1 Nerve Injuries

- Injuries to the superficial mucosal distal fibers of the mental nerve often occur during the mucosal incision.
- The long-term incidence of sensory loss of the mental nerve due to intraoperative alteration/ablation/injury is approximately 20%.
- Especially during chin wing surgery injuries of the mental and inferior alveolar nerve due to preparation and dissection at the mental foramen and the course of the alveolar canal

P. Kessler (✉)
Department of Cranio-Maxillofacial Surgery, Maastricht University Medical Center, Maastricht, The Netherlands
e-mail: peter.kessler@mumc.nl

N. Hardt (✉)
Kantonsspital Lucerne, Clinic and Policlinic of Cranio-Maxillofacial Surgery, Lucerne, Switzerland

P. Kessler et al. (eds.), *Illustrated Manual of Orthognathic Surgery*,
https://doi.org/10.1007/978-3-031-06978-9_45

can happen. Not only the neural structures but also the vascular content of the mandibular canal can be hurt.
- Injuries to the marginal mandibular branch of the facial nerve but also the facial artery can happen during the chin wing osteotomy.

Note
Nerve damage is possible due to:

- Incision.
- Periosteal dissection.
- Nerve retraction.
- Osteotomy.
- Application of osteosynthesis.
- Wound closure.

2 Intraoperative Tricks

- Prepare a wide, tension-free approach for the chin osteotomy.
- Clear exposure of the anterior and lateral mandibula to assess the extent and location of the chin deformity and to determine the position of the mental foramen.
- Atraumatic surgery to avoid severe postoperative edema of the lip and wound edges resulting in dehiscence of sutures and infection of the surgical site.
- If the osteotomy is to be placed distally of the mental foramen, the periosteum around the mental nerve should be sharply dissected, thus relieving the nerve to reduce the risk of nerve compression or avulsion.
- It is important that the chin osteotomy be placed 5 mm below the mental foramen to prevent injury to the anterior loop of the mental nerve as it ascends within the mandible channel before leaving the foramen.
- Rigid segment/chin fixation is achieved using microplates and screws.

3 Postoperative Complications

3.1 Early Postoperative Complications

- Excessive soft tissue swelling.
- Bleeding and hematoma.
- Damage to the lingual soft tissues.
- Injury of the genioglossus and geniohyoid muscles.
- Laceration of the sublingual and submental arteries with hematoma of the floor of the mouth—risk of airway obstruction due to hematoma of the floor of the mouth and bleeding into the tongue.

3.2 Late Complications

- Chin asymmetry.
- Unequal, asymmetrical contractions of the mental muscle.
- Chin ptosis with "dropping chin" phenomenon due to sagging of the mental muscle.

4 Conclusion

Various techniques for chin displacement exist. The technique itself is simple, the risks are well manageable. With careful execution of genioplasty, osteotomy of the chin is low-risk, circumscribed surgery. The chin position must be taken into account in every orthognathic surgical procedure. The chin position must not be neglected from an esthetic point of view [1–4].

References

1. Bell WH, Proffit WR, White RP. Surgical correction of dentofacial deformities, Band 1–3. Saunders; 1980.
2. Joos U, Delaire J, Scheibe B. Schilli W Funktionelle Aspekte der Kinnplastik. Fortschr Kiefer Gesichtschir. 1981;26:86.
3. Fonsecca RI, Marciani RD, Turvey TA. Oral and maxillofacial surgery. Saunders; 2009.
4. Hofer O. Die operative Behandlung der alveolären Retraktion des Unterkiefers und ihre Anwendungsmöglichkeit für Prognathie und Mikrogenie. Dtsch Zahn Mund Kieferheilk. 1942;9:142–4.

Part X

The Temporomandibular Joint

Introduction

46

Barbara Gerber and Nadeem Saeed

Contents

Abstract

The temporomandibular joint is a diarthrodial, bicondylar-type joint and unique in its rotational and translational movements; due to this it is known as a gingliomyoarthrodial joint. The internal fibrocartilage disc is attached to the condyle by ligaments that permit rotation during translational movements. The disc is thought to have several roles to include distribution of joint loads, joint stability in chewing, facilitating lubrication and nourishment of the joint surfaces and promoting growth of the condyle. Therefore, any change in the condyle/disc relationship could potentially lead to joint dysfunction and instability.

Operations on the upper and lower jaw, as well as corrections of malocclusions, have an impact on the temporomandibular joints. The temporomandibular joint shows a high degree of adaptability over the course of a lifetime but can also be damaged under certain circumstances. In addition, there are systemic diseases that affect the temporomandibular joint. The assessment of the temporomandibular joint from a structural and functional point of view is an essential part of diagnosis before treatment, but it also needs to be checked after the completion of orthodontic and orthognathic treatment.

Keywords

TMJ · TMD · Diagnosis in temporomandibular joint disorders · Classification of TMD · TMD clinical assessment · Management strategies · At-risk groups · Occlusion · Controversy

B. Gerber (✉)
Oxford University Hospitals, Oxfordshire, UK
e-mail: Barbara.Gerber@ouh.nhs.uk

N. Saeed
Oxford University Hospitals, Oxfordshire, UK

Great Ormond Street Hospital for Children, London, UK
e-mail: Nad.Saeed@ouh.nhs.uk

P. Kessler et al. (eds.), *Illustrated Manual of Orthognathic Surgery*,
https://doi.org/10.1007/978-3-031-06978-9_46

In order to discuss the impact of orthognathic surgery on the temporomandibular joint (TMJ) and any pre-existing or subsequent dysfunction, it is necessary to define what dysfunction of the TMJ encompasses. Temporomandibular dysfunctions (TMD) have a variety of different nomenclatures in the literature as well as numerous definitions. This contributes to, and highlights, the complexity of this topic and to the potential difficulty in devising management strategies to treat this condition.

1 Definition of TMD

TMD is a collective term used to describe a wide-ranging condition that involves a variety of signs and symptoms of the TMJ and its related structures [1]. Most common signs and symptoms include:

- Myalgia.
- Headaches.
- Facial/neck pain.
- Otalgia in the absence of aural disease.
- Joint noises.
- Limitation of mouth opening.

Additionally, there may be evidence of parafunctional habits, deviation of mouth opening and tenderness in the masticatory muscles. The etiology of this condition has remained a subject of much debate and controversy. It is likely multifactorial in nature from a biopsychosocial model with initiating, predisposing, and perpetuating factors [1]. Its reported incidence is 3–4% per annum (OPPERA study) with increasing prevalence in adults, peaking in the second and third decades until age 45 years [2]. Hence, it is likely that TMD will be encountered in patients who are undergoing orthognathic surgery (OGS).

2 Conclusion

The assessment of TMJ function and TMD is part of the preclinical assessment of all combined orthodontic-orthognathic treatments. The special anatomy and role of the TMJ must be regarded.

References

1. Durham J, Newton-John TR, Zakrzewska JM. Temporomandibular disorders. BMJ. 2015;350:1154.
2. Slade GD, Ohrbach R, Greenspan JD, Fillingim RB, Bair E, Sanders AE, Dubner R, Diatchenko L, Meloto CB, Smith S, Maixner W. Painful temporomandibular disorder: decade of discovery from OPPERA studies. J Dent Res. 2016;95(10):1084–92.

Diagnosis and Classification

47

Barbara Gerber and Nadeem Saeed

Contents

Abstract

In order to diagnose and characterize TMD, many indexes have been devised as standardized tools for clinical applications; one of the earliest was described by Helkimo (Sven Tandlak Tidskr. 1974;67(2):101–21). Subsequent indexes were developed for clinical research and this led to the RDC/TMD (Research Diagnostic Criteria for TMD); this has been further developed to the DC/TMD with a more clinical application (Schiffman E, Ohrbach R. J Am Dent Assoc. 2016;147(6):438–45).

Keywords

TMJ · TMD · Diagnosis in temporomandibular joint disorders · Classification of TMD · Wilkes classification · Disk dislocation

1 Diagnosis and Classification

The Wilkes classification is a commonly used clinical and radiographic index that not only includes TMD severity but also stages of TMJ internal derangement and disk-fossa relations. This classification is often used to guide treatment (Fig. 47.1).

Internal derangement (ID) includes clinical and radiologic disk displacement and can often be associated with TMD symptomatology. It is likely that TMJ ID is related to multiple factors including macro- and microtrauma but also systemic factors including hormonal, nutritional, and autoimmune variables. It is known that MRI findings do not always correlate with clinical symptomology [1] and therefore there

B. Gerber (✉)
Oxford University Hospitals NHS Foundation Trust, Oxfordshire, UK
e-mail: Barbara.Gerber@ouh.nhs.uk

N. Saeed
Oxford University Hospitals, Oxfordshire, UK

Great Ormond Street Hospital for Children, London, UK
e-mail: Nad.Saeed@ouh.nhs.uk

P. Kessler et al. (eds.), *Illustrated Manual of Orthognathic Surgery*,
https://doi.org/10.1007/978-3-031-06978-9_47

- Stage I: TMJ early opening click/no pain/no radiographic disc displacement
- Stage II: Joint sounds/pain with intermittent locking/episodes of pain/radiological disc displacement with reduction
- Stage III: As stage II, but with radiological disc displacement without reduction/multiple painful episodes/ restricted mobility
- Stage IV: Non-reducing anterior disc displacement/chronic and increasing functional disturbance/arthritic changes
- Stage V: Disc perforation or non-reducing disc displacement/osteoarthritis/grating, grinding symptoms/pain/restricted mobility/limited function

Fig. 47.1 Wilkes classification—adapted

must be elements of TMJ adaptation to account for this.

The TMJ articular surfaces have great potential for physiological adaptation to numerous functional procedures. During the course of a lifetime, progressive remodeling maintains a constant balance between shape and function. If the joint is exposed to nonphysiological effects, then the adaptive ability can be overcome, and can lead to permanent damage to the articular surfaces and potential condylar resorption. This total adaptive capacity can also be affected under normal conditions when it is weakened due to aging or numerous systemic disorders [2].

This adaption is supported anecdotally by the multitude of orthognathic procedures performed with only a small number of patients that present postoperatively with TMD and TMJ pathology. It is this ability of the TMJ that allows us to alter its position often without detrimental effects. However, there are still a cohort of patients that succumb to TMD and some of its more pathological effects, i.e., idiopathic condylar resorption (ICR).

2 Conclusion

TMJ disease can coexist with jaw deformity and undiagnosed or untreated disease can lead to unpredictable results with unfavorable outcomes in both functional and aesthetic terms. Decisions about the timing of intervention for TMJ disease in patients undergoing orthognathic treatment are dependent on the severity and onset of the disease process. Some dentofacial deformities are a result of TMJ disorders such as idiopathic condylar resorption or severe degenerative joint diseases.

References

1. Kircos LT, Orthendahl DA, Mark AS, Arakawa M. Magnetic resonance imaging of the TMJ disc in asymptomatic volunteers. J Oral Maxillofac Surg. 1987;45(10):852–4.
2. Ivkovic N, Racic M. Structural and functional disorders of the temporomandibular joint (internal disorders). In: Almasri MA, Kummoona R, editors. Maxillofacial surgery and craniofacial deformity–practices and updates. IntechOpen; 2018.

Clinical Assessment

48

Barbara Gerber and Nadeem Saeed

Contents

Abstract

It is standard that all patients requesting orthognathic treatment are subject to a thorough clinical examination as well as a pertinent history, symptom evaluation, treatment history, and outcome expectations. Included in this should be a TMJ history and examination, being mindful that certain dentofacial deformities can be related to a high risk of obstructive sleep apnea, and that these deformities may be as a result of a pre-existing TMJ disease process. Further screening should optionally be provided to include Stop-Bang scoring and an Epworth sleepiness scale. Assessment of medical comorbidities and nutritional status should also be standard practice.

Keywords

TMJ · TMD · Diagnosis in temporomandibular joint disorders · Classification of TMD · TMD clinical assessment · TMJ imaging

B. Gerber (✉)
Oxford University Hospitals, Oxfordshire, UK
e-mail: Barbara.Gerber@ouh.nhs.uk

N. Saeed
Oxford University Hospitals, Oxfordshire, UK

Great Ormond Street Hospital for Children, London, UK
e-mail: Nad.Saeed@ouh.nhs.uk

The clinical examination should include evaluation of the TMJ status and function, noting any positive findings to include:

- TMJ clicking/crepitus.
- Tenderness in the muscles of mastication.
- Deviation in mouth opening.
- Inter-incisal distance (if considered limited).

1 Imaging

- OPT/Lateral Cephalogram.
- CBCT/CT.
- MRI +/− contrast.

P. Kessler et al. (eds.), *Illustrated Manual of Orthognathic Surgery*,
https://doi.org/10.1007/978-3-031-06978-9_48

Included in every workup for orthognathic surgery are panoramic and cephalometric radiographs and dental study models (see: Chap. 7).

Plain radiographs may highlight significant TMJ abnormalities that can guide the clinician to consider further detailed imaging in the form of a CT for bony pathology. In addition, the oropharyngeal and nasal airway can also be evaluated if necessary from these scans. Significant clinical symptoms of ID may warrant additional MRI with or without contrast. This can help in quantifying the degree of synovitis, disk morphology, position, and effusions. MRI has shown to have a high sensitivity and specificity to clinical symptoms [1].

2 Conclusion

A thorough clinical assessment related to TMJ morphology and function is indicated in all orthodontic and especially orthognathic treatments.

Reference

1. Kumar R, Pallagatti S, Sheikh S, Mittal A, Gupta D, Gupta S. Correlation between clinical findings of temporomandibular disorders and MRI. Open Dent J. 2015;9:273–81.

Management Strategies

49

Barbara Gerber and Nadeem Saeed

Contents

Abstract

As with all patients once a diagnosis of the dentofacial deformity has been made, then treatment can proceed as per any other orthognathic strategy. The treatment of concomitant TMD should follow strategies aimed at the degree of TMD as per the Wilkes classification. Often TMD treatment occurs alongside presurgical orthodontics. Although controversial, there has been no clear evidence that orthodontic treatment nor the preceding malocclusion induces TMD (Sim et al. Korean J Orthod. 2019;49(3):181-187; Egermark et al. Angle Orthod. 2003; 73:109–115; McNamara et al. J Orofac Pain. 1995; 9:73–90).

Keywords

TMJ · TMD · Diagnosis in temporomandibular joint disorders · Classification of TMD · TMD clinical assessment · Wilkes classification · Management strategies · At-risk groups · Occlusion

1 TMJ Disease Prior to Commencement of Orthognathic Surgery

These patients should have a well-documented TMJ history and examination performed and treatment guided by their initial Wilkes staging [1].

B. Gerber (✉) · N. Saeed
Oxford University Hospitals, Oxford University NHS Foundation Trust, London, UK
e-mail: Barbara.Gerber@ouh.nhs.uk; Nad.Saeed@ouh.nhs.uk

P. Kessler et al. (eds.), *Illustrated Manual of Orthognathic Surgery*,
https://doi.org/10.1007/978-3-031-06978-9_49

- Wilkes I and II.
- Nonoperative modalities: physiotherapy, medical management (analgesia, muscle relaxants), jaw exercises, soft diet (when required).
- Wilkes III and IV.
- Initial nonoperative management, if unresponsive, then arthroscopy (lysis and lavage) prior to definitive surgery.
- Wilkes V.
- Combined TMJ replacement and orthognathic surgery. The TMJ complex is not stable enough to withstand orthognathic surgery alone.

It has been shown that arthroscopic treatment of Wilkes II–IV patients to be more than 80% successful and hence recommended as a simple intervention. For those that have no improvement in their symptoms it has been advocated by Wolford and Dhameja [2] that simultaneous disk repositioning and orthognathic surgery be performed. They reported good results with this approach as have other studies, with increased pain scores in those that didn't have simultaneous disc surgery [3]. This was noted particularly in those that had large mandibular advancements and long-standing (> 4 years) pre-existing TMD.

However, as we know that there will be some degree of TMJ repositioning after orthognathic surgery, it might be prudent to wait and assess any persistence of TMD ID postoperatively. It has been shown that in certain groups, orthognathic surgery alone has improved TMD symptomatology [4, 5].

If necessary, TMJ arthroscopy with disc repositioning and plication can be performed as a stand-alone procedure, to avoid open TMJ surgery, once full recovery from orthognathic surgery has been achieved. A simple flow diagram and treatment algorithm for patients with dentofacial deformity and TMD symptoms has been proposed by Nale [6]. Essentially this protocol suggests treatment of painful TMD is completed and stabilized prior to OGS (orthognathic surgery) or in severe disease concomitant surgeries undertaken (Fig. 49.1).

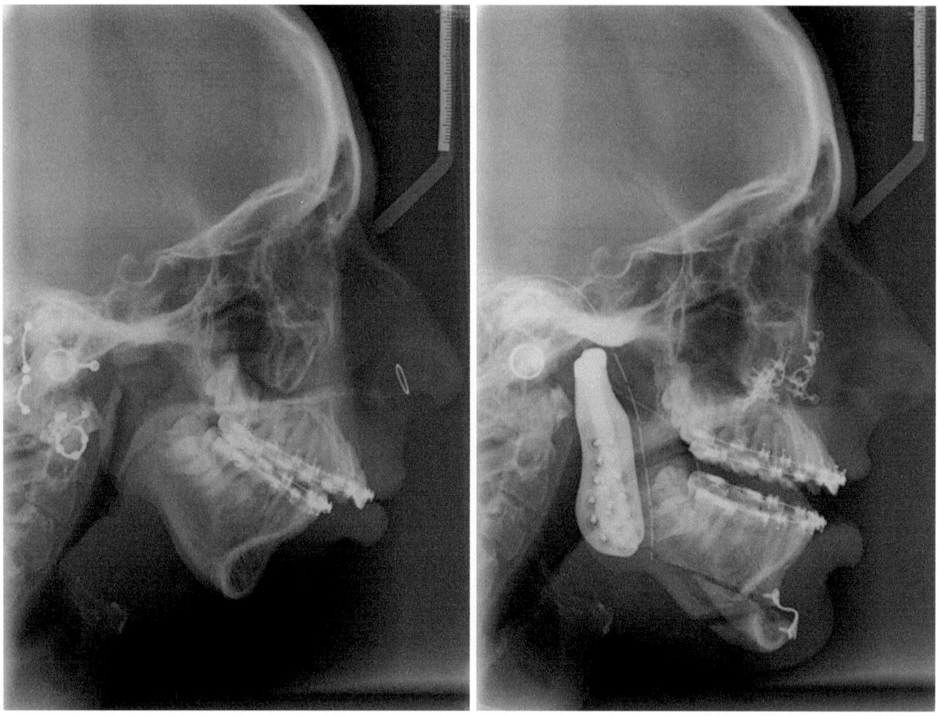

Fig. 49.1 Wilkes V TMJ with condylar resorption, sleep disordered breathing, poor facial aesthetics. Treated with combined counterclockwise Le Fort I osteotomy and bilateral TMJ replacement. Pre- and post-lateral cephalograms confirming airway changes, overjet change, lateral and frontal facial views

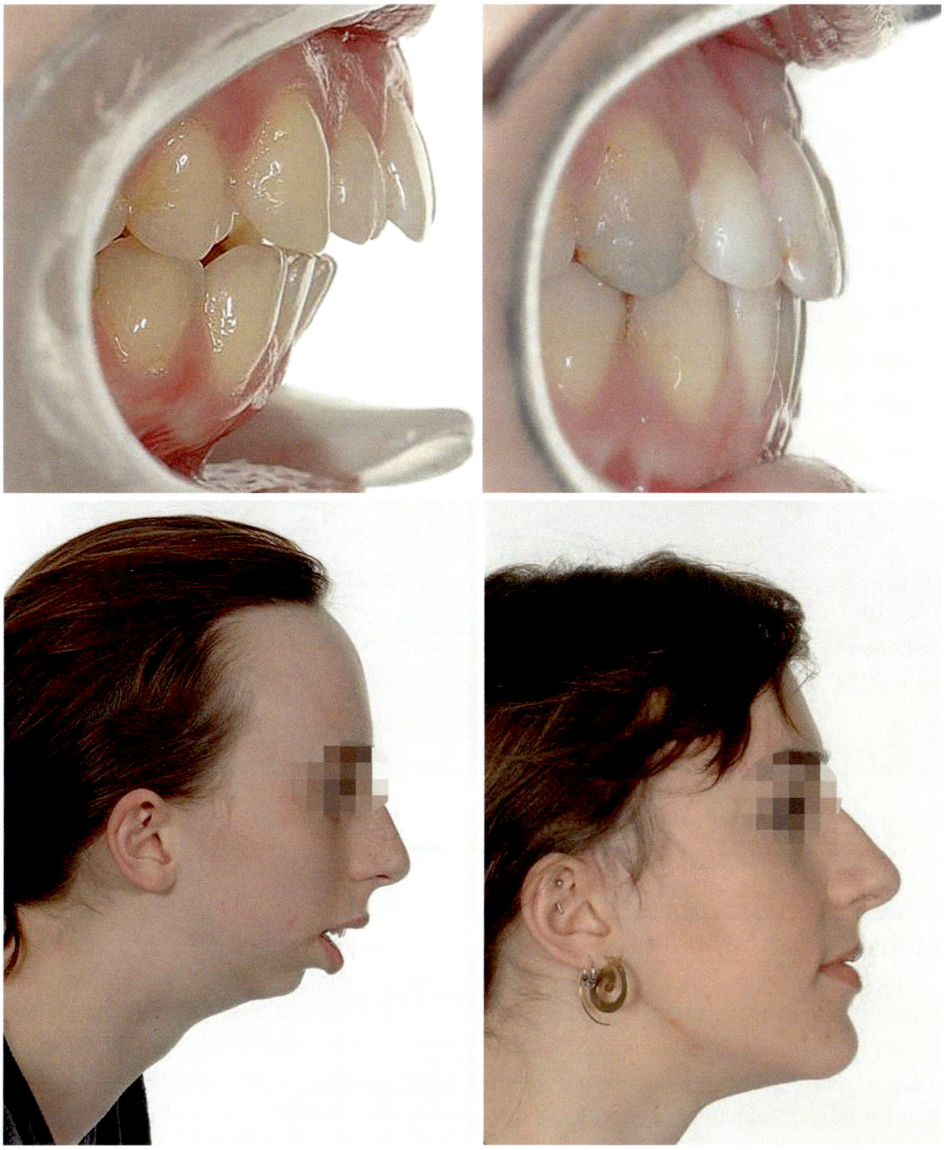

Fig. 49.1 (continued)

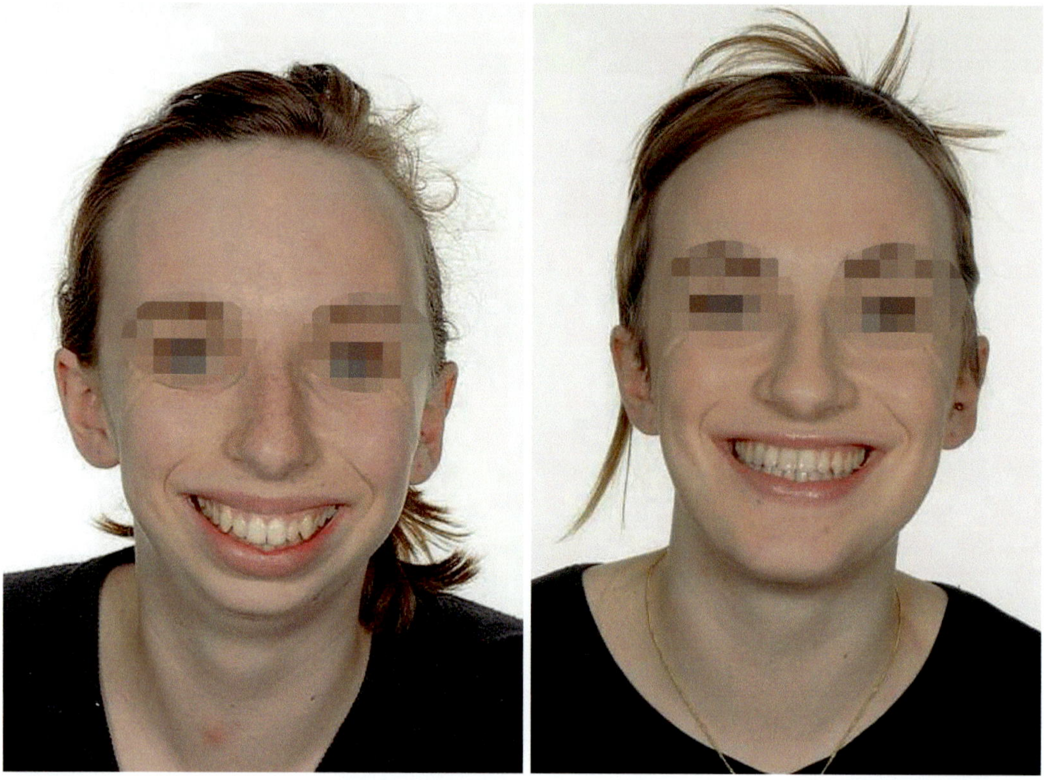

Fig. 49.1 (continued)

2 At-Risk Groups

There are a subset of patients that should be cautiously considered before the commencement of orthognathic surgery. They are known to have the potential for adverse outcomes if careful assessment and planning is not performed (Fig. 49.2).

It has been well documented that female patients with a high Frankfurt-Mandibular plane angle who have a class II skeletal relationship are at a higher risk of developing idiopathic condylar resorption (ICR) postoperatively and hence relapse. They should be closely counselled about this risk if a mandibular procedure is considered or alternative osteotomies recommended [7]. Much research has gone into understanding the etiology of this phenomenon with postulations around an estrogen-mediated process. Other contributing factors have included a diminished posterior face height, and posteriorly inclined condylar neck [8].

TMJ condylar resorption can also occur de novo without any preceding surgery, and the cause of this can be related to local, systemic, or idiopathic causes. The resorptive process is via cytokine-activated osteoblasts which promote osteoclast activity. This results in an enzymatic breakdown of hydroxyapatite and collagen [9]. Certain individuals may be predisposed to condylar resorption due to a multitude of factors. These can include gender, nutritional status, genetics, oral habits, and parafunction. As mentioned once the TMJ adaptive capacity is overcome then resorption or destruction of the articular structures can ensue.

It has also been suggested that those patients with pre-existing TMD that require counterclockwise rotation of the maxillomandibular complex

- ICR +/- TMD – female, Class II, large mandibular advancements, high angle
- Bilateral TMJ ID - cephalometric analysis has highlighted that such patients tend to have a short ramus, clockwise rotation of mandible, and retrognathic mandible (38)
- Counter-clockwise rotation movements in pre-existing TMD patients

Fig. 49.2 At-risk groups

are at risk of persistent and likely worsening TMD. This is due to the stretch on the pterygomasseteric muscles and stretch of the soft tissues. This movement theoretically increases the TMJ loading. In this instance, addressing the TMD prior to surgery would be advantageous and can provide a more stable outcome [10]. This surgical move has been shown to be as stable as conventional treatment that doesn't alter the occlusal plane.

3 Orthognathic Surgery Effects on TMD

The effects of OGS on the TMD has been frequently debated in the literature, and studies both advocating its beneficial effect and deleterious effects have been published. During orthognathic surgery, the condylar position is important to avoid relapse or subsequent malocclusion upon waking. Some surgeons have even advocated waking the patient intraoperatively to make sure the condyle is seated correctly and to avoid sag [11].

It has also been suggested that certain orthognathic surgical movements can potentiate postoperative TMD due to the torque placed on the potentially newly positioned condyle. Condylar shape is not uniform, and 3D volumetric analysis demonstrates that different skeletal relationships have different condylar morphologies [12]. The relevance of whether this contributes to TMD is unknown and certainly it is understood that the condylar position is altered after orthognathic surgery. The most noticeable change is in the early postoperative period (6 months) with a slow move to a position close to the preoperative status; however, it never fully returns to this original position [13].

Numerous studies have reported an overall improvement with OGS with both setback ([14–17]) and advancement procedures via a sagittal split osteotomy (SSO) [18] with relatively low incidence of asymptomatic patients developing TMD postoperatively [19].

It has been shown that disc position improves after mandibular advancement in class II patients as well as reducing excessive translation [20]. Also noted that in class II patients that underwent OGS have better quality of life scores and a reduction in chronic and articular pain when not associated with a psychosocial input [21]. This too is noted in the class III patient having had a SSO procedure [22].

Combined orthodontic and orthognathic treatment has generally been shown to have a positive treatment outcome with respect to TMD pain, having a frequency similar to a control group [4].

Of note different osteotomy procedures and types of fixation have an effect on the condylar position and hence the potential to produce postoperative changes [7]. The commonest types of mandibular osteotomy are the sagittal split osteotomy (SSO) and intraoral vertical ramus osteotomy (IVRO). It is likely that IVRO for setback procedures are better to reduce the risk of TMD as the condyle takes a more anterior-inferior position resulting from the lateral pull of the lateral pterygoid. This allows an increased joint space and recapture of an anteriorly displaced disc (see: Mandibular Prognathism—Class III Setback—Surgical Technique—IVRO).

However, the drawback of the IVRO is the need for a period of IMF and potential for longterm hypomobility of the joint. Overall numerous studies have demonstrated a low incidence of hypomobility and recovery up to 90–98% of the premorbid mouth opening [18]. In terms of fixation, there's some evidence to support the use of monocortical plate fixation over bicortical screws in the SSO [23] but that lag screws should be avoided due to their increase on lateral torque of the condyles. The miniplate is more forgiving than positional bicortical screws for condylar seating (see: Osteosynthesis for Sagittal Splitting).

4 TMD in the Postoperative Patient

In most cases, like TMD in the preoperative patient, treatment should be guided by the severity and degree of TMD as per the Wilkes classification. Time must be given for the effects of OGS to settle and any planned surgical intervention should allow recovery time. As always, nonoperative measures should initially be instituted for symptom control.

Intermaxillary fixation should be avoided in the immediate postoperative period as it's known that prolonged immobility of the TMJ can induce stiffness and may induce TMD and long-term hypomobility. The initial reduced mouth opening after orthognathic surgery is transient, and with encouragement the premorbid status can be achieved [18].

If patients go on to develop intractable TMD ID (Wilkes III), then they should be treated as per any other TMJ patient. This would include arthroscopy (lysis and lavage) and consideration for Level 3 arthroscopy (disc repositioning and plication) or open TMJ surgery. Open surgery prior to 6 months is not recommended as there will be ongoing adaption and the potential to worsen rather than relieve symptoms (Fig. 49.3).

Careful consideration must be given to the late postoperative patient that presents with a Wilkes V TMJ secondary to ICR. These patients will need a full workup and clear discussion about the expectations of future treatment. It is likely that they will have developed a change in occlusion, asymmetry, and possibly facial aesthetics.

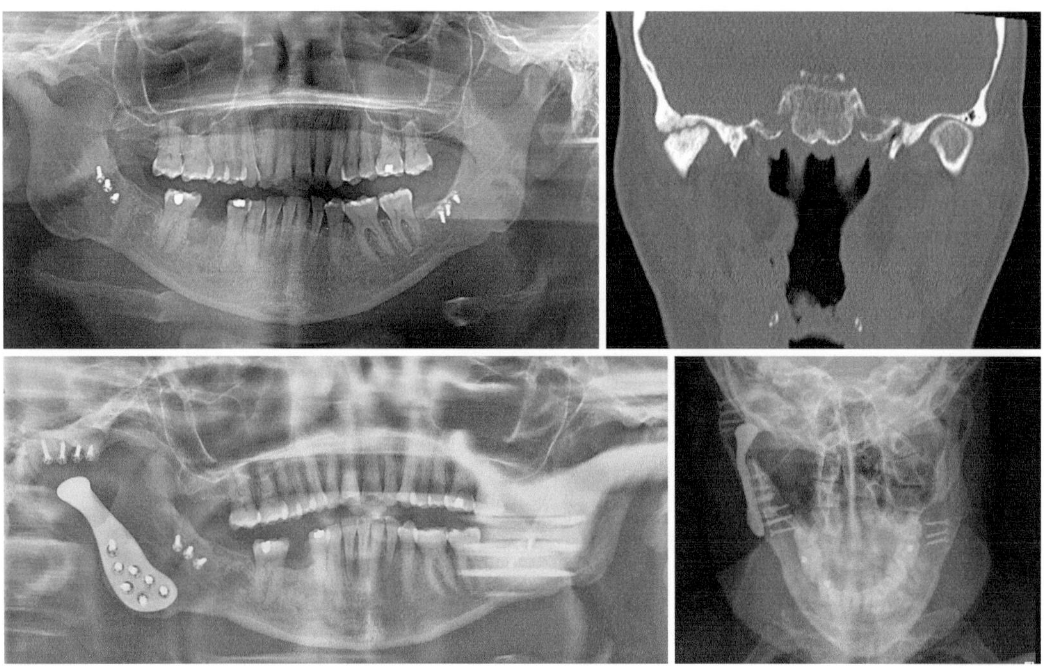

Fig. 49.3 Patient referred post BSSO advancement with bicortical screw fixation, and open disc plication only 3 months post-surgery due to TMJ pain. Fibrous ankylosis with restricted opening (15 mm) and degeneration at the time of referral treated with Right Total TMJ replacement restoring opening to 40 mm and pain reduction

Avoidance of future mandibular osteotomy procedures has been advocated but thought must also be given to TMJ replacement with an alloplastic joint. This allows a stable TMJ base if further orthognathic treatment is needed and desired.

5 Conclusion

The Wilkes classification helps to decide on adjuvant therapies and risks related to the TMJ and helps to select the best fitting therapy in orthognathic surgery.

References

1. Wilkes CH. Arthrography of the temporomandibular joint in patients with the TMJ pain-dysfunction syndrome. Minn Med. 1978;61(11):645–52.
2. Wolford LM, Dhameja A. Planning for combined TMJ arthroplasty and orthognathic surgery. Atlas Oral Maxillofac Surg Clin North Am. 2011;19(2):243–70.
3. Wolford LM, Reiche-Fischel O, Mehra P. Changes in temporomandibular joint dysfunction after orthognathic sugery. J Oral Maxillofac Surg. 2003;61:655–60.
4. Abramhamsson C, Henrikson T, Nilner M, Sunzel B, Bondemark L, Ekberg EC. TMD before and after correction of dentofacial deformities by orthodontic and orthognathic treatment. Int J Oral Maxillofac Surg. 2013;42(6):752–8.
5. Al-Moraissi EA, Wolford LM, Perez D, Laskin DM, Ellis E. Does orthognathic surgery cause or cure temporomandibular disorders? A systematic review and meta-analysis. J Oral Maxillofac Surg. 2017;75(9):1835–47.
6. Nale JC. Orthognathic surgery and the temporomandibular joint patient. Oral Maxillofac Surg Clin North Am. 2014;26:551–64.
7. Iguchi R, Yoshizawa K, Moroi A, Tsutsui T, Hotta A, Hiraide R, Takayama A, Tsunoda T, Saito Y, Sato M, Baba N, Ueki KJ. Comparison of temporomandibular joint and ramus morphology between class II and class III cases before and after bi-maxillary osteotomy. Craniomaxillofac Surg. 2017;45(12):2002–9.
8. Catherine Z, Breton P, Bouletreau P. Condylar resorption after orthognathic surgery: a systematic review. Rev Stomatol Chir Maxillofac Chir Orale. 2016;117(1):3–10.
9. Verhelst PJ, van der Cruyssen F, De Laat A, Jacobs R, Politis C. The biomechanical effect of the sagittal Split ramus osteotomy on the temporomandibular joint: current perspectives on the remodeling Spectrum. Front Physiol. 2019;10:1021.
10. Al-Moraissi EA, Wolford LM. Does temporomandibular joint pathology with or without surgical management affect the stability of counterclockwise rotation of the Maxillomandibular complex in orthognathic surgery? A systematic review and meta-analysis. J Oral Maxillofac Surg. 2017;75(4):805–21.
11. Politi M, Toro C, Costa F, Polini F, Robiony M. Intraoperative awakening of the patient during orthognathic surgery: a method to prevent the condylar sag. J Oral Maxillofac Surg. 2007;65(1):109–14.
12. Santander P, Quast A, Olbrisch C, Rose M, Moser N, Schliephake H, Meyer-Marcotty P. Comprehensive 3D analysis of condylar morphology in adults with different skeletal patterns–a cross-sectional study. Head Face Med. 2020;16(1):33.
13. Ma RH, Li G, Yin S, Sun Y, Li ZL, Ma XC. Quantitative assessment of condyle positional changes before and after orthognathic surgery based on fused 3D images from cone beam computed tomography. Clin Oral Invetig. 2020;24(8):2663–72.
14. Hu J, Wang D, Zou S. Effects of mandibular setback on the temporomandibular joint: a comparison of oblique and sagittal split ramus osteotomy. J Oral Maxillofac Surg. 2000;58:375–80.
15. Kerstens HC, Tuinzing DB, van der Kwast WA. Temporomandibular joint symptoms in orthognathic surgery. J Craniomaxillofac Surg. 1989;17:215–8.
16. Ueki K, Marukawa K, Nakagawa K, Yamamoto E. Condylar and temporomandibular joint disc positions after mandibular osteotomy for prognathism. J Oral Maxillofac Surg. 2002;60:1424–32.
17. White CS, Dolwick MF. Prevalence and variance of temporomandibular dysfunction in orthognathic surgery patients. Int J Adult Orthodon Orthognath Surg. 1992;7:7–14.
18. Jung HD, Kim SY, Park HS, Jung YS. Orthognathic surgery and temporomandibular joint symptoms. Maxillofac Plast Reconstr Surg. 2015;37:14.
19. Song YL, Yap AU. Orthognathic treatment of dentofacial disharmonies: its impact on temporomandibular disorders, quality of life and psychological wellness. Cranio. 2017;35(1):52–7.
20. Sharma R, Muralidharan CG, Verma M, Pannu S, Patrikar S. MRI changes in the temporomandibular joint after mandibular advancement. J Oral Maxillofac Surg. 2020;78(5):806–12.
21. Bergamaschi IP, Cavalcante RC, Fanderuff M, Gerber JT, Petinati MFP, Sebastiani AM, da Costa DJ, Scariot R. Orthognathic surgery in class II patients: a longitudinal study on quality of life, TMD, and psychological aspects. Clin Oral Investig. 2021;25(6):3801–8. Online ahead of print
22. Guo ML, Huang Z, Wang C, Wang YJ. Effect of bilateral sagittal split ramus osteotomy on temporomandibular joint symptom and condylar position in patients with skeletal class III malocclusion by cone beam computed tomography. Hua Xi Kou Qiang Yi Xue Za Zhi. 2020;38(5):519–24.

23. Ureturk EU, Apaydin A. Does fixation method affect temporomandibular joints after mandibular advancement? J Craniomaxillofac Surg. 2018;46(6):923–31.
24. Egermark I, Magnusson T, Carlsson GE. A 20-year follow-up of signs and symptoms of temporomandibular disorders and malocclusions in subjects with and without orthodontic treatment in childhood. Angle Orthod. 2003;73(2):109–15.
25. McNamara JA Jr, Seligman DA, Okeson JP. Occlusion, orthodontic treatment, and temporomandibular disorders: a review. J Orofac Pain. 1995;9:73–90.
26. Sim HY, Kim HS, Jung DU, Lee H, Han YS, Han K, Yun KI. Investigation of the association between orthodontic treatment and temporomandibular joint pain and dysfunction in the south Korean population. Korean J Orthod. 2019;49(3):181–7.

Controversy

50

Barbara Gerber and Nadeem Saeed

Contents

Abstract

The controversial topic of the association between malocclusion and TMD has been extensively discussed in the literature, often with contradictory results. The use of inconsistent terminology, within studies, makes this a difficult subject to compare.

Keywords

TMJ · TMD · Diagnosis in temporomandibular joint disorders · Classification of TMD · TMD clinical assessment · Management strategies · At-risk groups · Occlusion · Controversy

B. Gerber (✉) · N. Saeed
Oxford University Hospitals, Oxford University NHS Foundation Trust, London, UK
e-mail: Barbara.Gerber@ouh.nhs.uk; Nad.Saeed@ouh.nhs.uk

1 Occlusion, Orthodontics, and TMD

Many such studies discuss occlusion as a static phenomenon in relationship to TMD; however, as TMD is now accepted to be a multifactorial process, this binary relationship is unlikely to exist. Occlusion is most likely a complex pathway including a dynamic process of adaptation and a somatosensory process [1].

Longitudinal studies of adolescents with a variety of malocclusions have not shown an increase in the prevalence of TMD [2] and longstanding malocclusion and occlusal interferences have likely been subject to an adaptive process. The overriding consensus view is that malocclusion doesn't contribute to TMD [1, 3, 4].

That said, low levels of evidence have implicated some occlusal factors associated with TMD, including an overjet of >4 mm, unilateral posterior crossbite and retruded contact position, and intercuspidal position slides of greater than 1.75 mm.

P. Kessler et al. (eds.), *Illustrated Manual of Orthognathic Surgery*,
https://doi.org/10.1007/978-3-031-06978-9_50

However, no single occlusal factor was able to differentiate between TMD and healthy patients [5].

Some proponents suggest the use of therapies aimed at adjusting the occlusion in order to treat TMD, with some even advocating permanent occlusal adjustment. A Cochrane review showed there is no clear evidence that this contributes to the reduction or prevention of TMD [6]. In general, the literature suggests that occlusal equilibration or irreversible adjustment should not be used as a tool to treat TMD [7].

The role of orthodontic treatment has been cited as prevention, cure, and induction of TMD. The rationale behind these concepts were presumed to come from the idea that achievement of an ideal occlusal harmony or by repositioning the condyles in their optimal position, reduced the risk of TMD. However, opponents to this view considered orthodontics as a trigger for TMD [1]. It seems that overall orthodontic therapy has a neutral effect on TMD, neither as a cure nor as a prompt. In a literature review, it seems regardless of the type of orthodontic treatment plan used, including those with premolar extractions, none were associated with TMD [8].

2 Orthognathic surgery as a Treatment of TMD

There is very limited evidence to support orthognathic surgery as a treatment strategy for TMD as nearly all studies concentrate on the effects of surgery on TMD.

As most TMD symptoms (80–90%) can be treated effectively by simple measures, the use of orthognathic surgery as a treatment for TMD should be limited to those patients with a severely degenerative joint that require combined open surgery or joint replacement and orthognathic surgery.

To advocate OGS as treatment for TMD only, without concerns of a dentofacial disharmony would seem unwise.

3 Conclusions

The temporomandibular joint is known to be an adaptive joint in terms of its capability to withstand anatomical and physiological changes. It is this ability which allows most orthognathic surgery to have little impact on long-term TMJ health. In patients with mild TMD (Wilkes I/II), this should be treated conservatively prior to orthognathic surgery. Moderate (Wilkes III) or severe TMJ disease (Wilkes IV/V), or in patients with persistent issues, should be counselled as to the potential worsening of symptoms or offered concomitant open surgery or joint replacement. In moderate disease, the vast majority will settle and a wait-and-see policy should be adopted.

It should be noted that any individual propensity to develop TMD either as a pre-, intra-, or postoperative phenomenon will very much depend on a myriad of variables and the underlying biopsychosocial model of TMD must not be forgotten.

Orthognathic surgery and its relationship to the TMJ and TMD will continue to be a much investigated area, and ultimately the treatment of TMD due to this will always be via multiple treatment strategies.

References

1. Michelotti A, Rongo R, D'Antò BR. Occlusion, orthodontics, and temporomandibular disorders: cutting edge of the current evidence. World Fed Orthod. 2020;9:15–8.
2. Olliver SJ, Broadbent JM, Thomson WM. Occlusal features and TMJ clicking: a 30-year evaluation form a cohort study. J Dent Res. 2020;99(11):1245–51.
3. De Kanter RJAM, Battistuzzi PGFCM, Truin GJ. Temporomandibular disorders: "occlusion" matters! Pain Res Manag. 2018;2018:8746858.
4. Manfredini D, Lombardo L, Siciliani G. Temporomandibular disorders and dental occlusion. A systematic review of association studies: end of an era? J Oral Rehabil. 2017;44(11):908–23.
5. Al-Ani Z. Occlusion and temporomandibular disorders: a long-standing controversy in dentistry. Prim Dent J. 2020;9(1):43–8.
6. Koh H, Robinson PG. Occlusal adjustment for treating and preventing temporomandibular joint disorders. J Oral Rehabil. 2004;31(4):287–92.
7. Tsukiyama Y, Baba K, Clark GT. An evidence-based assessment of occlusal adjustment as a treatment for temporomandibular disorders. J Prosthet Dent. 2001;86(1):57–66.
8. Leite RA, Rodrigues JF, Sakima MT, Sakima T. Relationship between temporomandibular disorders and orthodontic treatment: a literature review. Dental Press J Orthod. 2013;18(1):150–7.

Index

P. Kessler et al. (eds.), *Illustrated Manual of Orthognathic Surgery*,
https://doi.org/10.1007/978-3-031-06978-9

GPSR Compliance

The European Union's (EU) General Product Safety Regulation (GPSR) is a set of rules that requires consumer products to be safe and our obligations to ensure this.

If you have any concerns about our products, you can contact us on ProductSafety@springernature.com

In case Publisher is established outside the EU, the EU authorized representative is:

Springer Nature Customer Service Center GmbH
Europaplatz 3
69115 Heidelberg, Germany

Batch number: 08204219

Printed by Printforce, the Netherlands